Benign Disorders and Diseases of the Breast

Benign Disorders and Diseases of the Breast:
Concepts and Clinical Management

L. E. HUGHES, MB, DS, FRCS, FRACS
Professor and Head of Department of Surgery

R. E. MANSEL, MB, FRCS
Senior Lecturer and Consultant Surgeon

D. J. T. WEBSTER, MD, FRCS
Senior Lecturer and Consultant Surgeon

University of Wales, College of Medicine
Heath Park, Cardiff, UK

With the collaboration of

I. H. GRAVELLE, BSc, MB, ChB, FRCP, FRCR, DMRD
Consultant Radiologist, University Hospital of Wales,
Heath Park, Cardiff, UK

Baillière Tindall
London   Philadelphia   Toronto   Sydney   Tokyo

Baillière Tindall	24–28 Oval Road
W.B. Saunders	London NW1 7DX, England

West Washington Square
Philadelphia, PA 19105, USA

1 Goldthorne Avenue
Toronto, Ontario M8Z 5T9, Canada

Harcourt Brace Jovanovich Group
(Australia) Pty Ltd
PO Box 300, North Ryde
NSW 2113, Australia

Harcourt Brace Jovanovich Japan, Inc.
Ichibancho Central Building, 22–1 Ichibancho
Chiyoda-ku, Tokyo 102, Japan

Typeset by Lasertext, Stretford, Manchester
Printed in Hong Kong

British Library Cataloguing in Publication Data
Benign disorders and diseases of the breast.
1. Women. Breasts. Diseases.
I. Hughes, L.E.
618.1'9

ISBN 0-7020-1290-4

Foreword

The clinical and scientific literature on the breast is voluminous and many books have been written on breast cancer, breast cancer research and cosmetic surgery. In contrast, there are no books devoted entirely to benign breast conditions, despite the fact that these will account for 90% of clinical presentations related to the breast. This book aims to make good the deficiency, particularly from the point of view of clinical management. It aims to give a comprehensive overview in relation to both broad physiopathological processes affecting the breast and details of clinical presentation and management. We do not attempt to deal with the subjects so generously covered in other books – breast cancer, breast cancer research and cosmetic surgery, except where they interact with benign breast disorders.

In spite of the paucity of books on the subject, the literature on benign breast disorders is vast – it would be impossible to cover it fully. We have tried to quote the papers which seemed to us to be most important – giving a mix of those which are historical, those which are seminal and those which report recent clinical advances. We have set the broad physiopathological processes in an historical context to highlight two centuries of major contributions, many of which had little recognition because of the preoccupation with cancer, with the result that conditions well described in the past have been 'rediscovered' at regular intervals.

Of recent years, there has been increasing recognition that many clinical presentations relate to normal processes, so that benign disorders, rather than diseases, of the breast is a concept which is gaining wide recognition. The concept has been taken further by some authors to suggest that most benign conditions are non-existent – particularly in relation to the condition known as fibroadenosis – but this does little to help women with genuine complaints or the fears that go with them. Benign presentations encompass a full spectrum from normality to disabling disease and we have tried to present this comprehensive approach and to introduce a terminology which is accurate in descriptive terms as well as pathogenesis and sufficiently broad to encompass a full spectrum from normality through benign disorder (aberrations) to benign disease. It is a brave person who puts forward a new terminology for benign breast disorder, yet no one can deny the need for a terminology which is both accurate and comprehensive.

A great many people come into contact with benign breast problems. General practitioners and general surgeons carry the brunt of the work in the UK, and endocrinologists and gynaecologists in some other countries. Yet general practitioners, plastic surgeons, radiologists, pathologists, radiotherapists and clinical oncologists all need an understanding of the processes affecting the breast and their clinical presentations and management. The development of national screening for breast cancer highlights the need for appreciation of the range of normality and minor aberrations in the breast. We have tried to cover the field for all these groups, to give a background understanding to the problem they will encounter in their clinical practice. Selective citation of literature has been inevitable, and for many less common conditions there is little guidance in the literature. Here we have based the recommendations on our experience in the specialized clinics for benign breast disorders which we have held in Cardiff for the last 17 years. It will be clear that many problems of management remain, and we hope that the survey of benign disorders and diseases of the breast given in this book will stimulate yet more research and clinical trials to answer remaining problems.

Acknowledgements

We owe a debt of gratitude to many people who have contributed to this book. Foremost are those research fellows who have been responsible for the day-to-day conduct of many studies and clinical trials in this department over the last 15 years: Paul Preece, John Wisbey, Nigel Pashby, Jonathan Pye, Sandeep Kumar, Anurag Srivastava, Barney Harrison, Paul Maddox and Graham Pritchard. Dr Huw Gravelle, Consultant Radiologist to the University Hospital of Wales, has provided a superb mammographic service throughout the period and has kindly provided the radiological illustrations throughout this book — in addition to those in Chapter 6. Co-operative studies with Dr Windsor Fortt of the Department of Pathology have provided most of the histological figures. Dr David Page, of Vanderbilt University, Nashville, Tennessee, gave much help and guidance in the preparation of Chapter 4. This book could not have been produced without the exceptional service given by the Department of Medical Illustration under Professor R. Marshall. The line drawings are by Peter Cox.

Our research has been supported over the years from many sources, including the Medical Research Council, Cancer Research Campaign, The Wellcome Trust and the pharmaceutical industry, including Efamol, Sandoz and Winthrop.

Mrs Edna Lewis has given voluntary service to the Mastalgia Clinic throughout most of its 15 years' existence.

The secretaries of the University Department of Surgery, Mrs Jackie Allen, Mrs Barbara Holland, Miss Mary Ryan and Mrs Enid Davies, have worked hard and long — far beyond the reasonable call of duty — to see this book typed through many drafts.

Above all we are grateful to our wives and families who have foregone so much over many years in the cause of research and the writing of this book.

Contents

Foreword   v
Acknowledgements   vi

1   **Problems of Concept and Nomenclature of Benign Disorders of the Breast**   1

The source of the problem   *1*
History   *2*

2   **Breast Anatomy and Physiology**   5

Development   *5*
Changes at puberty   *6*
Adult anatomy   *6*
Microscopic anatomy   *8*
Postmenopausal involution   *12*

3   **Aberrations of Normal Development and Involution (ANDI): A Concept of Benign Breast Disorders based on Pathogenesis**   15

The problems   *15*
Hormone-controlled processes of the breast   *16*
A framework based on pathogenesis   *19*
An extension of the concept of ANDI to include most benign breast disorders   *23*
Implications for the management of benign breast disorders   *24*

4   **The Epidemiology of Benign Breast Disease and Assessment of Cancer Risk**   27

Epidemiological studies of benign breast disorders   *27*
The cancer risk of benign breast disorders   *28*
Conditions without increased risk   *30*
Conditions with slightly increased risk (1.5–2 times)   *32*
Conditions with moderate increase in cancer risk (5 times)   *32*
Breast lesions associated with a high risk   *33*
Non-histological risk factors   *34*
New techniques for estimating risk   *34*
An outline of terminology and groupings of hyperplastic lesions of the breast   *35*
Lobular hyperplasia and neoplasia   *37*
Other epithelial hyperplasias   *37*

5   **The Approach to Assessment and Management of Breast Lumps**   41

Clinical assessment of a breast lump   *41*
Assessment using ancillary investigations   *43*
Management of nodularity   *44*
Features of individual lesions   *45*

Follow-up after assessment and/or benign breast biopsy   *46*
Management of recurrent lumps following biopsy   *47*
Breast masses in adolescence   *47*
Breast lumps in older women   *48*

6   **Breast Imaging Methods**   *49*

Techniques of proven value   *49*
Techniques of uncertain value   *53*
Mammography in benign breast disorders   *53*
Wolfe parenchymal patterns   *55*

7   **Fibroadenoma and Related Tumours**   *59*

Terminology   *59*
Fibroadenoma   *59*
Variations in histological appearance of fibroadenoma   *65*
Giant fibroadenoma – definition   *66*
Giant fibroadenoma of adolescence   *66*
Giant breast tumours of the perimenopausal period   *69*

8   **Breast Pain and Nodularity**   *75*

Historical note   *75*
Frequency of breast pain   *75*
Mastalgia in breast cancer   *76*
Classification   *76*
Aetiology of mastalgia and nodularity   *79*
Management of patients with mastalgia and nodularity
    of the breast   *82*
Treatment of non-cyclical mastalgia   *86*
Natural history of mastalgia   *87*
Recommended management   *87*
Conclusions   *90*

9   **Cysts of the Breast**   *93*

Pathology   *93*
Incidence   *94*
Pathogenesis   *94*
Aetiology   *96*
Clinical features   *96*
Investigation   *97*
Differential diagnosis   *97*
Management   *97*
Galactocele   *99*
Papillary tumours associated with macrocysts   *100*

10   **Sclerosing Adenosis**   *103*

Clinical presentation   *103*
Frequency of presentation   *104*
Radiological criteria   *104*
Pathological findings   *104*
Management   *104*

11 The Duct Ectasia/Periductal Mastitis Complex   107

Historical survey   *107*
Pathology of duct ectasia/periductal mastitis   *109*
Pathogenesis   *112*
The clinical spectrum of duct ectasia/periductal mastitis   *115*
Frequency of duct ectasia/periductal mastitis   *121*
Radiology   *121*
Management of duct ectasia/periductal mastitis   *122*
The consequences and results of operations
    for duct ectasia   *125*

12 Nipple Discharge   133

Incidence   *133*
Character and significance of discharge   *133*
Pathology underlying nipple discharge   *136*
Physical examination and investigation of
    nipple discharge   *138*
Management   *139*

13 Infection of the Breast   143

Lactational breast infection   *143*
Non-lactational breast abscess   *146*
Specific infections of the breast   *147*
Infections of associated structures   *149*

14 Disorders of the Nipple and Areola   151

Nipple inversion and retraction   *151*
Cracked nipples   *152*
Nipple crusting   *152*
Erosive adenomatosis   *152*
Syringomatous adenoma   *153*
Simple fibroepithelial polyp   *153*
Eczema   *153*
Leiomyoma   *154*
Traumatic lesions   *154*
Raynaud's phenomenon   *154*
Montgomery's glands   *154*
Sebaceous cyst of the nipple   *155*
Viral infections   *156*

15 Congenital and Cosmetic Aspects   159

Developmental anomalies   *159*
Hypertrophic abnormalities of the breast   *162*
Excessive postlactational involution   *164*
Cosmetic aspects   *164*

16 The Male Breast   167

Gynaecomastia   *167*
Other male breast disease   *172*

17   Miscellaneous Conditions   175

Trauma   *175*
Fat necrosis   *175*
Paraffinoma   *176*
Radiation damage   *177*
Lipoma   *177*
Adenolipoma (hamartoma)   *177*
Mondor's disease   *178*
Oedema of the breast   *178*
Fibrous disease of the breast   *179*
Fibromatosis (desmoid tumour)   *179*
Diabetes   *179*
Sarcoid   *180*
Amyloid   *180*
Granular cell myoblastoma   *180*
Vasculitis   *180*
Aneurysm of the breast   *180*
Infarction   *180*
Non-specific granulomatous disease   *181*
Collagenous spherulosis of the breast   *181*
Benign disorders of the breast in non-western
   populations   *181*
Artefactual disease of the breast   *181*
Mammalithiasis   *183*
Hidradenitis suppurativa of the breast   *183*

18   Operations   187

Needle biopsy   *187*
Open biopsy procedures   *189*
Removal of a fibroadenoma   *191*
Radiologically controlled biopsy   *192*
Removal of a giant fibroadenoma   *194*
Microdochectomy   *194*
Excision of mammary duct fistula   *196*
Major duct excision (Adair/Urban/Hadfield)   *198*
Drainage of a lactational breast abscess   *201*
Subcutaneous mastectomy in male patients   *202*
Subcutaneous mastectomy in women   *203*
Inverted nipple   *204*

Index   207

1 Problems of Concept and Nomenclature of Benign Disorders of the Breast

The Source of the Problem

The condition commonly called fibrocystic disease, or fibroadenosis of the breast, has been a clinical problem for centuries, as reflected in writings as early as those of Astley Cooper at the beginning of the nineteenth century. For patients it causes discomfort and anxiety which varies from nuisance value to serious interference with the quality of life. For clinicians, the condition causes a range of problems of diagnosis, assessment and management which are not always clearly recognized.

In the past, the clinical condition has been linked with a variety of histological appearances including fibrosis, adenosis and cyst formation; but these changes are increasingly recognized as lying within the range of histological appearance in the normal breast. Many authors have tried to determine and assess premalignant potential of fibrocystic disease but most attempts have resulted in confusion and frustration. Recent workers, especially Page[1], have shown that only a few specific histological patterns show an association with cancer and these show no consistent correlation with the clinical picture of fibrocystic disease. This poor correlation between histology and clinical symptoms led Love and her co-authors[2] to conclude that fibrocystic disease of the breast is a 'non-disease'. Their arguments are cogent in a histological context but this approach provides no satisfactory answer to the very common clinical problems of benign breast disorders, such as mastalgia and lumpy breasts. 'Disorder' is a better term than 'disease' because so many of these conditions lie within the spectrum of normality, but to dismiss the problem as a non-disease is far from satisfactory. 'Non-disease' is useful in conceptual terms by denying the loosely defined cancer risk, but does little to help the many women who suffer from a variety of physical symptoms – sometimes of distressing severity. The magnitude of the problem is escalating with the wider concern of women about breast disease and the wider introduction of breast screening programmes.

Benign conditions of the breast have always been neglected in comparison to cancer, despite the fact that only one out of ten patients presenting to a breast clinic suffers from cancer. This is not surprising in view of the emotional implications of breast cancer and its treatment, but it has meant that the study of the benign breast has been undeservedly neglected. Reported studies have been directed largely towards a possible relationship to cancer, rather than towards the basic processes underlying benign conditions.

This neglect is most evident in standard textbooks, because interest in benign processes can be found when studying historical reference material. Great names in surgery such as Hunter, Astley Cooper, Billroth, Cheatle, Semb, Bloodgood and Atkins appear in the literature. But whereas breast cancer has stimulated a continuous, on-going body of research – each new project building on the work preceding it – benign disease has been the subject of a relatively small number of isolated and unconnected projects, earlier related work having often been ignored. The sporadic nature of these investigations and the insularity of the resulting publications had led to much confusion which has had more serious consequences than neglect alone.

Each worker has tended to introduce his own terminology for a condition, either to stress a particular aspect that he has noted, or through ignorance of work that has gone on perhaps many years before. Table 1.1 illustrates this, showing

Table 1.1 Some of the names used for common benign breast disorders.

Cyclical nodularity
  Fibrocystic disease
  Fibroadenosis
  Cystic hyperplasia
  Hyperplastic cystic disease
  Schimmelbusch's disease
  Chronic cystic mastitis
  Cystic mastopathy

Duct ectasia/periductal mastitis
  Plasma cell mastitis
  Varicocele tumour
  Comedo mastitis
  Mastitis obliterans
  Secretory disease

Giant fibroadenomatous tumours
  Giant fibroadenoma
  Cystosarcoma phyllodes
  Phyllodes tumour
  Juvenile fibroadenoma
  Serocystic disease of Brodie

the large number of names which have been associated with just three conditions – so-called fibrocystic disease, duct ectasia and giant fibroadenomas. This list is by no means comprehensive; some 40 names have been used to describe the variety of conditions covered by the old term 'chronic fibrocystic disease', none of which can be considered satisfactory.

For reasons given throughout this book, they are better replaced by an inclusive term which will be both comprehensive and descriptive in the sense of pathogenesis. We suggest the term 'aberrations of normal development and involution' (ANDI) as the least complex term which meets these criteria. The multiplicity of names used in the past has led to confusion of communication, particularly when information is passed between pathologist, radiologist and surgeon, and even between surgeons themselves. Consideration from a historical point of view provides a clearer understanding of the present situation.

History

Sir Astley Cooper was an important early worker in this field. He described many aspects of benign breast disorders as well as malignant disease, in his monograph – *Illustrations of Diseases of the Breast*[3] – published in 1829. Among the conditions discussed are cystic disease, pain and fibroadenoma. He distinguished two main groups of patients with mastalgia – those with and those without a palpable tumour, which we might now better define as painful nodularity and non-

cyclical breast pain. He also laid much of the basis of the macroscopic anatomy of the breast in his book on the anatomy of diseases of the breast published in 1845. The French surgeon, Reclus, gave an excellent description of the clinical and pathological aspects of cystic disease in 1893[4], recognizing both the multiplicity and bilaterality of the cysts.

Many of the current problems in terminology and understanding derive from the publications of German surgeons in the late nineteenth century. Koenig[5] called the disease 'chronic cystic mastitis', because he believed it had an inflammatory basis. At the same time, Schimmelbusch[6] described the same condition, compounding the problem by calling it cystadenoma. Both authors gave the disease inexact names, and both gave incomplete descriptions of the pathology. Certainly they did not recognize the wide range of histological appearances found in these breasts, and they failed to recognize these as merely variants of normal processes within the breast.

There was an early reaction to this confusion. Cabot[7] questioned the inflammatory connotation of the term 'chronic cystic mastitis' and urged more precise terminology, but unfortunately it fell on stony ground. In the 1920s there were major studies by Semb in Norway[8] and Cheatle in the UK[9] and their disease descriptions and data are still worth serious study. However, Cheatle gave the name 'cystiphorous desquamative epithelial hyperplasia' to the clinical spectrum we have termed 'ANDI' in Chapter 3 and this can hardly be regarded as helpful. The tendency of the Scandinavians to use Semb's term 'fibroadenomatosis' also caused difficulty because of its obvious confusion with fibroadenoma[8]. In spite of detailed investigations, Cheatle and Cutler confused changes of cyclical nodularity with both duct ectasia and fibroadenomas[9] and the term they finally chose – 'mazoplasia' – is hardly evocative in a descriptive sense.

While most workers concentrated on the clinical problems of 'fibrocystic disease', some gave accurate descriptions of other benign breast conditions. The paper on 'the varicocele tumour' by Bloodgood is a striking account of the clinical and macropathological aspects of duct ectasia and its clinical variants (*see* Ref. 3, p. 130). The accuracy and detail of the observations come as a surprise to those who believe advances in medical understanding are recent.

Special clinics for breast disease set up by Atkins in London and Geschickter in the USA concentrated experience and allowed adequate documentation and assessment of the results of treatment for the first time. Both authors made many contributions to benign breast disorders[10, 11], but suffered equally from the limited knowledge at that time of basic pathology and endocrinology of the breast. Each unfortunately continued the use of the term 'chronic mastitis'. The 40 years since their contributions has seen an increasing momentum in investigation of benign breast conditions. Great benefit has derived from histological study of the normal breast and the development of hormonal estimations using radioimmunoassay. In particular, the autopsy study of Sandison[12] showed that most of the changes previously regarded as disease are so common as to be within the spectrum of normality and his work stimulated others to define the wide range of histological appearances of the normal breast. For example, Parks[13] studied both surgical and autopsy specimens and showed a gradation between normal lobules and fibroadenomata, and between involuting lobules and cyst formation. He also showed that papillary epithelial hyperplasia of the terminal ducts is so common in the premenopausal period as to be regarded as normal, and that these lesions regress without treatment after the menopause. While these writers have had a profound effect on the thinking of workers interested in breast disease, it is salutary to go back even further. In 1922, McFarland[14] wrote: 'The so-called chronic mastitis is not inflammatory, and is not a pathological entity; it is nothing but a result – or at most a perversion – of involution. The only difficulty lies in clearly defining when the process of involution can be said to become abnormal, when it is so diversified.'

Why has it taken so long to reach a reasonable understanding of the processes involved in benign breast conditions? The main stumbling block has been the failure to appreciate the range of basic physiological and structural changes within the normal breast – an organ dynamic throughout the reproductive period of life as it first develops, then undergoes repeated cyclical change and finally involutes. Because it is an organ under systemic hormonal influence, one would expect the breast to be uniform throughout in its appearance and behaviour, but this is not so. Like other endocrine target organs such as the thyroid, it varies greatly from one part to another, and end-organ response must be a factor in this variability. It has been usual practice to concentrate on the local findings as shown by biopsy, at one point in time when the patient presents with a clinical problem, assuming that the particular clinical condition at that time is directly associated with the local radiological and biopsy findings. It is tempting to ignore the findings of Parks and Sandison and others, that all these apparently specific findings are frequently found in asymptomatic breasts. So a particular clinical event that leads a patient to biopsy must be assessed against the background of this almost random variation in histological appearance which is a part of normality.

A further source of confusion has arisen from the association of radiological appearances with pathological descriptions, without adequate correlative studies to establish a relationship. A recent example has been the description of radiological density as 'dysplasia' in relation to Wolfe patterns – when detailed study can show that 'density' is unrelated to epithelial dysplasia[15]. The cause of the patient with benign breast problems will be best served by abandoning terminology which implies disease, and substituting terminology which reflects the normality of many of the underlying processes. The terminology should come from consideration of the basic physiological and pathological processes which lead a patient to present to a breast clinic.

Perhaps the reason for persisting and increasing confusion is an unwillingness to be sufficiently radical in moving away from the ideas which do not fit in with present knowledge. Not only must the concept of fibrocystic disease as a clinical concept or a histopathological entity be done away with, it must be replaced with an accurate concept and terminology consistent with present knowledge.

These basic aspects of the non-malignant breast are considered in Chapter 3.

REFERENCES

1. Page D. L., Vander-Zwag R., Rogers L. W., Williams L. T., Walker W. F. & Hartmann W. H. Relationship between component parts of fibrocystic disease complex and breast cancer. *Journal of the National Cancer Institute* 1978; **61**: 1055–1063.
2. Love S. M., Gelman R. S. & Silen W. Fibrocystic 'disease' of the breast. A non disease. *New England Journal of Medicine* 1982; **307**: 1010–1014.
3. Cooper A. *Illustrations of Diseases of the Breast.* London, Longmans, 1829.
4. Reclus P. Maladie Kystique De La Mammelle. *La Semaine Medicale* 1893; **13**: 353–354.
5. Koenig P. Mastitis chronica cystica. *Centralblatt für Chirurgie* 1893; **20**: 49–53.
6. Schimmelbusch C. Das Fibroadenom der Mamma. *Archiv für Klinische Chirurgie* 1892; **64**: 102–116.
7. Cabot R. C. Irritable breasts, or chronic lobular mastitis. *Boston Medical and Surgical Journal* 1900; **CXLIII**: 555–557.

8. Semb C. Pathologico-anatomical and clinical investigations of fibroadenomatosis cystica mammae. *Acta Chirurgica Scandinavica Supplementum* 1928; **64**(10): 1–484.

9. Cheatle G. L. & Cutler M. *Tumours of the Breast.* London, Edward Arnold, 1931.

10. Atkins H. J. B. Chronic mastitis. *Lancet* 1938; i: 707–712.

11. Geschickter C. F. *Diseases of the Breast,* 2nd edn. Philadelphia, J. B. Lippincott & Co., 1945.

12. Sandison A. T. An autopsy study of the human breast. *National Cancer Institute Monograph No. 8,* US Dept Health, Education and Welfare, 1962.

13. Parks A. G. The microanatomy of the breast. *Annals of the Royal College of Surgeons (England)* 1959; **25**: 295–311.

14. McFarland J. Residual lactation acini in the female breasts. Their relationship to chronic cystic mastitis and malignant breasts. *Archives of Surgery* 1922; **5**: 1–64.

15. Mansel R. E. Gravelle I. H. & Hughes L. E. The interpretation of mammographic ductal enlargement in cancerous breasts. *British Journal of Surgery* 1979; **66**: 701–702.

2 Breast Anatomy and Physiology

Development

The prepubertal breast is identical in both sexes and consists of a number of small ducts embedded in a collagenous stroma. The ducts develop *in utero* from an ectodermal mammary ridge which invades the epidermis at the seventh embryonic week and progresses to a budding stage at the twelfth week. The mammary ridge extends from the base of the upper limb bud to the base of the lower limb bud (Figure 2.1). The epithelial bud then branches and canalizes between weeks 13 and 20 to form the 15–20 major ducts found in the adult breast. The major ducts at this stage only have small vesicles at the distal ends and no lobular development is visible. The increasing development of the foetal breast parenchyma induces considerable growth and specialization of the surrounding stroma. A comprehensive three-layer vascular network forms at the 9–10 week budding stage and eventually produces a cylindrical vascular envelope around each of the major ducts[1]. From the tenth week *in utero* to birth a series of developments occur. Ingrowth of connective tissue gives rise to partitions between each of the end-vesicles (primitive alveoli) and acts as a framework for the adult segmental pattern. Specialized fat cells also invade the matrices between the blood vessels and fibrous septae. Externally the nipple is small and flattened and no aveolar development has occurred, although rudimentary sebaceous glands and Montgomery's tubercles are present. The circular interlacing smooth muscle fibres that give the nipple its erectile properties are already developed at this stage. All the above changes are completed by the time of birth and essentially no further development occurs until puberty.

At the time of birth, transient secretory changes occur in the new-born breast which give rise to the clinical entities of 'witches' milk' or 'neonatal mastitis'. In late pregnancy the high levels of

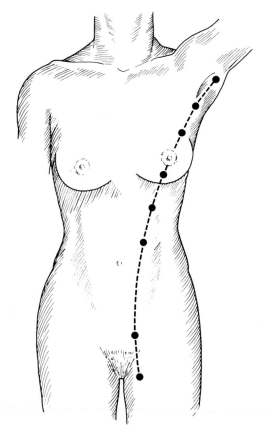

2.1 *The extent of the foetal mammary ridge. Accessory nipples or breasts are usually found along this line (see Chapter 15).*

luteal and placental hormones in the mother's blood cross the placenta into the foetal circulation and cause stimulation of the foetal breast. This primes the primitive foetal end-vesicles for milk production in an analogous fashion to the adult female breast in late pregnancy. Birth inevitably causes separation of the maternal and foetal circulations resulting in a rapid fall in circulating sex steroids in the baby's blood, whereas prolactin secretion is maintained by the baby's pituitary. These conditions correspond once more to the maternal situation and result in secretion of colostrum which can be expressed from the nipple in 80–90% of new-born breasts of either sex. The new-born prolactin levels then decline and the secretion dries up over the next few weeks. Thus the secretion of colostrum and the swelling of the new-born breast are both normal physiological events and should not be considered as due to disease unless they become persistent.

Changes at Puberty

The next series of steps in development are activated at puberty in the female and follow the well-ordered sequence described by Marshall and Tanner[2] and Zacharias et al[3] (Figure 2.2). The first change (at about the age of 10 years) is growth of the mammary tissue beneath the areola with enlargement of the areolar area producing the characteristic swelling known as the breast bud or mound. This development is often asymmetrical. At 12 years the nipple begins to grow outwards and the breast elevation increases, but there is no distinct separation between nipple and areola. Between the ages of 14 and 15, increasing subareolar growth leads to elevation of the areola above the breast outline giving the 'secondary mound'. The familiar shape of the adult resting breast is then attained by a recession in the level of the areola to that of the surrounding breast leaving the nipple projecting.

The exact physiological mechanisms that trigger and control the changes of puberty are not fully understood but recent advances in radio-immunoassay have clarified some of the issues. The primary event in the initiation of puberty is the increasing secretion of follicle stimulating hormone (FSH) and luteinizing hormone (LH) from the anterior pituitary in reponse to increasing stimulation by the hypothalamus. Detectable levels of FSH and LH are found in prepubertal children showing that some hypothalamic activity is present even in young children but, as maturation proceeds, this hypothalamic activity increases dramatically. This is probably due to a change in frequency of the pulsatile secretion of the gonadotrophin releasing factors[4]. The increased FSH/LH causes activation of primordial ovarian follicles and secretion of oestrogen which is responsible for the first stages of breast development. Oestrogen induces duct sprouting and branching but lobular development at this stage consists only of small buds. Adult levels of progesterone are required for further development of the lobular component. Oestrogen also induces connective tissue and vascular growth which is required for the support of the new ducts. In the early stages of puberty, ovarian cycles are frequently anovular and luteal function is poor, resulting in an oestrogen-dominated milieu; conse-quently ductal growth predominates. When ovulating cycles begin, luteal function improves, the increased output of progesterone balances the oestrogen and results in differentiation of the terminal ductular buds to produce adult lobules. These differential growth patterns associated with the two major ovarian steroids have been studied principally in animals[5, 6], but appear to be true also for the human. Insulin, growth hormone, corticosteroids and prolactin are also required for optimal growth of the breast but only play minor roles.

Adult Anatomy

The adult female breasts lie on each side of the anterior thorax with their bases extending from about the second to the sixth ribs. Medially the breasts reach the sternal edge and laterally the mid-axillary line and extend up into the axilla via a pyramidal-shaped axillary tail (Figure 2.3). The breast lies on a substantial layer of fascia overlying the pectoralis major muscle in the superomedial two-thirds and the serratus anterior muscle in the lower outer one-third. This extent is greater than that of the breast given in many descriptions, and is important for matching in cosmetic and reconstructive surgery. The precise position of the nipple areolar complex varies widely with the fat content of the breast and the age of the woman. The nipple extends about 5–10 mm above the level of the areolar skin and is covered with rugose skin which is variably pigmented (Figure 2.4). The surface of the areola shows a number of small protuberances which are the openings of Montgomery's glands: modified large sebaceous glands which lubricate the areolar skin during suckling. Craigmyle suggests that each Montgomery's tubercle is an aposebaceous unit as the

2.2 *The stages of breast development at puberty. (a) Breast bud elevation; (b) growth and protrusion of the nipple; (c) elevation of the secondary areolar mound; (d) regression of the areolar mound to the level of the general breast contour.*

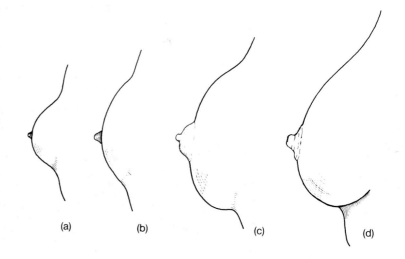

(a)   (b)   (c)   (d)

sebaceous gland openings surround the orifices of the apocrine glands which are readily found in the areolar skin[7]. The nipple and areolar skin are rich in smooth muscle fibres which are responsible for nipple erection.

Vascular Anatomy

The blood supply is from the axillary artery via its thoracoacromial, lateral thoracic and subscapular arteries, and from the subclavian artery via the internal thoracic (mammary) artery. The internal thoracic artery supplies three large anterior perforating branches through the second, third and fourth intercostal spaces. Perforating branches from the anterior intercostal arteries also come through these spaces more laterally. The veins form a rich subareolar plexus and drain to the intercostal and axillary veins and to the internal thoracic veins.

Lymphatics of the Breast

The lymphatic drainage of the breast is of great importance in the spread of malignant disease of the breast but of lesser importance in benign breast disease. Several lymphatic plexi issue from the parenchymal portion of the breast and the subareolar region and drain to the regional lymph nodes, the majority of which lie within the axilla. The majority of the lymph from each breast passes into the ipsilateral axillary nodes along a chain which begins at the anterior axillary (pectoral) nodes and continues into the central axillary and apical node groups. Further drainage occurs into the subscapular and interpectoral node groups. A small amount of lymph drains across to the opposite breast and also downwards into the rectus sheath. Some of the medial part of the breast is drained by lymphatics which accompany the perforating internal thoracic vessels and drain into the internal thoracic group of nodes in the thorax and on into the mediastinal nodes. The older accounts of breast lymphatics derived from dissection studies have been clarified and superseded by dynamic studies *in vivo*[8].

Nerve Supply

The innervation of the breast is principally by somatic sensory nerves and autonomic nerves accompanying the blood vessels. In general, the areola and nipple are richly supplied by somatic sensory nerves while the breast parenchyma is mostly supplied by autonomic supply which appears to be solely sympathetic. No parasympathetic activity has been demonstrated in the

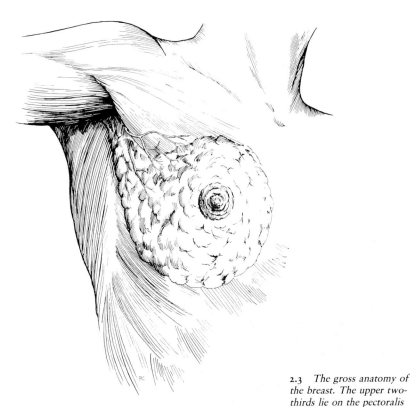

2.3 *The gross anatomy of the breast. The upper two-thirds lie on the pectoralis major and the lower one-third on the serratus anterior. Note the prolongation of the upper outer quadrant into the axilla.*

breast[9]. Detailed histological examination has failed to show any direct neural end-terminal connections with breast ductular cells or myoepithelial cells suggesting that the principal control mechanisms of secretion and milk ejection are humoral rather than nervous mechanisms. It is interesting that the areolar epidermis is relatively poorly innervated whereas the nipple and lactiferous ducts are richly innervated; these findings are supported by the clinical findings of poor appreciation of light touch and two-point discrimination over the areola. The rich nipple innervation is thought to be the basis of the well-known suckling reflex whereby a neural afferent pathway causes rapid release of both adenohypophyseal prolactin and neurohypophyseal oxytocin on suckling.

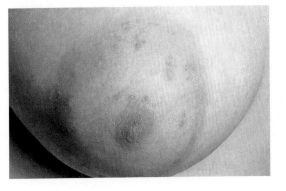

2.4 *The normal nipple and areola. The pinker areolar skin is clearly demarcated from the surrounding breast skin and shows several small nodules which are the openings of Montgomery's tubercles.*

The somatic sensory nerve supply is via the supraclavicular nerves (C3, C4) superiorly and laterally from the lateral branches of the thoracic intercostal nerves (third to fourth). The medial aspects of the breast receive supply from the anterior branches of the thoracic intercostal nerves which penetrate the pectoralis major to reach the breast skin. A major supply of the upper outer quadrant of the breast is via the intercostobrachial nerve (C8, T1) which gives a large branch to the breast as it traverses the axilla.

Fascia of the Breast

The fascial framework of the breast is important in relation to clinical manifestations of disease and surgical technique. Because the breast develops as a skin appendage, it does so within the superficial fascia, such that the superficial part of the superficial fascia forms an anterior boundary and the deep layer of the superficial fascia forms a posterior boundary. In between, condensation of this interlobar fascia gives rise to the pyramidal-shaped ligaments of Cooper, called suspensory ligaments because they provide a supporting framework to the breast lobes. They are best developed in the upper part of the breast and are connected to both pectoral fascia and skin by fibrous extensions. In spite of these fibrous extensions, the superficial layer of superficial fascia gives a plane of dissection between the skin and breast. (The small subcutaneous fat lobules are readily differentiated from the much larger mammary fat lobules.) Likewise, the retromammary space provides a ready plane of dissection between the deep layer of superficial fascia and the deep fascia of pectoralis major and serratus anterior. This structural fascial support is so intimately connected to interlobular and intralobular fascia with their enclosed ductal units, that no ready plane of dissection exists within the breast substance and all surgery must be carried out by sharp dissection. The skin overlying the breast has been shown to vary in thickness from 0.8 mm to 3 mm on mammograms of normal breasts and tends to decrease with increasing breast size[10].

Microscopic Anatomy

The adult resting breast has a branching major duct system leading to terminal ductal–alveolar (lobular) units (TDLU) (Figure 2.5). Histological sections cut the three-dimensional lobules in several planes giving rise to a sponge-like appearance on section (Figure 2.6a). The tree-like branching structure of breast ductules is very nicely shown

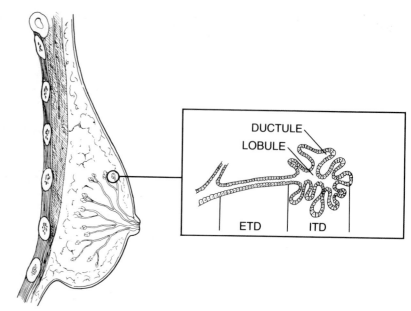

by the technique of microradiography, which has been developed in Cardiff for small pieces of breast tissue (Figure 2.6b). The ductal and alveolar epithelium are similar in structure and consist of two layers of cells, the basal cells being cuboidal and the surface cells being cylindrical with their long axes at right angles to the duct wall. Surrounding the ductal and alveolar walls is a discontinuous fenestrated layer of contractile myoepithelial cells. The myoepithelial cells contract in response to oxytocin stimulation and are responsible for the ejection of milk from the expanded TDLU of pregnancy into larger ducts. Light microscopy has shown some variation in the epithelial cells and two main cell types have been described by Bassler[11]. The more numerous basal cells have a light cytoplasm and were called clear basal B-cells by Bassler, who thought they might function as stem cells for differentiation into myoepithelial cells or the second cell type (A-cells). The darker A-cells are luminal cells which have an eosinophilic cytoplasm packed with ribosomes which are responsible for the darker appearance under the microscope. Bassler[11] postulated that the dark A-cells develop from the clear B-cells under the influence of oestrogen and migrate towards the luminal surface where they engage in secretory activity. A number of dark cells show regressive changes and are then shed as cellular debris into the lumen. Some dark A-cells which have large membrane-bound vesicles containing lipid have been described as 'foam cells'; these may represent phagocytic histiocytes[12].

Ultrastructural studies show that breast epithelial cells have well-developed luminal microvilli and complex interdigitating basal laminae with prominent desmosomes at intercellular bound-

2.5 *Cross-section of the breast to show the ductal and lobulo-alveolar structure. The expanded diagrams show the schematic structure of the terminal ductal lobular unit (TDLU). ETD = extralobular terminal ductule; ITD = intralobular terminal ductule.*

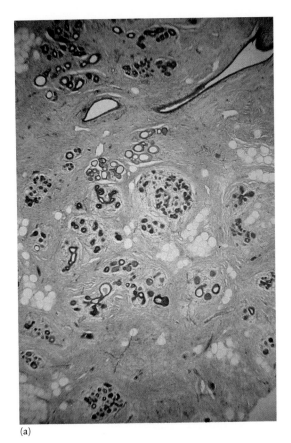

(a)

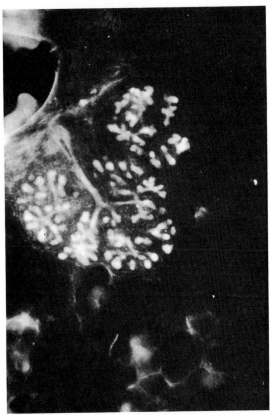

(b)

aries. Cytoplasmic densities have been shown to vary in the same way as observed in light microscopy, in that a population of pale and dark cells can be identified[13-15]. Ozzello[13] also describes an intermediate cell which may represent Bassler's postulated stem cell. As might be expected, myoepithelial cells contain well-marked contractile myofilaments and cilia running parallel to the long axis of the cell. Myoepithelial cells are closely related to the basement membranes of the luminal epithelial cells and to the basal lamina, to which they are attached by numerous hemidesmosomes. Ultrastructural studies have revealed the unsuspected complexity of the epithelial stromal junction (ESJ) which is the crucial interface across which all nutrients must reach the breast ductal cells[14, 16]. The ESJ consists of a complex intertwining of fibroblasts, elastic fibres and endothelium and it is possible that the cause for some of the puzzling aspects of benign breast disease may lie in disorders of this region.

The Breast Stroma

Careful histological study by Parks has shown the heterogeneity of connective tissue in the breast[17]. The intralobular and periductal connective tissue is probably as important in physiological terms as the interlobular Cooper's ligaments in structural terms, although it must be admitted that our knowledge of the physiology of the lobular stroma is still rudimentary. The segmental and interlobular fascia is dense and reticular, while the periductal and intralobular stroma is much looser – a contrast between loose and dense reminiscent of the papillary and reticular layers of the dermis – the tissue from which the breast arises. The interlobular fascia often shows a large amount of fatty infiltration, especially in the larger breast. Further differences can be detected between periductal and lobular stroma. Periductal connective tissue is found as a cuff of loose stroma around the ducts in which run the lymphatic vessels. It is more cellular (fibrocytes) than the supporting fibrous tissue and contains a considerable amount of elastic tissue, which tends to increase with age and parity. The lobular stroma is even more loose, more vascular, more cellular and markedly mucoid – a structure which facilitates expansion of the developing acini in pregnancy. The lobule contains no elastic tissue and this fact is helpful to the pathologist in differentiating lesions arising from the lobule from those arising from ducts. Lobular stroma, and probably periductal stroma, is under hormonal influence, but little is known about the detailed hormonal responsiveness of this tissue.

Durnberger *et al*[18] have shown that the differentiation of the mammary epithelial bud in the male foetal rodent occurs in response to a transient increase in testosterone secretion which does not affect the mammary ductular epithelium directly but is mediated by the surrounding stromal fibroblasts. Recent work from the authors' own laboratories has shown that human breast fibroblasts are highly stimulatory to human breast cancer cells in an *in vivo* nude mouse xenograft model[19]. These experiments point to a major regulatory role for breast fibroblasts in epithelial cell growth.

Cyclical Changes in Breast Epithelium

The normal ovulatory menstrual cycle of females produces distinct changes in primary target organs such as endometrium and vagina, and it would not be surprising to find some readily observable changes in the breast. Definite proof of changes has not emerged in most studies and many pathologists doubt that clear histological changes can be detected in breast tissue taken at different phases of the cycle. An early report by Rosenberg[20] suggested that epithelial proliferation and stromal oedema could be documented at various phases of the menstrual cycle; these studies were based on postmortem material and lacked clear documentation on the menstrual cycle. Later reports have not found clear changes and Haagensen[21] emphatically states that he was unable to confirm any cyclical variation in the number of acini per lobule – despite a search for the purported specific changes. A recent paper by Vogel *et al*[22] also suggested that specific changes were seen which correlated with the phase of the menstrual cycle although an unspecified inter- and intra-observer variation was admitted. Fanger and Jung Ree[23] studied the ultrastructural characteristics of breast tissue at different phases of the menstrual cycle and described two different types of cell – phase I and phase II – which were seen in the preovulatory and postovulatory phases of the cycle, respectively. Masters *et al*[24] reported on increased labelling index (thymidine uptake) during the luteal phase of the cycle, suggesting increased DNA synthesis.

The conflicting views regarding histological change during the menstrual cycle reflect the paucity of knowledge of the normal physiology of the human breast and further work is needed to clarify the issue. Whatever the evidence is for histological change, there is clearly documented evidence that breast volume measured by water displacement methods increases during the luteal phase of the cycle and falls at menstruation[25]. These changes are noticed by a large number of women and may be explained by vascular or lymphatic changes without requiring obvious

changes in breast histology. Anderson *et al* have shown that mitosis (cell growth) and apoptosis (cell death) occur in definite biorhythms with a 3-day difference between the peak of mitosis which occurred on day 25 and peak of the apoptosis which occurred on day 28[26]. There was no correlation with parity or contraceptive pill use, but the cyclicity of apoptosis declined with age. These authors conclude that the factors promoting breast cell apoptosis are not clear.

Changes of Pregnancy and Lactation
Anatomy

The greatly increased levels of luteal and placental sex steroids, with the addition of placental lactogen and chorionic gonadotrophin, in pregnancy cause a remarkable increase in lobuloalveolar growth. Prolactin levels also increase progressively throughout pregnancy but this hormone appears to be mainly concerned with milk production at the end of pregnancy after the preceding hormones have primed the breast by inducing marked proliferative changes. Chronologically the changes are shown in Table 2.1.

Table 2.1 Changes during pregnancy.

Week	Change
0	Resting breast approx 200 g in weight
1–4	Ductular sprouting/lobular formation
5–8	Breast enlarges/vascular engorgement/areolar pigmentation/predominant lobular formation
>12	Large alveoli with single epithelial cell layer. Beginning of colostrum formation
>20	Alveolar dilatation/colostrum formation. New capillary formation/myoepithelial cell hypertrophy
Term	180% increase of mammary blood flow Weight approx 400 g Fat droplet accumulation in alveolar cells

After Vorherr[27].

Histologically, the most remarkable features are the great predominance of dilated alveoli and the conversion of the resting two-layer epithelium to a monolayer within the alveoli (Figure 2.7).

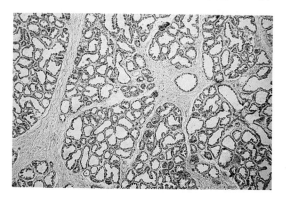

2.7 *Histological section (H & E) of lactating breast showing grossly dilated acini lined by a low cuboidal epithelium. Note the high ratio of epithelium to stroma.*

The large ducts maintain their two-layer configuration.

Physiology

Basal prolactin levels increase from the non-pregnant level of 10 ng/ml to peak values of over 200 ng/ml at week 40, postpartum prolactin levels fall over the next 4 weeks to around 20 ng/ml but are immediately elevated to about 10 times basal levels on suckling the infant. Although, as previously described, some colostral secretion is visible in the breast before term, the process of milk production proper begins 2–5 days after birth. The change from colostrum to milk is caused by high levels of prolactin maintained against a rapidly falling level of ovarian and placental sex steroids.

Prolactin is the primary stimulant for galacto-poiesis and has been shown to have a variety of actions on breast tissue, which would contribute to milk production[28]. The increased mitosis required for alveolar growth and early colostrum production is stimulated primarily by ovarian and placental sex steroids, placental lactogen, cortisol and growth hormone with the placenta supplying the bulk of the sex steroids and lactogenic factors. Although some milk protein and fat synthesis is seen from mid-pregnancy onwards, the full lactogenic stimulation of prolactin is inhibited by the high levels of circulating sex steroids. Birth and the consequent loss of the placenta reverses the inhibition and full milk production then begins. The predominant role of prolactin in lactopoiesis is illustrated by the fact that ovariec-tomized women and animals can successfully breast-feed.

Established Lactation

Once established, lactation will continue almost indefinitely provided the milk is regularly removed from the breast. After 48 hours of milk stagnation, milk synthesis begins to fall rapidly[1, 29].

During milk secretion, alveolar cells change shape and histological appearance. During active lactation, the upper part of the cell breaks away or is extruded and the cell changes from a columnar shape to a low cuboidal shape. Thus milk secretion is an apocrine and merocrine type secretion as only part of the cell is lost. The fat globules in milk are surrounded by a membrane which is presumably derived from the luminal cell membrane of the alveolar cell. Following secretion, resynthesis of milk proteins such as lactalbumin and casein and milk fats occurs and the cell begins to elongate. Prolactin is the primary stimulant for lactose synthesis by stimulation of lactose synthetase and protein synthesis by stimulation of nuclear RNA polymerase. Lactose synthesis takes place in the Golgi apparatus and the cell becomes large and swollen with secretory products[30, 31]. Secretion then takes place with fats and protein being excreted by apocrine secretion, lactose by merocrine secretion and inorganic ions by a combination of active transport and diffusion[26]. The cycle of extrusion and resynthesis then restarts.

The active transport processes across the luminal cell (the blood–milk barrier) are of considerable interest as recent studies of cyst fluids suggest that different morphological types of epithelium may differ in the handling of ions[32].

Excretion of Drugs into Milk

Another important area is the transport of drugs from the mother's blood into the milk and hence into the infant. This subject is not well documented and the passage of many drugs into human milk is unknown or fragmentary[33]. As in other body cells, most small water-soluble molecules may pass through aqueous 'pores' in the cell membrane whereas larger molecules have to be transported actively. In general approximately 1% of the ingested dose will appear in the milk. Most drugs taken in normal therapeutic doses will be harmless to the infant due to the low concentration in human milk. Some agents however may be toxic especially if an excess dose is taken by the mother. Documented adverse effects in breast-fed infants are shown in Table 2.2, but these side-effects only occurred after the mother had taken an excessive dose of the drug shown.

Thus, few drugs are likely to cause major problems to the breast-fed infant, but where

Table 2.2 Adverse effects of drugs excreted in human milk.

Drug	Adverse effect in breast-fed infant
Alcohol	Vomiting, drowsiness
Barbiturates	Sleepiness
Diphenylhydantoin	Vomiting, tremors
Dihydroxyanthraquinone	Diarrhoea
Ergot alkaloids	Nausea, vomiting, diarrhoea
Dextroamphetamine	Tremor, insomnia
Bromide	Rash, drowsiness
Thiouracil, iodine	Hypothyroidism, goitre
Metronidazole	Anorexia, vomiting, blood dyscrasia
Tetracycline	Teeth staining
Reserpine	Nasal stuffiness
Sulphonamides	Jaundice
Anticoagulants	Bleeding

After Vorherr[27].

potentially dangerous drugs are being taken in high dosage, bottle-feeding should be advised. Otherwise a commonsense approach with close observation of the infant should be advised as the potential benefits of breast-feeding usually outweigh possible adverse effects of the drug passage in the milk.

Postlactational Involution

Postlactational involution starts on weaning and is initiated by local mechanical factors causing alveolar distension and capillary obstruction. The one-layer secretory alveolar cells regress and reform the two-layered epithelium characteristic of the resting breast. This process is facilitated by cell death and phagocytosis performed by invasion of the alveoli by histiocytes. A lymphocytic infiltrate is also characteristic, but connective tissue regression is limited. The branching alveolar structures become fewer in number but the ductular structure remains mostly intact – this is the fundamental difference between postlactational and postmenopausal involution, where both lobules and ductules are reduced in number. The ducts become smaller although some secretion remains persistently in the duct lumen in the postlactational breast and can be aspirated or expressed from the nipple in most parous women[34]. The fluid aspirated from 61% of women is of sufficient volume to study the cellularity and hormone content[34].

Postmenopausal Involution

This process can be divided into a preclimacteric phase starting at about the age of 35 and a postmenopausal phase starting at the time of the menopause. The predominant feature is regression of the glandular epithelium and adjacent connective tissue with gradual replacement by fat. In the preclimacteric phase, there is a gradual loss of lobules and infiltration by round cells and the specialized loose connective tissue around the lobules changes into dense collagen. In the postmenopausal phase, the typical outline of a lobule is lost and is replaced by dense collagen containing a compressed epithelial remnant. Lobular involution may proceed to formation of microcysts which may be mistaken for cystic disease microscopically. The essential difference between the two conditions is the preservation of the specialized lobular stroma in the former[35]. Stromal changes dominate and fat deposition accelerates and connective tissue regression is marked. The end result is that the branching major duct system is visible, but very few lobules can be seen and these are embedded in dense fibrotic capsules unlike the loose stroma surrounding the lobules in the breasts of younger women. Some lobules may develop into microcysts by dilatation, possibly due to obstruction of the terminal ductule and interlobular connective tissue is greatly reduced. Externally these changes produce the shrunken, pendulous breast of the old woman and, when mammography is performed, are responsible for good contrast of parenchyma to fat obtained on mammograms of the older breast. Variations of this process are responsible for many of the clinical presentations and histological appearances of benign breast disease and are discussed fully in the next chapter.

REFERENCES

1. Dabelow A. Die Milchdruse In: Bagman W (ed.) *Handbuch der mikroskopischen Anatomie des Merchen*, Vol 3, Part 3, *Haut und Sininesorgane*, Berlin, Springer-Verlag, 1957, pp 277–485.
2. Marshall W. A. & Tanner J. M. Variations in pattern of pubertal changes in girls. *Archives of Diseases of Childhood* 1969; 44: 291–303.
3. Zacharias L., Wurtman R. J. & Schatzoff M. Sexual maturation in contemporary American Girls. *American Journal of Obstetrics and Gynecology* 1970; 108: 833–846.
4. Wildt L., Marshall G. & Knobil E. Experimental induction of puberty in the infantile female rhesus monkey. *Science* 1980; 207: 1373–1375.
5. Hadfield G. & Young S. The controlling influence of the pituitary on the growth of the normal breast. *British Journal of Surgery* 1958; 46: 265–273.
6. Topper Y. J. & Freeman C. S. Multiple hormone interactions in the developmental biology of the mammary gland. *Physiological Reviews* 1980; 60: 1049–1106.
7. Craigmyle M. B. L. *The Apocrine Glands and the Breast*. Chichester, John Wiley & Sons, 1974.
8. Turner-Warwick R. T. The lymphatics of the breast. *British Journal of Surgery* 1959; 46: 574–582.
9. Vorherr. H. *The Breast: Morphology, Physiology and Lactation*. New York, Academic Press, 1974.
10. Wilkson S. A., Adams E. J. & Tucker A. K. Patterns of breast skin thickness in normal mammograms. *Clinical Radiology* 1982; 33: 691–693.
11. Bassler R. The morphology of hormone-induced structural changes in the female breast. *Current Topics in Pathology* 1970; 53: 1–89.
12. Toker C. Observations on the ultrastructure of a mammary ductule. *Journal of Ultrastructure Research* 1967; 21; 9–25.
13. Ozzello L. Epithelial–stromal junction of normal and dysplastic mammary glands. *Cancer (Philadelphia)* 1970; 25: 586–600.
14. Stirling J. W. & Chandler J. A. The fine structure of the normal, resting terminal ductal–lobular unit of the female breast. *Virchows Archiv Abteilung A Pathologische Anatomie und Histologie* 1976; 372: 205–226.

15. Ahmed A. In: *Atlas of the Ultrastructure of Human Breast Diseases*, Edinburgh, Churchill Livingstone, 1978, pp 1–26.

16. Stirling J. W. & Chandler J. A. The fine structure of ducts and subareolar ducts in the resting gland of the female breast. *Virchows Archiv Abteilung A Pathologische Anatomie und Histologie* 1977; **373**: 119–132.

17. Parks A. G. The micro-anatomy of the breast. *Annals of the Royal College of Surgeons* 1959; **25**: 295–311. (Wrongly numbered as 235–251.)

18. Durnberger H., Heuberger B., Schwartz P., Wasner G. & Kratochwil K. Mesenchyme-mediated effects of testosterone on embryonic mammary epithelium. *Cancer Research* 1978; **38**: 4066–4070.

19. Horgan K., Jones D. L. & Mansel R. E. Mitogenicity of human fibroblasts in vivo for human breast cancer cells. *British Journal of Surgery* 1987; **74**: 227–229.

20. Rosenberg A. Ueber menstruelle, duch das corpus luteum bedingte mammaryranderungen. *Frankfurt Zeitschrift für Pathologie* 1922; **27**: 466–506.

21. Haagensen C. D. *Diseases of the Breast*, 3rd edn. Philadelphia, Saunders, 1986, pp 50–54.

22. Vogel P. M., Georgiade N. G., Fetter B. F., Vogel F. S. & McCarty K. S. The correlation of histologic changes in the human breast with the menstrual cycle. *American Journal of Pathology* 1981; **104**: 23–34.

23. Fanger H. & Jung Ree H. Cyclical changes of human mammary gland epithelium in relation to the menstrual cycle – an ultrastructural study. *Cancer* 1974; **34**: 574–585.

24. Masters J. R. W., Drife J. O. & Scarisbrick J. J. Cyclic variation of DNA synthesis in human breast epithelium. *Journal of the National Cancer Institute* 1977; **58**: 1263–1265.

25. Milligan D., Drife J. O. & Short R. V. Changes in breast volume during normal menstrual cycle and after oral contraceptives. *British Medical Journal* 1975; **iv**: 494–496.

26. Anderson T. J., Ferguson D. J. P. & Raab G. M. Cell turnover in the 'resting' human breast: influence of parity, contraceptive pill, age and laterality. *British Journal of Cancer* 1982; **46**: 376–382.

27. Vorherr H. Puerperium: Maternal involutional changes and lactation. In: Posinsky J. J. (ed.) *Davis' Gynecology and Obstetrics*, Vol 1, Chap 20. New York, Harper, 1972, pp 1–46.

28. Cowie A. T. Induction and suppression of lactation in animals. *Proceedings of the Royal Society of Medicine* 1972; **65**: 1084–1085.

29. Zilliacus H. Physiologie und Pathologie des Wockenbettes. In: Kasero O. *et al* (eds.) *Gynakologie und Geburtshilfe*, Vol II. Stuttgart, Thième, 1967, pp 966–997.

30. Turkington R. W. Measurement of prolactin activity in human serum by the induction of specific milk proteins in mammary gland in vitro. *Journal of Clinical Endocrinology Metabolism* 1971; **33**: 210–216.

31. Turkington R. W., Brew K., Vanaman T. C. & Hill R. C. The hormonal control of lactose synthetase in the developing mouse mammary gland. *Journal of Biological Chemistry* 1968; **243**: 3382–3387.

32. Dixon J. M., Miller W. R., Scott W. N. & Forrest A. P. M. The morphological basis of human cyst populations. *British Journal of Surgery* 1983; **70**: 604–606.

33. Editorial. Drugs and breast feeding. *British Medical Journal* 1979; **i**: 642.

34. Petrakis N. L. Physiologic, biochemical and cytologic aspects of nipple aspirate fluid. *Breast Cancer Research and Treatment* 1985; **8**: 7–19.

35. Azzopardi J. G. In: Bennington J. L. (ed.) *Major Problems in Pathology*, Vol II, *Problems in Breast Pathology*, Chap 2. London, W. B. Saunders, 1979, pp 8–22.

3 Aberrations of Normal Development and Involution (ANDI): A Concept of Benign Breast Disorders based on Pathogenesis

The management of benign breast conditions is critically dependent on an understanding of the normal and histological processes within the breast, and the aberrations which lead to clinical presentation.

In our experience, most of the confusion discussed in Chapter 1 arises from considering symptoms or histological appearances in isolation. Breast disorders are better assessed in terms of dynamic processes, because clinical syndromes are more readily related to pathogenesis than static histology. Each major clinical presentation can be assessed in relation to pathogenesis, which involves a number of processes within the breast. Each process encompasses a spectrum which extends from normality – as assessed by frequency within the general population and minimal symptoms – through to a benign breast disorder – less common and with modest to severe symptoms. With some processes, the spectrum extends further to encompass manifestations sufficiently infrequent and/or severe to be designated disease.

Most processes can be related to the dynamic changes occurring in the normal breast throughout reproductive life, and hence we would suggest the generic term 'aberrations of normal development and involution' (ANDI), on which cyclical changes are superimposed. This is in keeping with the concept that many of the disorders can be regarded as 'non-disease'[1], but allows a more individual assessment of each clinical problem within the normal-to-disease spectrum, essential for clinical understanding and rational management.

The first step towards the development of management guidelines is to define the problems in current clinical practice and then to produce solutions of pragmatic value to patient care. The problems straddle clinical and pathological aspects and many arise through the interrelationship of the two.

The Problems

Nomenclature

The situation has been beset by multiple loose terminology, as set out in Chapter 1. Each worker in the past has tended to introduce his own terminology, reflecting his own ideas of disease and its underlying pathology, without linking it to earlier studies. At first the terms were mainly clinical, e.g. 'chronic mastitis', but later reflected biopsy appearance, e.g. fibrocystic disease, of symptomatic lesions without appreciating the range of histological appearance in patients without symptoms. This leads on to the second problem.

The Borderline between Normal and Abnormal

Many organs under endocrine control show a wide range of appearances associated with cyclical or pulsed hormonal secretion. This is especially true in females where cyclical changes are set against a background of the broader changes of development and involution at the extremes of reproductive life, and particularly so in the breast. Most of these cyclical changes show a spectrum which on occasions may extend outside the normal range. Clearly it is important to try to define the point, even if blurred, at which the transmutation to abnormality occurs.

Correlation of Clinical Symptoms and Signs with Histological Changes

In the past, a patient with a local clinical abnormality has been subjected to biopsy and the local histological changes correlated with that clinical episode. This ignores the fact that the classic changes of 'fibrocystic disease', including fibrosis, adenosis, cyst formation and lymphocytic infiltration, may be seen in the asymptomatic breast, and ignores the dynamic changes within the breast from month to month. Thus, a second biopsy from breast tissue a few centimetres away which is clinically identical might show quite different histological changes, while a biopsy of the same site a few months later (if that were possible!) might show different histology with the same clinical signs or vice versa. Hence, the histological features of individual clinical lesions must be assessed against the broad spectrum of histological change which might be seen within a 'normal' breast, symptomatic or not. Failure to do so leads to confusion of significance – as an example, 'fibroadenosis' is a clinical condition which has no distinct radiological or pathological counterpart; yet it has repeatedly been correlated with cancer, a very distinct condition with clearly defined radiology, pathology and outcome. Only lesions which are definite clinical and pathological entities, e.g. a macrocyst, can be assessed from both points of view. Terms such as 'fibroadenosis' or 'fibrocystic disease' are misleading, because they imply that these histological patterns are abnormal and that they correlate with clinical conditions.

The Assessment of Premalignant Potential

This aspect has understandably dominated the efforts of breast surgeon and pathologist alike. Both have been frustrated by the three factors discussed above and it is not surprising that attempts to assess premalignant potential have given almost infinitely variable results from one study to another. Confusion of nomenclature is particularly great when discussing the epithelial hyperplasias. Because of their pre-cancerous association, the use of different terms in different countries has lead to serious misunderstanding, compounded by failure to define the borderline between normal and abnormal.

Where do the answers to these problems lie? First, in defining the range of normality, both in terms of clinical symptoms and signs, and of histological appearance. Secondly, recognizing that breast problems may be clinical, physiological or histological, and each problem may sometimes reflect only one of these three: sometimes more than one. But clinical, physiological and histological aspects should be correlated only where there is clear evidence that they are significantly and causally associated. Thirdly, by providing a comprehensive framework within which individual clinical or histological situations can be placed so that they are seen within an overall context. This must allow precise placement of a problem within the overall framework but also encompass the necessity to decide whether an individual clinical situation lies within the normal or abnormal end of the spectrum of a particular process.

The main physiopathological processes in the breast are only three in number: conditions related to development, cyclical change and involution of lobules; duct ectasia/periductal mastitis; epithelial hyperplasias. These physiopathological processes are more easily classified than the clinical presentations which arise from them, so they are first outlined. This provides a framework into which the clinical presentations can be placed. This is followed by the implications for management of this pathogenesis orientated approach.

Pathogenesis, clinical presentation and management are set out in this chapter only in conceptual terms. The detailed pathology and management are given in the rest of the book. We hope readers will persevere with the concepts of this chapter – we believe it makes detailed assessment and management of individual clinical problems so much easier.

Hormone-controlled Processes of the Breast

Consideration of the normal processes going on within the breast throughout a woman's life, provides an understanding of the pathogenesis of many of the benign breast disorders and diseases. These have often been regarded as abnormal in the past but are better regarded as variations within the spectrum of normal behaviour and appearance and, in particular, without any intrinsic premalignant potential.

Breast Development

The premenstrual breast consists of a few ducts only. The striking feature of the perimenarchal development of the breast is the addition of lobular structures to the already developing duct system. The lobules develop particularly during early reproductive life: 15–25 years of age. This explains the frequency of fibroadenoma during early and mid-reproductive life, for it is a condition analogous to gross hypertrophy of a lobule. Until the age of about 35 years, the luteal phase is also associated with enhanced acinar sprouting from the ductules.

A distinctive element of the lobule is its highly specialized connective tissue, and the close interaction between epithelium and connective tissue separated only by a basement membrane. This lobular connective tissue is pale and loose (Figure 3.1) with mononuclear infiltrate and differs notably from the much less interesting and urbane interlobular fibrous stroma (*see* Chapter 2).

Cyclical Change

Both epithelial and stromal elements of the lobule are under hormonal control and there is evidence that the two work in tandem. In fact, normality seems to be very much dependent on a normal, balanced relationship between both elements. It is likely that interference with the close relationship of the two elements is responsible for many of the conditions which are often included under the term 'benign breast disease'. The changes occurring with each menstrual cycle have been summarized by Vorrher[2] (*see* Chapter 2). Although the specificity of these changes during the menstrual cycle is questioned, this is less important for present discussion than the fact that these differing appearances are seen within the normal breast during reproductive life.

The cyclical changes are associated with clinical symptoms of heaviness and fullness that are not associated with detectable histological change, but for which a hormonal basis is being elucidated through recent studies. Superimposed on the cyclical changes are the much more radical effects

of pregnancy and lactation. With the repeated development and involutional changes of menstruation and pregnancy occurring throughout 40 years of reproductive life, there is abundant opportunity for minor aberrations to occur.

When one studies a section of normal breast from a patient who has no breast complaint or overt clinical disease on examination, the striking feature is the wide spectrum of histological appearance. Figure 3.2 is from an asymptomatic patient in her thirties, and within a small area may be seen well-developed lobules, poorly developed lobules, dilated ducts and normal ducts, lobule-deficient fibrous tissue and fatty tissue. These normal appearances provide the elements – 'fibrosis' and 'adenosis' – which have been documented as the histological appearance of biopsies taken from patients with nodular breasts. It has not always been appreciated that the same changes may be evident elsewhere in the same breast – where there is no clinical complaint.

The variability of appearance within the normal breast is illustrated following pregnancy. Under the intense hormonal stimulation associated with pregnancy, a uniform pattern of lobular development and maturation is seen (Figure 3.3), but postlactational involution is patchy (Figure 3.4). With such variable involution following the total stimulation of pregnancy, it is not surprising that the more minor cyclical changes with menstruation can, compounded over a long period, produce marked differences in structure and appearance of various areas of the breast tissue on a purely random basis.

Breast Involution

Involution starts quite early and changes are obvious by 35 years of age and often earlier. Thus cyclical change and involution run in tandem for 20 years or more, increasing the chance of aberration of normality – as reflected in the high

3.1 *The perimenarchal breast, showing lobular development. The pale, loose lobular connective tissue contrasts with the denser interlobular fibrous stroma.*

3.2 *A section from a 'normal' asymptomatic breast. It shows a wide variety of histological appearances–the changes commonly ascribed to 'fibrocystic disease'.*

3.1

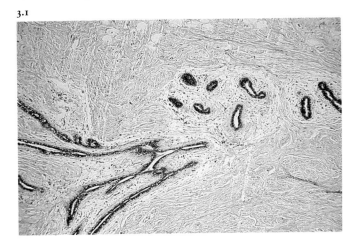

3.2

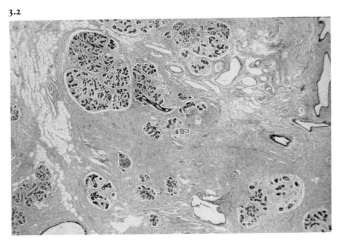

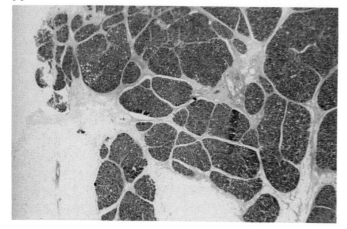

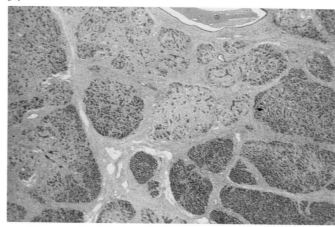

frequency of presentation to a breast clinic during this period. The changes progress over the next 15–20 years. The involution affects the lobules particularly and is much dependent on the relationship between the epithelium and specialized stroma of the lobule. Figure 3.5 shows an involuting breast; an orderly regression of lobules and surrounding fibrous tissue is obvious. During this process of lobular involution, the loose hormone-responsive intralobular connective tissue is replaced by the more standard interlobular type of fibrous tissue. If this replacement is well co-ordinated with the regression of epithelial tissue, the uniform picture of involution shown in Figure 3.5 is seen. Eventually, by the time the menopause has been reached and passed, involution is extensive (Figure 3.6) with only a few ducts remaining, and no evidence of lobular structures. But it does not always happen in that way, and minor aberrations of this process are very common during a period of fluctuating involution extending over 20 years. The exact mechanism of this involution is not well understood, but it appears that normal epithelial involution of the lobule is dependent on the continuing presence of the specialized stroma around it. Should the stroma

disappear too early, the epithelial acini remain and may form microcysts. These are obviously a prime target for macroscopic cyst formation if obstruction of the draining ductule occurs. Microcystic formation is very common in normal breasts (Figures 3.7 and 3.8) as demonstrated by Parks[3] and, in this process of cystic lobular involution, microcysts may appear even though there is still specialized stroma present. Presumably this arises from minor obstruction to the duct by kinking or compression from fibrous tissue, or perhaps by vigorous secretion from still active epithelial tissue. (It is interesting that the lobular vein exits from the lobule alongside the ductule so venous compression readily occurs.) As long as some of the specialized stroma remains, the lobule can still involute normally in spite of these microcysts. But should the specialized stroma disappear early then further cystic change is likely (Figure 3.9). Mechanical duct obstruction leading to macrocysts (Figure 3.10) is almost bound to occur in a proportion of lobules, because there are many possible mechanisms: from internal blockage by epithelial cells or debris, through simple kinking and angulation to strangulation by the surrounding maturing fibrous tissue.

3.3   A section of a normal pregnant breast, showing extreme, uniform lobular development.

3.4   Histological section from a postlactational breast. Involution is patchy, varying from marked to negligible.

3.5   Section from a normal involuting breast. The orderly regression of both epithelial and stromal elements of the lobule is obvious. The lobular stroma has been replaced by fibrous tissue, and there is little residual epithelial tissue.

3.6   A section of post-menopausal breast, showing advanced lobular involution.

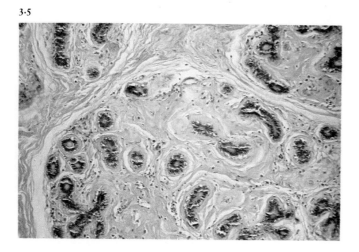

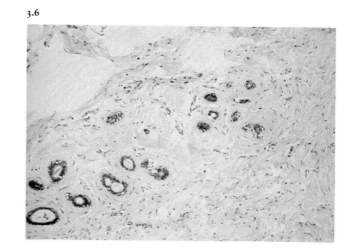

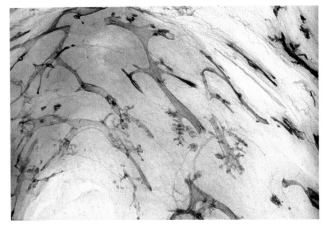

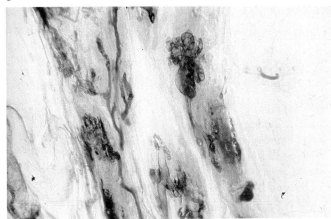

Thus three periods occur and overlap: lobule development 15–25 years, cyclical change 15–50 years, involution 35–50 years. Each period has its own clinical presentations, but overlapping and interacting processes also lead to complex clinical situations.

A Framework based on Pathogenesis

This is set out in simplest form in Table 3.1, which deals with the commoner clinical benign breast disorders. The largest group of disorders are covered by the concept of ANDI. Together with duct ectasia/periductal mastitis and epithelial hyperplasia, a framework is provided for considering the whole spectrum of benign breast disorders.

An important point of the classification is the replacement of the term 'disease' by 'disorders' in the interpretation of benign breast disease (BBD). This does not mean that there is no benign breast disease, but recognizes that most breast complaints are due to disorders based on the normal processes of development, cyclical change and involution. Such disorders occasionally extend to the frankly abnormal and then may

Table 3.1 A broad classification of benign breast disorders.

1. ANDI (aberration of normal development and involution.)
    Development
        Adolescent hypertrophy
        Fibroadenoma
    Cyclical change
        Mastalgia
        Clinical nodularity
    Involution
        Cyst formation
        Sclerosing adenosis
2. Duct ectasia/periductal mastitis
3. Epithelial hyperplasias
4. Conditions with well-defined aetiology, e.g.
    Lactational abscess
    Traumatic fat necrosis

3.7 Involuting, postmenopausal breast studied by a thick section technique.

3.8 Involuting breast showing microcystic lobular involution.

rightly be considered as benign breast disease. The borderline within the spectrum is determined largely by frequency and by the problems it causes to patients and clinicians; it is not a well-defined cut-off point. Conditions which affect a large percentage of the population must be regarded as normal, or at most as a disorder. The concept that conditions such as fibroadenoma and duct ectasia lie within the normal range is foreign to

3.9 A further stage in the evolution from microcystic involution to macrocyst formation.

3.10 In a fully developed macrocyst, the bands in the wall reflect the origin from gross distension of a number of acini (ductules) within a single lobule.

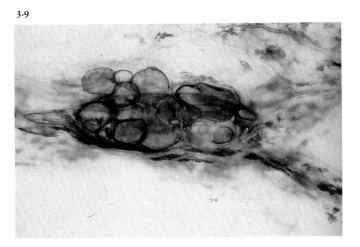

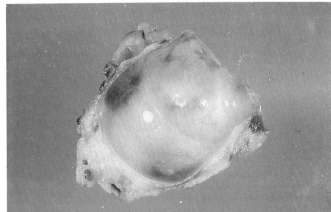

conventional teaching in pathology and surgery. Hence we give the reason in some detail.

ANDI

Disorders of Development

Fibroadenoma
Since it can be shown that fibroadenomas arise from lobules, it is not surprising that these are seen predominantly during the 15 to 25-year period, even though they may not be diagnosed until later, when postpregnancy or involutional changes facilitate clinical recognition in the softer drooping involutional breast. The use of elastic stains allows differentiation of ductal from lobular tissue – showing that each fibroadenoma develops from a single lobule, although adjacent lobules may be incorporated. What is the evidence to support the contention that fibroadenoma should be placed in the benign breast disorder side of ANDI rather than be regarded as a neoplasm? Parks[3] showed that hyperplastic lobules, histologically identical to clinical fibroadenomas, are present so commonly as to be regarded as normal; they can probably be found in all breasts if they are sought sufficiently carefully. A full spectrum can be found between these hyperplastic lobules and clinical fibroadenomas, which do not show the inexorable growth typical of true neoplasms. They usually grow to 1 or, at most, 2 cm in diameter and then stay constant in size. They show hormonal dependence similar to normal lobules by lactating during pregnancy (Figure 3.11) and will involute to be replaced by hyaline connective tissue in concert with the rest of the breast in the perimenopausal period. These hormonal responses are much more complete than those usually seen in benign tumours. Rarely, a fibroadenoma will continue to grow to a size of 3 cm, although this is sufficiently common to be regarded as within the normal spectrum.

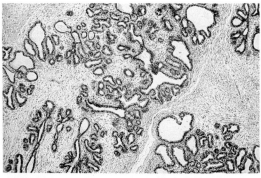

3.11 *A fibroadenoma removed in the postpartum period. It shows lactation similar to the normal breast, indicating that fibroadenomas respond readily to normal physiological stimuli.*

Growth beyond 5 cm is sufficiently uncommon in Western populations as to justify being regarded as a disease – giant fibroadenoma (though some authorities would require a 10 cm diameter before moving into the disease category).

Adolescent hypertrophy
This condition is associated with gross stromal hyperplasia at the time of breast development. The aetiology is unknown, and this is not surprising because so little is known about the control of breast stroma – important though this is. Nevertheless, it is likely that there is a hormonal basis to the condition – a view supported by recent reports that danazol (an antigonadotrophin) may have a beneficial effect. The continuous spectrum from hypoplasia of the breast through to massive hyperplasia justifies its classification under ANDI, and unilateral hypoplasia and breast asymmetry presumably have a related pathogenesis.

Disorders of Cyclical Change

Mastalgia and nodularity
Premenstrual enlargement and postmenstrual involution of the breast occurring with each cycle is so commonly associated with discomfort and nodularity as to lie firmly within the spectrum of normality. In more gross cases, it is associated with the clinical entities of cyclical mastalgia and cyclical nodularity. No histological basis has been defined for these changes, and attempts to demonstrate oedema as the obvious cause of cyclical nodularity have so far been unsuccessful. We have used the term 'cyclical pronounced mastalgia' or 'severe painful nodularity' to differentiate the disorder from the more common physiological discomfort and lumpiness. A duration of painful nodularity of more than one week of the cycle is a useful definition for differentiation from normal discomfort. This is the clinical presentation often termed 'fibrocystic disease', an unfortunate term because it is not necessarily associated with fibrosis or cysts. The lack of histological correlation has led to the suggestion that it is a non-disease – a concept which is not accepted by those unfortunate women who suffer from its more severe manifestations. Their objection to the concept of 'non-disease' is supported by recent hormonal studies[4] which show an underlying physiological abnormality demonstrated by excess prolactin release from the pituitary following stimulation of the hypothalamic pituitary axis. These findings stress the importance of taking a broad view of benign breast disorders, avoiding undue emphasis on non-specific histological changes and giving due attention to significant physiological changes. It is likely

that subtle stromal and epithelial changes accompany physiological variations in more severe cases of cyclical nodularity and mastalgia, but this has not yet been studied properly. Certainly there is poor correlation between cyclical mastalgia and nodularity and the histological appearance of fibrosis, adenosis and cyst formation commonly regarded in the past as disease.

Painful nodularity of the predominantly cyclical phase of reproductive life (20–35 years) merges into and overlaps those symptoms which are more typically part of the involutional phase, especially cyst formation and sclerosing adenosis. All have been lumped together as fibrocystic disease (or fibroadenosis) in the past, but the clinical problems and management differ.

ANDI: Disorders of Involution

Cyst formation

The desirable integrated involution of stroma and epithelium outlined earlier in this chapter is not always seen, and minor aberrations of the process are understandably common during a period of fluctuating involution extending over 20 years. The exact mechanism of this involution is not well understood[5], but it appears that the normal epithelial involution of the lobule is dependent on the continuing presence of the specialized stroma around it. If the stroma disappears too early, the epithelial acini remain and may form microcysts, setting the pattern for macrocyst development by obstruction of the efferent ductule as discussed above. This concept of the macrocyst as being an involutional aberration (and hence part of ANDI), rather than a disease, fits in with their common occurrence and the fact that they are so frequently multiple and subclinical.

The fact that macrocysts appear to develop in two directions – apocrine and non-apocrine cysts[6] – is something which is as yet poorly understood, but the evidence is strong that both develop from a common origin of microcystic involution[7].

Sclerosing adenosis

This condition may be considered as an aberration of either the cyclical or the involutional phase of breast activity because it can show histological changes which are both proliferative and involutional. This illustrates the complexity on the one hand, but the simplicity of concept on the other, of regarding these as aberrations of so many interacting normal processes. When one considers the complex interrelationship of stromal fibrosis and epithelial regression occurring during involution, superimposed on cyclical changes of ductal

sprouting, it is not surprising that this complex picture, in which epithelial acini are strangled and distorted by fibrous tissue, should arise. It is surprising that it does not occur more commonly.

Thus, all the changes described can be considered as minor aberrations of the normal dynamic processes of breast development, cyclical change and involution. They are best regarded as benign breast disorders occasionally moving, by virtue of extreme severity, into the spectrum of abnormality to become benign breast disease.

Duct Ectasia and Periductal Mastitis

The second major group of benign breast disorders consists of those associated with duct ectasia and periductal mastitis. The pathogenesis of duct ectasia/periductal mastitis is obscure. The classic theory, proposed by Haagensen[8] regards duct ectasia (dilated ducts) as being the primary event, leading to stagnation of secretion, epithelial ulceration and leakage of duct secretions containing chemically irritant fatty acids into periductal tissue to give a chemical inflammatory process. This view was developed and graphically illustrated by Ewing[9] (Figure 3.12). This secondary inflammation is then seen as leading to periductal fibrosis, with subsequent fibrous contraction and nipple retraction. However, this classic view does not meet all facets of the clinical picture. In particular, the age distribution is wrong. Duct ectasia with nipple discharge is commonest in the perimenopausal age group, much later than the inflammatory complications which classically occur in an earlier age group – and are not uncommon in the twenties and thirties. An alternative theory to explain this discrepancy sees the primary process as periductal mastitis – perhaps on an autoimmune basis – leading to weakening of the muscle layer of the ducts and secondary dilatation. We think it likely that both processes may occur separately or in conjunction, thus explaining the wide spectrum of clinical behaviour in this condition. Two other concepts need to be fitted into the overall picture. First, periductal fibrosis can occur in the absence of duct ectasia or of inflammation[10] and probably represents part of the normal involutional process in the breast. Secondly, there is increasing evidence of a bacterial role in severe forms of periductal mastitis, although at present this would appear to be secondary rather than primary.

The wide variety of clinical symptoms associated with this condition – nipple discharge, nipple retraction, inflammatory masses and abscesses (sterile or bacterial) – can best be explained and

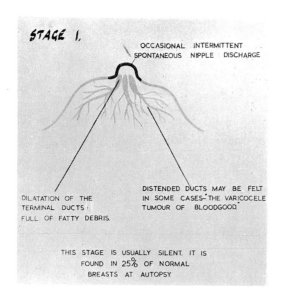

STAGE I.

OCCASIONAL INTERMITTENT
SPONTANEOUS NIPPLE DISCHARGE

DILATATION OF THE
TERMINAL DUCTS:
FULL OF FATTY DEBRIS.

DISTENDED DUCTS MAY BE FELT
IN SOME CASES - THE VARICOCELE
TUMOUR OF BLOODGOOD.

THIS STAGE IS USUALLY SILENT. IT IS
FOUND IN 25% OF NORMAL
BREASTS AT AUTOPSY

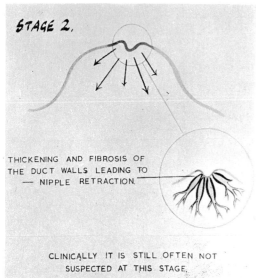

STAGE 2,

THICKENING AND FIBROSIS OF
THE DUCT WALLS LEADING TO
— NIPPLE RETRACTION.

CLINICALLY IT IS STILL OFTEN NOT
SUSPECTED AT THIS STAGE.

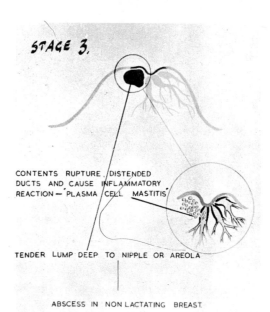

STAGE 3,

CONTENTS RUPTURE, DISTENDED
DUCTS AND CAUSE INFLAMMATORY
REACTION — 'PLASMA CELL MASTITIS'

TENDER LUMP DEEP TO NIPPLE OR AREOLA

ABSCESS IN NON LACTATING BREAST.

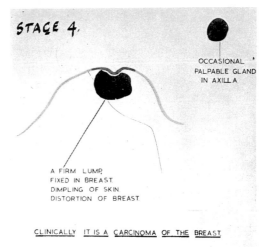

STAGE 4.

OCCASIONAL
PALPABLE GLAND
IN AXILLA

A FIRM LUMP,
FIXED IN BREAST.
DIMPLING OF SKIN.
DISTORTION OF BREAST.

CLINICALLY IT IS A CARCINOMA OF THE BREAST

3.12 *Diagrammatic representation of the older view of the sequence of pathogenesis of duct ectasia and periductal mastitis (from Ewing[9], with permission of* Journal of the Royal College of Surgeons (Edinburgh).*)*

understood by accepting more than one process in the pathogenesis.

Epithelial Hyperplasia

The third element of the benign breast disorder complex – epithelial hyperplasias – has given rise to most confusion and problems in management. Many people would see this lying firmly on the side of disease rather than disorder, but a number of studies have shown that this is not so with simple hyperplasias. Parks[3] showed that lobular and intraductal papillary hyperplasia is common in the premenopausal period and tends to regress spontaneously after the menopause, and hence should be regarded as an aberration of normal involution. Kramer and Rush[11] found in their autopsy study that 59% of women over the age of 70 exhibited some degree of epithelial hyperplasia. Sloss et al[12] concluded from their autopsy study that 'the mere presence of blunt

duct adenosis, apocrine epithelium and intra-ductal epithelial hyperplasia in the breast of women is insufficient to warrant such tissue being called disease'. Hence the simple epithelial hyperplasias may be placed firmly within the concept of benign breast disorder. However, careful studies by Page et al[13] and Wellings and Jensen[14] have shown that the other ends of the spectrum – atypical lobular hyperplasia and atypical ductal hyperplasia – particularly as seen in the terminal duct lobular unit (TDLU), is sufficiently commonly associated with malignancy as to be regarded as an associated or a premalignant condition. Hence, epithelial hyperplasias with marked atypia belong firmly under the column of benign breast disease. There is at present insufficient evidence to allow a firm opinion as to whether conditions we have placed under the benign breast disorder column present a continuous spectrum with the implication that the 'disorders' move to 'disease'. They may be entirely separate processes and certainly, at the present time, no such progression of hyperplasias to cancer *in situ* should be assumed – it should be left as an open question. This controversial area is discussed more fully in Chapter 4.

An Extension of the Concept of ANDI to include most Benign Breast Disorders

In the foregoing discussion benign breast disorders have been divided into the three groups: ANDI, duct ectasia/periductal mastitis and epithelial hyperplasia. But in fact a case can be made for most, if not all, conditions placed under the benign breast disorder column, including duct ectasia, mild periductal mastitis and benign hyperplasias, to be regarded as aberrations of normal development and involution. Provided the underlying associations and pathogeneses are clearly understood, it matters little and, as long as the terms are specifically descriptive in a pathological and/or clinical sense, there should be little confusion regarding their aetiology, significance and management. However, conditions such as duct ectasia and epithelial hyperplasias have such a fixed place in medical concept that it is probably best to continue to regard them as specific conditions, and retain the term 'ANDI' to cover the well-recognized conditions of fibroadenoma, adolescent hypertrophy, cyclical mastalgia and nodularity, cyst formation and sclerosing adenosis.

Nevertheless, some of the less common benign breast disorders fit well into the concept of aberrations of normality and it is useful to consider the arguments for including them within this framework (Table 3.2). Briefly, these arguments are as follows:

1. *Nipple inversion*: an aberration of normal development of the terminal ducts, preventing the normal protrusion of ducts and areola.

2. *Mammary duct fistula*: nipple inversion predisposes to terminal duct obstruction, leading to recurrent subareolar abscess and mammary duct fistula – the usual form of periductal mastitis seen in younger women.

3. *Epithelial hyperplasia of pregnancy*: marked hyperplasia of the duct epithelium occurs in pregnancy, and the papillary projections sometimes give rise to bilateral bloody nipple discharge – a condition which is always benign when occurring in pregnancy.

4. *Benign duct papilloma* is a common condition during the period of cyclical activity and shows minimal if any malignant potential. It is reasonable to regard it as an aberration of cyclical epithelial activity.

For similar reasons it might be considered logical to extend the concept of aberration of normality to encompass adenosis as a manifestation of involution.

Table 3.2 A framework of pathogenesis for the classification of benign breast disorders.

Reproductive period	Normal process	Benign breast disorder	Benign breast disease
Development	Ductal development	Nipple inversion Single duct obstruction	Mammary duct fistula
	Lobular development Stromal development	Fibroadenoma Adolescent hypertrophy	Giant fibroadenoma (Severest form)
Cyclical change	Hormonal activity	Mastalgia Nodularity Focal Diffuse	(Severest form)
	Epithelial activity	Benign papilloma	
Pregnancy and lactation	Epithelial hyperplasia	Blood-stained nipple discharge	
	Lactation	Galactocele and inappropriate lactation	
Involution	Lobular involution	Cysts and sclerosing adenosis	
	Ductal involution Fibrosis Dilatation	Nipple retraction Duct ectasia	Periductal mastitis with suppuration
	Micro papillomatosis	Simple hyperplasias	Lobular hyperplasias with atypia Duct hyperplasias with atypia Intracystic papilloma

Implications for the Management of Benign Breast Disorders

If follows from the foregoing that most of the conditions listed under benign breast disorders (see Table 3.1) can be regarded as minor aberrations of normality and hence not demanding active specific treatment. We believe this to be the case, and any active management of these conditions should be based on considerations such as accurate diagnosis, patient concern and interference with quality of life. No treatment is required based solely on inherent pathological significance. This concept of management is outlined here; details of management are given in the appropriate chapter.

Adolescent Hypertrophy

In its more severe forms, treatment is indicated because of psychological and physical morbidity from the size and weight of the breast. It is the degree of this morbidity that determines treatment with hormonal or surgical therapy.

Fibroadenoma

Because fibroadenoma is a benign and self-limiting condition in the vast majority of cases, a clinically typical fibroadenoma in a patient younger than 25 years can be safely left untreated. We have followed this policy for many years for very small lesions, or for second lesions after surgical excision of a fibroadenoma, without cause for regret. The case for this policy is strengthened by the incidence of hypertrophic scars in young girls. Over the age of 25, the diagnosis can never be certain and biopsy is usually indicated for accuracy of diagnosis. Clinical diagnosis is particularly difficult during the second half of reproductive life, because a fibroadenoma is incorporated within the evolving processes of cyclical change and involution, frequently losing its classic characteristics of well-defined lobularity and mobility. Diagnosis then comes as a surprise following biopsy for dominant nodularity. Conservative therapy over the age of 25 carries a considerable risk of missing a carcinoma.

Inverted Nipple

This is the failure of development of major ducts, and it is unlikely that any treatment short of severing the ducts will give a long-term satisfactory result. Hence treatment is related to the patient's view of the cosmetic deformity, and recommended only after recognizing the uncertain long-term results of minor surgical procedures for this condition, and the consequences of total duct division for cosmesis and lactation if the defect is to undergo total correction.

Cyclical Mastalgia and Nodularity

It is generally accepted that these manifestations are physiological, and that most cases can be treated by adequate reassurance. But the view that the most severe cases – those lasting perhaps 2 weeks or more of the menstrual cycle – interfere so much with the quality of life as to merit consideration as 'dis-ease' is confirmed by the high incidence of hormonal abnormalities in these patients. There is equally strong evidence that they are not psychologically based, and hence endocrine related treatment is appropriate in those cases severe enough to warrant therapy[15].

Cysts

Macrocysts and microcysts are so common as to require no active treatment other than that to allow diagnosis and allay patient concern. It is now well established by practice that simple cysts are satisfactorily treated by aspiration – a policy that might have been predicted from the ANDI concept. The recent differentiation of cysts into apocrine and non-apocrine[6] does not at present alter this conservative therapeutic approach, because any cancer risk is very small, if it exists at all.

Sclerosing Adenosis

This condition causes diagnostic problems to surgeons, radiologists and histopathologists and sometimes problems to the patient in the form of a lump or pain. It requires no treatment other than careful exclusion of cancer, although it sometimes requires symptomatic treatment for pain.

Postmenopausal Nipple Retraction

The only importance of this is to recognize that it may be caused by the simple involutional process of periductal fibrosis. It requires no active management other than exclusion of cancer. In our experience, nipple retraction is more commonly due to ductal fibrosis than to cancer, and fortunately the diagnosis is easily made in older patients because the postmenopausal breast lends itself to accurate mammography.

Duct Ectasia/Periductal Mastitis Complex

Duct ectasia and mild periductal mastitis cause little clinical upset and require no therapy other than reassurance, when the nipple discharge is typically creamy and opaque. When suppuration supervenes in periductal mastitis, therapy appropriate to a disease state is indicated – drainage, antibiotics and eradication of the underlying cause.

Epithelial Hyperplasia

Epithelial hyperplasias without atypia fall into the category of benign breast disorder, having no significant cancer risk, and required no specific management. With atypical hyperplasias, a disease state exists and special consideration should be given to assessment of cancer risk, as defined particularly by Page[13].

REFERENCES

1. Love S. M., Gelman R. S. & Silen W. Fibrocystic 'disease' of the breast – A non disease. *New England Journal of Medicine* 1982; **307**: 1010–1014.
2. Vorherr H. *The Breast. Morphology, Physiology and Lactation.* New York, Academic Press, 1974.
3. Parks A. G. The microanatomy of the breast. *Annals of the Royal College of Surgeons* 1959; **25**: 295–311.
4. Kumar S., Mansel R. E., Hughes L. E., Edwards C. A. & Scanlon M. F. Prediction of response to endocrine therapy in pronounced cyclical mastalgia, using dynamic tests of prolactin release. *Clinical Endocrinology* 1985; **23**: 699–704.
5. Azzopardi J. G. *Problems in Breast Pathology.* London, W. B. Saunders, 1979.
6. Miller W. R., Dixon J. M., Scott W. N. & Forrest A. P. M. Classification of human breast cysts according to electrolyte and androgen conjugate composition. *Clinical Oncology* 1983; **9**: 227–232.
7. Dixon J. M. Scott W. N. & Miller W. R. An analysis of the content and morphology of human breast microcysts. *European Journal of Surgical Oncology* 1985; **11**: 151–154.
8. Haagensen C. D. Mammary duct ectasia – a disease that may simulate carcinoma. *Cancer* 1951; **4**: 749–761.
9. Ewing M. Stagnation in the main ducts of the breast. *Journal of the Royal College of Surgeons (Edinburgh)* 1963; **8**: 134–144.
10. Davies J. D. Inflammatory damage to ducts in mammary dysplasia: a cause of duct obliteration. *Journal of Pathology* 1975; **117**: 47–54.
11. Kramer W. M. & Rush B. F. Mammary duct proliferation in the elderly – a histological study. *Cancer* 1973; **31**: 130–137.
12. Sloss P. T., Bennett W. A. & Clagett O. T. Incidence in normal breasts of features associated with chronic cystic mastitis. *American Journal of Pathology* 1957; **33**: 1181–1191.
13. Page D. L. Vander-Zwag R., Rogers L. W., Williams L. T., Walker W. F. & Hartmann W. H. Relationship between component parts of fibrocystic disease complex and breast cancer. *Journal of the National Cancer Institute* 1978; **61**: 1055–1063.
14. Wellings S. R., Jensen H. M. & Marcum R. G. An atlas of subgross pathology of the human breast with reference to possible pre-cancerous lesions. *Journal of the National Cancer Institute* 1975; **55**: 231–273.
15. Pye J. K., Mansel R. E. & Hughes L. E. Clinical experience of drug treatments for mastalgia. *Lancet* 1985; **ii**: 373–377.

4 The Epidemiology of Benign Breast Disease and Assessment of Cancer Risk

The epidemiological aspects of breast cancer have been widely studied and a large number of epidemiological associations, such as age, race and age at first pregnancy are well recognized. In contrast, there has been little study of the epidemiology of benign breast conditions, although there have been some attempts to correct this deficiency recently.

Previous efforts have concentrated on the relationship of 'fibrocystic disease' and cancer, and studies have been carried out for many decades, but until recently no consensus has emerged. Because different studies report widely varying estimates of the cancer risk of benign breast disorders, it is no surprise that the confusion felt by the individual clinician is eventually transmitted to the patient, who is all too often left without clear advice regarding prognosis and follow-up. Many of the contradictions in the literature are due to badly designed studies, performed on selected populations with poorly defined diagnostic groups, as discussed in Chapter 1. The seemingly random results are thus understandable. There are many different aspects of risk for each individual patient, such as family history, personal reproductive history and, if the patient has undergone biopsy, histology. All of these need to be taken into account and studies to quantitate these risks have been commenced over the last decade.

The epidemiological aspects of breast cancer are outside the scope of this book. The epidemiology of benign breast disorders and their relation to cancer risk are considered here.

Epidemiological Studies of Benign Breast Disorders

General Population Incidence

One of the most valuable studies in this area has come from Vancouver[1]. A 23-year prospective study of 726 nurses showed that 215 (30%) had reported breast symptoms requiring medical advice and 107 (14%) had had a biopsy with a histological report of benign breast disease during the follow-up period. The likelihood of having a benign biopsy was associated with a previous history of premenstrual pain or swelling, lack of oral contraceptive use and a family history of both benign and malignant breast disease. The high awareness of breast cancer among nurses would almost certainly influence these results.

Fewer biopsies for benign breast disease were performed in long-term oral contraceptive users in the large prospective Oxford–FPA study[2], particularly for fibroadenoma and histologically confirmed cystic disease. This study also provides data on other risk factors for biopsy. It showed that the risk of having a breast biopsy was much lower in obese women. It was suggested that this was due to the greater difficulty of feeling a small dominant lump in a large breast. Several factors were found to be associated with increased risk of biopsy, including previous history of breast symptoms and family history. However, these would tend to sway the clinician towards biopsy of a doubtful lump and this in part may explain the observed association.

A recent prospective study carried out from our department of the prevalence of breast symptoms in a South Wales working female population of 820 women, showed that 40% experienced at least mild mastalgia and 10% had had a previous benign biopsy.

A number of other epidemiological studies of BBD – both descriptive and analytical – have been reviewed in a paper by Cook and Rohan[3]. Unfortunately, these studies tend to rely on clinical diagnosis or use non-specific terms such as 'fibrocystic disease', so their value is limited.

Epidemiological studies of histological patterns have come largely from autopsy series[4]. These have clear limitations from an epidemiological viewpoint, but provide some useful guidelines[5].

They confirm the high incidence of simple hyperplasias in non-selected hospital death populations, with figures reported as high as 69%.

The Contraceptive Pill and Benign Breast Disorders

The widespread use of oral contraceptives among modern women has prompted numerous detailed studies of possible effects on benign and malignant breast disease. Worries of thromboembolic complications have prompted the use of pills with lower doses of both the oestrogen and progestogen component of the formulation, so that earlier studies are not necessarily relevant to the pills in current common use. Nevertheless, most results of large epidemiological surveys have shown that BBD is reduced in long-term pill users. The Oxford–FPA study[2], and the Royal College of General Practitioners study[5] both clearly show a reduction in the risk of biopsy for BBD in long-term pill users. These findings have been confirmed in other studies[6] and the protective effects appear to relate to the progestogen component of the pill. Because women taking a modern oral contraceptive pill appear to have a lower incidence of benign breast disorders (of the ANDI group), patients with such disorders need not discontinue their current oral contraceptive.

One aspect causing controversy is the effect of the pill on different types of hyperplasias. Some workers have reported that all types are reduced by pill usage, others have suggested that benign hyperplasias are decreased but the atypical hyperplasias are unchanged or increased. Anderson et al[7] studied the mitosis and apoptosis (cell death) rates in women on oral contraceptives and non-users and found no significant differences between the two groups. This subject is reviewed in the paper by Cooke and Rohan[3] and clearly further work is required.

Some concern has been expressed regarding breast cancer risk in women who start the pill before their first full-term pregnancy. Recent large case-control studies suggest a small increase of × 2.5 in early pill users, but the formulations studied were of the high dose type and are probably not relevant to modern pill users[8]. The Committee on Safety of Medicines has reviewed all the recent literature and has concluded that no change in current policy is indicated[9]. Because women taking a modern oral contraceptive long term should have a lower incidence of BBD, patients with BBD need not discontinue their current oral contraceptive on diagnosis of their condition.

The Effect of Public Health Education on Referral Rates

In the UK, a general practitioner will see an average of 13 patients with breast problems each year[10]; an overwhelming majority will be benign. Pain is the commonest presentation (47%) followed by lump (35%). Similar results were obtained in the study from Southampton[11] and the results did not differ from a study 10 years earlier[12]. In the Edinburgh study[10], these rates were not influenced by a local health education campaign, which might have been expected to result in a large increase. Likewise, the percentage of patients requiring referral by the GP for specialist consultation did not change during the education period.

Other Epidemiological Factors Affecting the Incidence of BBD

These have been discussed in the review by Ernster[13]. Women of high socio-economic class and those with a maternal history of cancer are liable to an increased risk of biopsy for benign disorder, although this may involve factors related to concern or awareness. Some cancer risk factors – such as age of menarche, age at first childbirth, nulliparity etc. – have been reported by some workers as showing no relation to BBD, and by others to be positively associated. The balance of evidence seems to be in favour of no association, and this has also been the case for relationship between age at first birth and risk of benign breast disorder subclassified by the degree of histological atypia.

The Cancer Risk of Benign Breast Disorders

Recent Studies

With such a high incidence in unselected hospital autopsy series of histological abnormalities in the breast, it will clearly be difficult to assign a cancer risk to many of these histological patterns. However, a number of important studies have appeared recently.

Perhaps the first very important paper was that of Wellings et al[14]. This looked at the incidence of benign histological lesions in cancerous breasts, suggesting that the coexistence of benign and malignant is probably significant, although a concurrent study of this nature cannot give definitive data of value equal to that obtained from prospective studies. The particular significance of their work was the careful description and definition of histological patterns. Using a detailed, subgross slicing technique, they suggested that most hyperplastic lesions seen in the breast originate from the terminal ductal-lobular unit (TDLU; see Figure 2.4) and proceeded to either a lobular or ductal type of hyperplasia, which they designated type A and B, respectively.

This was followed shortly by a similar important study of Page et al[15], who likewise produced a detailed descriptive classification of proliferative lesions of the breast. Their study was much more powerful in having a prospective element. A second recent publication[16] reports a series of over 10 000 biopsies with a follow-up rate greater than 90%. Their detailed findings are discussed below in relation to the American College of Pathologists (ACP) document.

A third study from Cardiff[17], followed 778 patients with symptomatic benign breast disorders for a minimum of 14 years. It illustrates some of the problems of translating risk factors of benign breast disorders into practical terms. Only 22 of their 770 symptomatic patients developed breast cancer, considered to be three times the background risk (although the control cancer incidence was taken from national statistics which may not be fully validated). Only 1 in 30 of the 326 patients from the series undergoing biopsy developed cancer, so a totally predictive histological marker would have only a low power of prediction of cancer arising within 14 years of follow-up. This study also indicates the difficulties of follow-up by clinical examination in an unselected series of symptomatic benign breast cases, as about 11 000 clinic visits per year would have been required to see each patient annually and pick up two cancers. Indeed this paper concludes that regular follow-up of patients with benign breast disease is not worth while.

The American Cancer Society Consensus Statement

This statement produced for the American Cancer Society by the College of American Pathologists[18] (Table 4.1), draws heavily on the findings of Page's group[16] and is careful to assign specific terminology to the histological categories. However, it must be accepted that assessment of these patterns embraces a considerable subjective element so that even experienced pathologists may differ in their assessment of individual lesions. The questions of assessment and definition are discussed more fully at the end of this chapter.

This consensus statement is based solely on

Table 4.1 Relative risk for invasive breast carcinoma based on pathological examination of benign breast tissue (American College of Pathologists Consensus Statement)[15].

No increased risk

Adenosis, sclerosing or florid	Hyperplasia (mild 2–4 epithelial cells in depth)
Apocrine metaplasia[a]	Mastitis (inflammation)
Cysts macro[a] and/or micro	Periductal mastitis
Duct ectasia	Squamous metaplasia
Fibroadenoma	
Fibrosis	

Slightly increased risk (1.5–2 times)

Hyperplasia, moderate or florid, solid or papillary.
Papilloma with a fibrovascular core[a]

Moderately increased risk (5 times)

Atypical hyperplasia
    Ductal
    Lobular

Insufficient data to assign a risk

Solitary papilloma of lactiferous sinus
Radial scar lesion

[a] The risk of these conditions is more controversial than sugested by this statement – for details see text.

histological findings on biopsy and stresses the importance of specifying the component elements of benign breast disorders we have included under the umbrella of ANDI (Chapter 3). However, there is no reason to believe that their relative risk assessment may not be applied to clinical conditions, provided this is limited to those conditions where the gross and histological diagnosis are clearly related, e.g. duct ectasia or lactational mastitis. With other conditions, risk must be assessed on biopsy material.

The simplest approach to the discussion of subsequent cancer risk of benign breast disorders is a pragmatic one, discussing the risks and management of individual patients in relation to the diagnostic groups listed in Chapter 3 and described in succeeding chapters, dealing with them as they present in clinical practice. Non-histological risk factors, in particular family history of breast cancer, must also be taken into consideration.

One problem relates to the fact that the diagnosis of some conditions, e.g. fibroadenoma in young girls and macroscopic cysts, is often made clinically and the conditions managed without obtaining biopsy material for histological study. Similarly, a patient with mastalgia or cyclical nodularity will not need a biopsy, but may still wish to have an assessment of cancer risk. The incidental finding of a specific hyperplasia in a biopsy performed for a dominant lump also requires assessment. Thus, in practice, both clinical and histological aspects must be taken into consideration, although histological findings will take precedence if available. Conditions are discussed in three risk groups according to the ACP consensus statement – no increased risk, slight and moderate increase. However, the risk of individual lesions is sometimes more controversial than the statement suggests and our own assessment is given in some detail in each section.

Conditions without Increased Risk

There is general agreement that the malignant potential of most conditions in the galaxy of benign breast disorders is very low (less than 1.5 times normal) or equivalent to the background population risk.

ANDI

Fibroadenoma

Fibroadenomas are not premalignant and the evidence suggests that most fibroadenomas would involute by hyalinization if they were not removed. Carcinoma arising in a fibroadenoma is a very rare event and has been estimated at 1 in 1000 fibroadenomas by Azzopardi[19]. These tumours are usually lobular in type, as would be expected from the lobular origin of fibroadenoma. Most reports show no increased cancer risk in patients followed up after excision of a fibroadenoma. Semb[20] failed to find a single case of carcinoma in his series of 142 patients with fibroadenoma followed up from 4 to 27 years post-operation. A second study by Oliver and Major[21] of 175 patients reported 1 case of carcinoma in 4–25 year follow-up. In our follow-up of 369 cases of fibroadenoma followed for 1–10 years, only 2 cases of cancer were detected, both in the opposite breast.

Roberts et al[10] showed a slight increased risk for fibroadenoma, but interpretation of this study is complicated by the fact that all patients in their clinic – irrespective of diagnosis on biopsy – showed this degree of increased risk, raising the possibility that the figures used for population cancer incidence may be faulty. In practical terms, the balance of evidence is in keeping with the view expressed in the consensus statement and patients who have had their fibroadenomas excised do not require routine follow-up other than the common sense approach of self-examination.

However, because simple fibroadenoma occurs in a young population, lifetime follow-up would be necessary to provide definitive guidance and such long-term data are not available at present.

Blunt Duct Adenosis and Sclerosing Adenosis

These are both histological appearances of ANDI and do not carry an increased cancer risk[15, 22]. These lesions are usually found incidentally in a biopsy performed for a dominant lump and require no follow-up.

Mastalgia and Cyclical Nodularity

These are aberrations of normality and therefore should not be labelled as a 'disease'. These clinically diagnosed conditions are not associated with any specific histology and, by definition, they will have the same cancer risk as the normal population, unless a biopsy has been performed which shows an incidental histological marker of risk. The cancer risk of an individual patient suffering from the symptoms must be calculated from the individual risk factors defined in this chapter.

Macroscopic Breast Cysts

The consensus statement places all forms of cysts in the 'no increased risk' group without comment. However, the subject is more controversial than this suggests and requires more detailed discussion. Attention has been focused on gross cystic disease because it is a common benign breast condition which is often found coexisting in cancerous breasts and it appears around the age that cancer becomes common. It is important to specify 'gross cystic disease' as defined by Haagensen et al[22] to denote macroscopic cysts which can be felt, aspirated, or seen at operation in contradistinction to microscopic cysts which are impalpable and only found in association with other pathology in the breast. Many studies have reported the incidence of cystic disease in cancerous breasts, but most have found that cysts are just as common in non-cancerous breasts studied at autopsy as in cancerous breasts. Thus, gross cysts taken in isolation from hyperplastic lesions do not appear to be commoner in cancerous breasts. Many investigations have examined the question of subsequent breast cancer development after a diagnosis of cystic disease in 'prospective' studies dating as far back as 1940, but as Azzopardi[19] points out: 'These studies are in reality mostly retrospective observation studies and suffer from a variety of methodological and statistical errors which give rise to varying estimates of increased risk.' Also many of these studies were carried out before the specific histological subgroups detailed above had been described adequately and so many of the series have failed to identify accurately those histological patterns which would influence subsequent cancer rates. Davis et al[23] in 1964 reviewed the results of six studies and found a 2.6 times increase in cancer risk in the published works and a 1.73 times increase in their own material. However, Haagensen et al[22] and Azzopardi[19] both concluded that none of the earlier studies was valid because of poorly defined pathology or invalid statistics. Nevertheless, Haagensen et al[22] describe a relative risk of three times for his private patients with gross cystic disease and two times for his public patients. This work has been criticized on the basis that it has been reported only in his monograph, and not in a refereed journal. Page's study[15] in over 4000 women found that cysts alone had a risk of only 1.2 times, i.e. not significantly different from normal. However, the most recent work suggests Haagensen may be right.

Apocrine Metaplasia

Apocrine metaplasia or pink cell change is such a common finding in the breast that it has long been considered to be of no importance in cancer risk. It is very commonly seen in cysts. However, recent detailed studies have suggested that apocrine metaplasia may be an indicator of increased risk when it is present in biopsies. Page showed a 2.7 times increase in risk for papillary apocrine change[15] and Roberts reported a 6.9 times increase for pink cell metaplasia[17]. This suggests some increase in cancer risk, but it should be noted that Page's finding of increased risk applies only to women over the age of 45 years and was present in his earlier study. A similar analysis of their larger series is awaited with interest. These studies have been supported by Haagensen's long-term follow-up of his series of gross cystic disease[22], where an increased risk of six times was noted in patients with gross cysts who had apocrine metaplasia on their biopsies in addition to the cyst. Patients without apocrine metaplasia had a lower risk of subsequent breast cancer. Haagensen also believed that many established breast cancers arise from apocrine-like cells.

These studies suggest that apocrine metaplasia in association with cystic disease and papillary apocrine change by itself are associated with a small increase in risk but further work is needed to clarify this issue. It is noteworthy that the consensus statement attaches no increased risk to apocrine metaplasia. Any significance attached to apocrine metaplasia in breast cysts is difficult to apply in practice as most breast cysts are treated by aspiration and no histology is available to assess the presence of apocrine metaplasia. New research techniques of biochemical evaluation of breast cyst fluid may solve this problem and these are discussed later in this chapter. In summary, the balance of evidence at the present time suggests that cysts alone carry no significant increase in risk – any such risk is associated only with coexisting apocrine histological change and probably only in women over the age of 45 years. Hence, currently patients with gross cysts treated by aspiration need not be followed up regularly unless a biopsy has shown significant associated histology findings.

Duct Ectasia/Periductal Mastitis

There is no evidence that duct ectasia or periductal mastitis predisposes to subsequent development of cancer, although we are not aware of any formal follow-up study and some degree of duct ectasia is so common in the general population that it will often coexist with other conditions carrying their own risk factors. Despite the stasis of duct content which must occur after total duct excision operations, there is no evidence that this is associated with increased cancer risk. Follow-up data presently available cannot be regarded as definitive, although we have no evidence to suggest that long-term follow-up is necessary.

Simple Epithelial Hyperplasia

Focal–Solitary Duct Papilloma

Solitary intraduct papilloma presenting as nipple discharge with or without a subareolar mass is usually considered to be a benign condition which carries no increased risk of breast cancer. A clear distinction must be made between the solitary intraductal papilloma and the much rarer (by a factor of 10) multiple intraduct type, which probably does carry an increased cancer risk[22]. The differences between these two types are discussed later in this chapter. Prolonged follow-up is not regarded as necessary if the surgeon and pathologist are happy that the papilloma is indeed a solitary one and has been excised by microdochectomy. However, Table 4.1 shows that the recent consensus statement from the American College of Pathologists[18] puts papilloma with a fibrovascular core in the moderate risk group (1.5–2 times).

This conclusion seems surprising in relation to the general clinical view given above, but is perhaps less surprising when we consider the long running controversy on this subject, reviewed by Azzopardi[19]. Once again the basic defect is the lack of large series of well-defined cases followed up for life. At present it is reasonable to treat cases as having no increased risk, or a risk so little increased that long-term follow-up is unnecessary.

Non-focal-epithelial Hyperplasia

The work of Page and others shows that mild epithelial hyperplasia (defined in the consensus statement as more than two but not more than four epithelial cells in depth) does not carry an increased risk. For notes on the nomenclature and groupings of hyperplasias, see p. 35.

Conditions with Slightly Increased Risk (1.5–2 times)

Moderate or florid hyperplasia without atypia is considered to carry this slight increase in risk of later developing cancer. This accurate characterization of risk is crucially dependent on assessment of the pattern of hyperplasia by the histopathologist. Such accuracy of assessment of benign and malignant patterns, and of the gradation between the extremes, as used in the ACP consensus statement, depend heavily on the work of Azzopardi and Page. It is essential that each individual case be discussed by the pathologist and clinician to ensure that the pathologist's interpretation is understood by the clinician. It is important that the pathologist uses standard terminology such as that of Page's group, and that the clinician has an understanding of the spectrum and patterns of hyperplasia and of modern terminology. This is discussed at the end of this chapter.

It is important to realize that minor degrees of hyperplasia are common and have no increased risk of breast cancer, so that the term 'hyperplasia' does not itself indicate an increase in risk. When the cytology and architecture change to move closer to that of intraduct or lobular carcinoma *in situ* then the risk of subsequent malignancy increases. The description and definition of the limits of each stage of increasing hyperplasia is difficult and a subject of considerable debate. Several grading systems with different names have been described by different pathologists, but it should be appreciated that the process is a continuum rather than a series of well-defined stages. The principal systems are outlined in Table 4.2 with approximate levels of equivalent severity of change indicated. The diagnostic features of each grade are outside the scope of this work and lie in the province of detailed pathology textbooks. The interested reader is referred to the works by Azzopardi[19], Black and Chabon[41], Wellings *et al*[14] and Dupont and Page[15, 16]. It is particularly important to note that the use of the word atypical (or atypia) differs between Page's group and the other workers, hence the presence of some overlap

Table 4.2 Classification of hyperplasias.

Black and Chabon[41]	Wellings *et al*[14]	Dupont and Page[15,16]	Risk
Grade 1	ALA-I	Minimal	None
Grade 2	ALA-II	Mild hyperplasia with atypia	None
Grade 3	ALA-III	Moderate and florid hyperplasia without atypia	Slight increase
Grade 4	ALA-IV	Florid hyperplasia with atypia	Moderate increase
Grade 5	ALA-V	Ca *in situ*	High

in the comparability of lesions III and IV (Table 4.2) and Page's hyperplasias with and without atypia. It is inevitable that some borderline cases will be graded differently by different pathologists, hence the importance of understanding the spectrum of appearance.

Intraduct hyperplasia without evidence of atypia (often called epitheliosis or papillomatosis) is a lesion which is commonly seen in biopsies undertaken for a dominant lump and was present in 22% of putatively normal breasts in a postmortem study[4]. It is clear that malignancy is not inevitable even in those patients with a pathological state which carries a high risk. This histological entity has caused endless debate among pathologists and interpretation of published series has been difficult due to imprecise definition of this term. Recent careful histopathological studies by Page's group[15] have shown an increased risk of subsequent breast cancer if atypia or atypical lobular hyperplasia was present in the biopsy (discussed below), but the risk was not increased where the hyperplasia was cytologically and morphologically bland. He further showed that a family history of breast cancer in a first-degree relative in a patient showing hyperplasia with atypia increases the relevant risk from 5 to 11 times[16]. Because the distinction between the degrees of hyperplasia is made on the fine morphological and cytological detail, it is important that the surgeon encourages his pathologist to produce clear descriptive reports which specify the situation of epithelial changes along the spectrum from normal through hyperplasia to atypias, rather than use ill-defined general terms such as 'chronic mastopathy' or 'fibrocystic disease'.

Conditions with Moderate Increase in Cancer Risk (5 times)

This group includes lobular and ductal hyperplasias with atypia. The quantitation of risk has been derived particularly from the work of Page's goup[15]. The risk of lobular hyperplasia with atypia has been found to be 6 times in women aged less than 45 and 3 times in older women. This risk estimate has been validated by a further study[17] which set the risk at 6.4 times normal.

Page's group found the risk of ductal hyperplasia with atypia to be 2.6 times, and papillary apocrine change to be 2 times normal so that ductal hyperplasia lies more in the slightly increased risk group (less than the corresponding patterns with assessment of lobular hyperplasia). This may reflect the greater difficulties associated with ductal hyperplasia – Azzopardi does not consider the case for an increased risk for ductal hyperplasia with atypia to be established. Hopefully, the situation with ductal hyperplasia will be clarified in the next few years; meanwhile, it is reasonable to see the ductal hyperplasias as lying mainly within the mildly increased risk group, but also straddling the moderate increased risk goup where there is a considerable degree of atypia.

It is of interest to note that these levels of risk are lower than nearly all of the earlier studies employing less critical pathology.

Breast Lesions Associated with a High Risk

The two entities of lobular carcinoma *in situ* (LCIS) and ductal carcinoma *in situ* (DCIS) are cytologically cancers and not strictly within the remit of benign breast disease. However, because both may be treated by local excision and require follow-up, the risk of cancer has to be quantified. These two lesions are uncommon and rarely present as a clinical mass or with nipple discharge. LCIS is normally discovered as an incidental finding on about 0.8% of benign biopsies and DCIS is commonly seen in cancerous breasts as an associated finding. However, DCIS alone is presenting with increasing frequency as a mammographic abnormality discovered during routine screening of well women.

LCIS has generally been considered to be malignant, and is thus commonly treated by mastectomy, although Haagensen uses the term 'lobular neoplasia' for LCIS in order to denote its relatively favourable prognosis due to absence of microscopic invasion and lack of metastatic potential[24]. The main problem with LCIS is that it is multicentric and frequently bilateral.

Of 172 biopsy-treated cases reviewed in the literature by Anderson[25], 15% developed ipsilateral carcinoma and 9% developed contralateral carcinoma with a mean follow-up of 10 years, while his personal series showed rates of 20% and 9% respectively, with a mean follow-up of 16 years. Haagensen's figures[22] are similar and he advocates careful follow-up on the grounds that bilateral mastectomy is too high a price to pay for carcinoma that is going to occur in a maximum of 25% of women after a long interval. He states that his patients have invariably chosen follow-up when given the full information on risk of subsequent breast cancer.

Ductal carcinoma *in situ* (DCIS) represents the extreme end of the spectrum of intraduct hyperplasia (epitheliosis in British literature and papillomatosis in American literature) and, as pointed out by Wellings, probably arises in the terminal ductal–lobular unit (TDLU). Wellings suggests that the process develops along a continuous path from simple hyperplasia to DCIS. He grades hyperplasias with varying degrees of cellular atypia and microarchitectural abnormality from I to V. Grades I and II represent mild hyperplasia while grade V is DCIS. However, Azzopardi argues that the link between these grades has not been fully established and that most difficult cases of severe hyperplasia can be split into one of two broad groups, either DCIS or severe (but benign) intraduct hyperplasias. Azzopardi argues that the clinical importance of atypical hyperplasia with atypia is not fully established, although Page's study now gives strong support to its importance as an intermediate risk factor between simple hyperplasia and cancer *in situ*.

Established DCIS is most commonly seen in breast ducts adjacent to an established cancer. The detailed criteria for the diagnosis of DCIS are well discussed in a paper by McDivitt et al[26] and should be read by those needing further information, as should Azzopardi's detailed discussion. Because DCIS is firmly placed towards the cancer end of the spectrum, management is usually by some form of mastectomy as advocated by Haagensen et al[22], but an alternative approach is to perform a wide excision or quadrantectomy of the affected portion of the breast. This tissue is then sectioned carefully and, if the DCIS is found to be multicentric, mastectomy is performed. No further procedure is performed if the original area of the DCIS is the only focus in all the biopsied material. This approach is based on the fact that DCIS tends to fall into two distinct populations – focal and multicentric – with little tendency for the first to proceed to the second. The patient having wide excision only is then followed carefully as for the severe hyperplasia patients with monthly self-examination, yearly clinical examination and biennial mammography. Certainly these patients are at considerable risk of developing subsequent invasive cancer with figures of up to 67% for ipsilateral disease and 17% for contralateral disease being quoted in a recent editorial[27], although this editorial does not make the important distinction between small unifocal areas and widespread multifocal change. Along with LCIS, the only totally logical surgical prophylactic approach would be bilateral mastectomy, although DCIS is less commonly a bilateral disease. Most surgeons adopt the compromise of unilateral mastectomy or wide excision and watch policy. A trial of the different types of primary therapy for DCIS is currently being run by the European Organisation for Research and Treatment of Cancer (EORTC) and the results of this randomized trial should give important new information in due course.

Non-Histological Risk Factors

Study of the epidemiology of breast cancer has revealed a few personal and familial risk factors which can be elicited on the initial history. The increased risk from each of these factors is relatively weak with only a few reaching a relative risk higher than four, approximately the risk for a contralateral breast cancer. These factors have recently been summarized by Kalache[28] who states that only two such factors reach a relative risk of four: a family history of premenopausal bilateral breast cancer and a previous cancer in the other breast. Three other demographic factors of risk are obvious: female vs male, old vs young and North European/American vs Asian, but clearly these features are of no help in the management of the individual patient. Thus the effect of the history on the management of patients with benign beast disease is simply that a family history in a mother or a sister (especially if premenopausal) should encourage follow-up and heighten the suspicion of the clinician towards any questionable dominant lump or borderline histology. Family history is a highly significant additive risk factor once atypical hyperplasia has been demonstrated in a biopsy (see above).

Radiology

Much interest in the last decade had been focused on the role of mammography of the benign breast in determining the cancer risk for individual patients. Wolfe has proposed an apparently simple classification of mammograms based on parenchymal patterns which he considers will divide pa-tients into high- and low-risk groups with the high-risk groups having as much as a 12-fold increase in risk, and the higher-risk group (DY pattern) a relative risk as high as 27[29]. However, this concept has run into fierce criticism recently and, although parenchymal patterns seem to have some interesting correlations with other non-radiological risk factors[30], many studies have failed to confirm Wolfe's original observations[31]. It must be said that all of these studies are retrospective and therefore subject to sampling errors, although a recent report from the Netherlands[32] is a prospective case-control study. A recent paper reviewed the publications on this subject and concluded that there is likely to be some increased risk associated with the DY pattern, but not to the degree reported by Wolfe[33]. A recent prospective study of a screened population from the island of Guernsey showed that Wolfe's DY pattern was associated with an increased risk of subsequent breast cancer but only gave a four times risk which is one-sixth of that proposed by Wolfe[34]. Until further prospective studies of this pattern are published, it must be concluded that benign mammographic parenchymal patterns are unproven as a predictor of increased cancer risk and no therapeutic recommendation should be made based solely upon the pattern. Our policy is to note the pattern, but we do not allow the report to alter our management policy as outlined above. We are currently prospectively investigating the value of Wolfe patterns in a cohort of 5000 women, but as the numbers of incident cancers are still small, we cannot as yet give a definite answer.

New Techniques for Estimating Risk

It will be clear from the preceding discussions of borderline or premalignant histology that pathological estimations of risk are not easy and depend crucially on the experience and knowledge of the individual pathologist. Also, a section of breast tissue – hopefully representative – is required to make the assessment of risk. There is no reason to believe that the clinical presentations that induce a surgeon to perform a biopsy will be associated with high-risk pathology as most of the hyperplastic lesions with atypia are found incidentally at biopsy for a condition such as dominant nodularity. This situation has been summarised by Sloane[35] when he said: 'Effective screening is the major problem as several clinicopathological studies suggest that the lesions with the greatest potential for neoplastic change usually produce no premonitory symptoms and are discovered incidentally.' An ideal method of risk estimation should be accurate in its prediction, be able to be performed on readily accessible body constituents – preferably blood or urine – and should not depend on subjective interpretation. No such marker has been discovered to date.

There are some recent interesting studies on risk factors which are currently research procedures but which throw some new light on the problem. Many of these studies have examined breast cyst fluid which is accessible by aspiration and is commonly available as some 7% of women have gross cystic disease. Studies of ionic concentrations[36], steroids[37] and proteins[38] have shown interesting differences in cyst fluids taken from different patients. Bradlow[36] has shown that patients with gross cysts fall into three broad groups with either a high or low potassium to sodium ratio (K^+/Na^+ ratio) and a small intermediate group where Na^+ and K^+ are approximately equal, i.e. the K^+/Na^+ ratio$=1$. He has also shown[37] that breast cyst fluid contains elevated levels of androgens suggesting a selective secretory mechanism by the cyst lining cells. Taken alone, these observations are interesting but not necessarily important, but, when linked with a series of new studies linking biochemistry of the cyst with its morphology, these ideas become profoundly interesting. Dixon et al[39] showed that apocrine cysts with a low Na^+/K^+ ratio (or high K^+/Na^+) are predominantly lined by tall apocrine epithelium and are not large 'tension' cysts with flattened epithelium. This is particularly interesting because of the work discussed earlier in this chapter linking the presence of apocrine metaplasia or papillary apocrine change with increased cancer risk. Also Wellings et al[14] showed an increased incidence of apocrine cysts in cancerous breasts and breasts contralateral to cancer, but a low incidence in autopsy breasts. Thus, it is possible that a simple estimation of the ionic content of breast cyst fluid will give some indication of risk in patients with palpable cysts. However, the evidence to date is only circumstantial and no increased cancer risk has been documented in a prospective series of patients selected on the basis of cyst fluid ion content.

Haagensen et al[38] have isolated an interesting glycoprotein from breast cyst fluid with a molecular weight of 15 000 (GCDFP-15) and has developed an antibody against it for use in an immunoperoxidase system. This antibody stains apocrine cells in apocrine cysts, and apocrine carcinomas and has recently been reported to stain lobular carcinoma in situ[40] but does not stain normal lobules. A radio-immunoassay is currently being developed to study the presence of GCDFP-15 in sera of women with benign and malignant breast disease. These studies all raise the hope of a better marker of premalignant risk in the not-too-distant future and results are awaited with interest.

An Outline of Terminology and Groupings of Hyperplastic Lesions of the Breast

These lesions have given rise to more confusion than any other aspect of benign breast disorders. This has resulted largely from confusion of definition and terminology, compounded by a natural tendency for clinicians to relate terms such as 'hyperplasia' or 'dysplasia' to cancer. The recent histopathological studies discussed earlier in this chapter have led to a much clearer understanding of significance and a better definition of patterns and terminology. We here attempt to give a simplified summary. The term 'hyperplasia' implies a benign condition – it does not signify cancer or cancer risk. Hyperplasias with atypia tend to be associated with a small or moderate increase in cancer risk. The term 'cancer in situ' is used for those patterns which imply a high risk of malignancy.

Structural Patterns – Organoid and Non-organoid

Hyperplasias are divided into organoid and non-organoid. Organoid hyperplasias are those in which different elements combine to form an organized structure, such as a lobule in adenosis. Thus, in organoid hyperplasias, existing lobules hypertrophy or new ducts and/or lobules are formed. The structure will show the normal lumen of the lobular acinus lined by its two-layer epithelium and surrounded by a loose lobular stromal tissue.

In the non-organoid form (epitheliosis or papillomatosis), the hyperplasia is of a single tissue, i.e. a single cell type, forming masses or sheets of cells without forming a new fully developed structure. Both organoid and non-organoid may be present in combination, i.e. when epitheliosis invades (or develops within) the lobular structure of adenosis. Sclerosing adenosis is considered to be an intermediate condition between organoid and non-organoid.

Recently there is a move towards discarding both the British term 'epitheliosis' and the corresponding American term of 'papillomatosis', and replace both with the simple term 'hyperplasia'.

Organoid Hyperplasia – Blunt Duct Adenosis

This is the prime example of a simple organoid hyperplasia. Many pathologists regard it as so common as to be a normal process – Haagensen states that it is 'normally seen in the breasts of modern women'. It arises by hypertrophy of existing lobules or the development of new lobular structures. The appearance is that of a group of alveolar type structures with a normal two-cell layer lining and surrounded by typical loose lobular stroma, although different lobular elements may be affected to a different degree. The condition has a spectrum, which merges with normal at one end while at the other end there is marked hypertrophy with enlarged lobules and dilatation of the lumen. There are a number of variants, including a microcystic variety where cystic dilatation of the glandular lumen takes place.

Sclerosing Adenosis

This may be regarded as an intermediate form – although the two-layer alveolar structure persists, there is marked hypertrophy of the myoepithelial element which distorts the lobular architecture so much as to mimic cancer.

These are generally considered to be of little importance *per se* in relation to cancer risk although epitheliosis may be superimposed. In this case the significance of the lesion would be that of the worst 'pattern', i.e. the epitheliosis.

Non-organoid Hyperplasia (Epitheliosis, Papillomatosis)

In this condition (Figures 4.1–4.4), a hyperplasia of the lining epthelium occurs giving rise to solid or semisolid sheets of a predominantly single cell type which fill small ducts and lobules. Hyperplasia may occur anywhere in the ductal system in the breast from within the lobule to the nipple ducts, but it is generally agreed that most significant hyperplasias arise in the smallest ducts of the TDLU from whence it may spread into the small ducts or into the lobule. Significant hyperplasias tend to take one or two forms – ductal or lobular. In British literature, the term 'epitheliosis' has been applied to hyperplasias

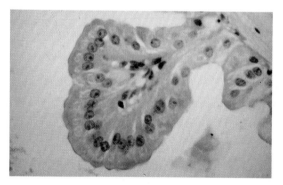

4.1 *An example of apocrine metaplasia within a cyst. This shows the large eosinophilic, cytologically regular apocrine cells projecting as a papillary tuft with a stromal core.*

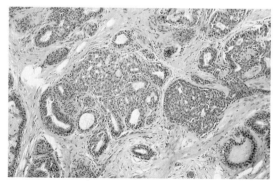

4.2 *Hyperplasia: This demonstrates the filling of ductules with cells which on high power were seen to be cytologically normal. The general architecture of the TDLU can still be seen despite the filling and distension of ducts by cells.*

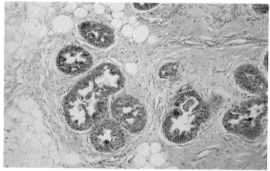

4.3 *Atypical ductal hyperplasia. The duct is not plugged with cells but the hyperplasia shows much more darkly staining epithelium, due to increased nuclear size and pleomorphism of the nuclei. The diagnosis of atypical changes was made on the basis of the cytology of the cells studied at high power.*

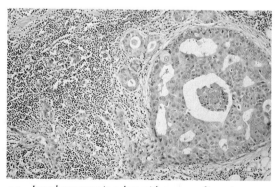

4.4 *Intraduct cancer in a duct with an area of invasive cancer around the duct. These two conditions frequently coexist as noted in the text (p. 33). Note the large paler cells of the intraduct cancer with spaces in the epithelium giving a rather cribriform appearance. There is a small area of central necrosis.*

severe enough to be considered significant, particularly when of the ductal type. In American literature the term 'papillomatosis' has been used for the same condition. This is confusing because the term is also used to describe a different condition – multiple intraduct papillomas. Hence the tendency to discard both terms – epitheliosis and papillomatosis. Neither term is used in the ACP consensus document which uses the term 'hyperplasia'.

Assessment of Hyperplasia

Grading

In early stages of hyperplasia the cells may be layered just three or four cells high; later they may fill the lumen or even distend it greatly. The hyperplasia may be graded on this basis, e.g. two to four epithelial cells in depth would be mild, more than four cells deep is moderate. Other pathologists use different gradings, e.g. mild is an increased number of epithelial cells without occluding the lumen; in moderate cases, the lumen is just occluded; in severe or florid hyperplasia, the duct is distended. This grading is distinct from cytological grading where individual cells are assessed.

Cellular Organization

The cells within hyperplasia show a varying degree of organization (Figures 4.2–4.4) and this is used in assessing the severity of the lesion in relation to malignant potential. For example, in benign hyperplasia the cells tend to be arranged parallel along their long axes (streaming) and the spaces within the sheet are irregular and crescentic. Necrosis is unusual.

Cytological Detail

The cytological characteristics of the cells are assessed separately – hyperplasia does not imply atypia, although the more florid the hyperplasia, the more likely it is to be associated with cellular atypia. The features assessed include characteristics such as nuclear size, pleomorphism and hyperchromatism.

Assessment of Future Risk of Malignancy

All the above features may be taken into account as discussed earlier in this chapter. As yet, there is unfortunately no agreed method for assessing these factors. Some workers assess each separately to give a form of scoring, while Page gives greatest emphasis to an overall pattern which resembles cancer in situ, but without sufficient features to merit this appellation. Thus his assessment of atypia is based on this pattern recognition, rather than a progressive scoring technique. The risks attached to these hyperplasias have been discussed earlier in this chapter. Much progress has been made in the last decade and further consensus conferences will undoubtedly lead to more agreement and uniformity.

Lobular Hyperplasia and Neoplasia

This is a pattern distinguished particularly by the histological character of the cells – the lobules are packed and distended by small uniform cells, with rare mitoses and little tendency to necrosis. It appears to start in the acini and proceed to the ductules of the TDLU, and may then involve the large ducts, characteristically by pagetoid spread. This is in contrast to ductal hyperplasias, which tend to start in the ductal portion of the TDLU, and spread by luminal extension down the duct and/or into the lobule. Lobular hyperplasia is assessed in similar fashion to ductal hyperplasia. Lobular neoplasia is often described as of three grades: lobular carcinoma in situ, lobular carcinoma in situ with invasion and invasive lobular carcinoma with no residual in situ disease. Because the in situ form carries such a good prognosis, Haagensen prefers the term 'lobular neoplasia', because he believes it to be treated more appropriately by wide local excision than mastectomy. It is disease predominantly of premenopausal women and it appears that most lobular neoplasia regresses after the menopause. However, it tends to multifocal, bilateral and associated with later development of invasive cancer. Such invasive cancers are long delayed, also bilateral and of good prognosis.

Other Epithelial Hyperplasias

Papillary Lesions (see also Chapter 12)

A papilloma is an epithelial lesion whose branches have a fibrovascular core. It may be macroscopic or microscopic, single or multiple, benign or malignant (papillary carcinoma when it loses its regular fibrovascular core).

Macroscopic Intraductal Papilloma

This is the typical lesion of the large subareolar ducts, usually 4–5 mm in diameter, presenting with bloody nipple discharge. It may be multiple in the sense of two to three similar papillomas lying adjacent in the one duct. Much less commonly, multiple papillomas may be seen as many large papillomas – often reaching a centimetre or so in diameter and hence readily palpable. These affect more than one duct system in the breast and occur peripheral to the subareolar region.

It is generally considered that solitary intraductal papilloma is a benign condition which does not evolve into papillary carcinoma, such carcinomas arising *de novo*[19].

The condition of multiple large duct papillomas is probably different, Haagensen reporting a distinct association with cancer. The rarity of the condition means that literature is sparse.

Microscopic papilloma

These occur in the smaller ducts of the breast in two forms: apocrine and non-apocrine. Apocrine papillary change is so common as to be regarded by most workers as normal (Figure 4.1). Non-apocrine, micropapillomas are less common but are frequently seen in the premenopausal breast. Parks[42] considered that they could regress spontaneously after the menopause.

Juvenile papillomatosis[43]

This is a breast tumour characterized by atypical hyperplasia and multiple cysts. The primary distinguishing feature is the young age of the patient – the mean age of 180 patients recorded in a registry of the condition was 23 years with a range of 12–48. There is a considerable tendency for the patient to develop breast cancer later and an excess incidence of breast cancer in relatives – suggesting a possible genetic element. The term 'papillomatosis' in this condition seems to be the American usage of epitheliosis, rather than true papillomas.

Figures 4.1–4.4 show the range of appearances from simple apocrine metaplasia through hyperplasia without atypia, hyperplasia with atypia and intraduct cancer. Detailed assessment requires high power microscopy – these low power photomicrographs merely illustrate the general appearances.

REFERENCES

1. Hislop T. G. & Elwood J. M. Risk factors for benign breast disease: a 30 year cohort study. *Canadian Medical Association Journal* 1981; **124**: 283–291.

2. Vessey M. P., McPherson K. & Doll R. Breast cancer and oral contraceptives: findings in the Oxford–FPA contraceptive study. *British Medical Journal* 1981; **282**: 2093–2094.

3. Cooke M. G. & Rohan T. E. The patho-epidemiology of benign proliferative epithelial disorders of the female breast. *Journal of Pathology* 1985; **146**: 1–15.

4. Sandison A. T. An autopsy study of the adult human breast. *National Cancer Institute Monograph* No. 8, US Dept Health, Education and Welfare, 1962; pp 31–43.

5. Royal College of General Practitioners. Breast cancer and oral contraceptives: findings in Royal College of General Practitioners Study. *British Medical Journal* 1981; **282**: 2089–2093.

6. Ory H., Cole P., MacMahon B. & Hoover R. Oral contraceptives and reduced risk of benign breast diseases. *New England Journal of Medicine* 1976; **294**: 419–422.

7. Anderson T. J., Ferguson D. J. P. & Raab G. M. Cell turnover in the 'resting' human breast: influence of parity, contraceptive pill, age and laterality. *British Journal of Cancer* 1982; **46**: 376–382.

8. McPherson K., Vessey M. P., Neil A., Doll R., Jones L. & Roberts M. Early oral contraceptive use and breast cancer: Results of another case control study. *British Journal of Cancer* 1987; **56**: 653–660.

9. Asscher A. W. Oral contraceptives and breast cancer. *Lancet* 1987; ii: 1267.

10. Roberts M. M., Elton R. A., Robinson S. E. & French K. Consultations for breast disease in general practice and referral patterns. *British Journal of Surgery* 1987; **74**: 1020–1022.

11. Nichols S., Waters W. E. & Wheeler M. J. Management of female breast disease by Southampton general practitioners. *British Medical Journal* 1980; **281**: 1450–1453.

12. Bywaters J. L. The incidence and management of female breast disease in a general practice. *Journal of the Royal College of General Practitioners* 1977; **27**: 353–357.

13. Ernster V. L. The epidemiology of benign breast disease. *Epidemiological Review* 1981; **3**: 184–202.

14. Wellings S. R., Jensen H. M. & Marcum R. G. An atlas of subgross pathology of the human breast with special reference to possible precancerous lesions. *Journal of the National Cancer Institute* 1975; **55**: 231–273.

15. Page D. L., Vander Zwaag R., Rogers L. W., Williams L. T., Walker W. E. & Hartmann W. H. Relation between component parts of fibrocystic disease complex and breast cancer. *Journal of the National Cancer Institute* 1978; **61**: 1055–1063.

16. Dupont W. D. & Page D. L. Risk factors for breast cancer in women with proliferative breast disease. *New England Journal of Medicine* 1985; **312**: 146–151.

17. Roberts M. M., Jones V., Elton R. A., Fortt R. W., Williams S. & Gravelle I. H. Risk of breast cancer in women with a history of benign disease of the breast. *British Medical Journal* 1984; **288**: 275–278.

18. Winchester D. P. ACP consensus statement. The relationship of fibrocystic disease to breast cancer. *American College of Surgeons Bulletin* 1986; **71**: 29–31.

19. Azzopardi J. G. In: *Major Problems in Pathology* Vol II, *Problems in Breast Pathology*. London, W. B. Saunders, 1979.

20. Semb C. Pathologico-anatomical and clinical

investigations of fibroadenomatosis cystica mammae and its relation to other pathological conditions in the mamma, especially cancer. *Acta Chirurgica Scandinavica* 1928; (Suppl 10), **64**: 1–484.

21. Oliver R. L. & Major R. C. Cyclomastopathy: a physio-pathological conception of some benign breast tumours, with an analysis of four hundred cases. *American Journal of Cancer* 1934; **21**: 1–85.

22. Haagensen C. D., Bodian C. & Haagensen D. E. *Breast Carcinoma, Risk and Detection*. London, Saunders, 1986, pp. 83–105.

23. Davis H. H., Simons M. & Davis J. B. Cystic disease of the breast: relationship to carcinoma. *Cancer* 1964; **17**: 957–978.

24. Haagensen C. D., Lane N., Lattes R. & Bodian C. Lobular neoplasia (so-called lobular carcinoma in situ) of the breast. *Cancer* 1978; **42**: 737–769.

25. Andersen J. A. Lobular carcinoma in situ of the breast. An approach to rational treatment. *Cancer* 1977; **39**: 2597–2602.

26. McDivitt R. W., Holleb A. I. & Foote F. W. Prior breast disease in patients treated for papillary carcinoma. *Archives of Pathology* 1968; **85**: 117–124.

27. Editorial. Intraduct cancer of the breast. *Lancet* 1984; **ii**: 24.

28. Kalache A. Risk factors for breast cancer: a tabular summary of the epidemiological literature. *British Journal of Surgery* 1981; **68**: 797–799.

29. Wolfe J. N. Risk for breast cancer development determined by mammographic parenchymal pattern. *Cancer* 1976; **37**: 2486–2492.

30. De Waard F., Rombach J. J., Collette H. J. A. & Slotboom B. Breast cancer risk associated with reproductive factors and breast parenchymal patterns. *Journal of the National Cancer Institute* 1984; **72**: 1277–1282.

31. Egan R. L. & Mosteller R. C. Breast cancer mammography patterns. *Cancer* 1977; **40**: 2087–2090.

32. Verbeek A. L. M., Hendricks J. H. C. L., Peters P. H. M. & Sturmans F. Mammographic breast pattern and the risk of breast cancer. *Lancet* 1984;

i: 591–593.

33. Boyd N. F., O'Sullivan B., Fishell E., Simor I. & Cooke E. Mammographic patterns and breast cancer risk. Methodologic standards and contradictory results. *Journal of the National Cancer Institute* 1984; **72**: 1258–1259.

34. Gravelle I. H., Bulstrode J. C., Bulbrook R. D., Wang D. Y., Allen D. & Hayward J. L. A prospective study of mammographic parenchymal patterns and risk of breast cancer. *British Journal of Radiology* 1986; **59**(701): 487–491.

35. Sloane J. P. Precancerous changes in the breast. In: Carter R. C. (ed.), *Precancerous States*. London, Oxford University Press, 1984.

36. Bradlow H. L., Skidmore F. D., Schwartz M. K. & Fleischer M. Cation levels in human breast cyst fluid. *Clinical Oncology* 1981; **7**: 388–390.

37. Bradlow H. L., Rosenfeld R. S., Kream J., Fleischer M., O'Connor J. & Schwartz M. K. Steroid hormone accumulation in human breast cyst fluid. *Cancer Research* 1981; **41**: 105–107.

38. Haagensen D. E., Mazoujian G., Dilley W. G., Pedersen C. E., Kister S. J. & Wells S. A. Breast gross cystic disease fluid analysis. 1. Isolation and radioimmunoassay for a major component protein. *Journal of the National Cancer Institute* 1979; **62**: 239–247.

39. Dixon J. M., Miller W. R., Scott W. N. & Forrest A. P. M. The morphological basis of human breast cyst populations. *British Journal of Surgery* 1984; **70**: 604–606.

40. Eusebi V., Betts C., Haagensen D. E., Gugliotta P., Bussolati G., & Azzopardi J. G. Apocrine differentiation in lobular carcinoma of the breast. *Human Pathology* 1984; **15**: 134–140.

41. Black M. M. & Chabon A. B. In situ carcinoma of the breast. In: Sommers S. C. (ed.) *Pathology Annual*. New York, Appleton-Century-Crofts, 1969, pp. 185–210.

42. Parks A. G. The micro-anatomy of the breast. *Annals of the Royal College of Surgeons (England)* 1959; **25**: 295–234.

43. Rosen P. P., Holmes G., Leser M. L., Kinne D. W. & Beatle E. J. Juvenile papillomatosis and breast carcinoma. *Cancer* 1985; **55**: 1345–1352.

5 The Approach to Assessment and Management of Breast Lumps

It is fortunate that, although there are many causes of lumps in the breast (Table 5.1), very few diagnoses cover the large majority. There are two major problems of diagnosis: first to decide whether the lump is within or outside the spectrum of normality and, secondly, if abnormal, whether it is benign or malignant.

Table 5.1 Causes of lumps in the breast.

Normal structures	ANDI
Normal nodularity[a]	Fibroadenoma[a]
Prominent fat lobule[b]	Cyclical nodularity[a]
Prominent rib[b]	Cyst[a]
Intramammary lymph node[c]	Galactocele[c]
Edge of biopsy wound[b]	Sclerosing adenosis[b]
Accessory breast[c]	Stromal fibrosis[c]

Inflammatory
Chronic infective abscess[c]
Fat necrosis[c]
Foreign body granuloma[c]
Mondor's disease[c]

Tumours	
Benign	*Intermediate*
Duct papilloma[b]	Phyllodes tumour[c]
Giant fibroadenoma[c]	Carcinoma *in situ*[b]
Lipoma[c]	
Granular cell myoblastoma[c]	

Malignant
Primary tumours[a]
Secondary tumours[c]

Lesions of the nipple and areola	Lesions of the skin
Squamous papilloma[b]	Sebaceous cyst[b]
Leiomyoma[c]	Hydradenitis[c]
Retention cyst[c]	Benign and malignant skin
Papillary adenoma[c]	Tumours[c]

Frequency of presentation as a lump: [a]common; [b]less common; [c]rare.

Until recent years, clinical assessment was not only the mainstay of diagnosis of breast lumps, but usually the only assessment prior to surgical excision or mastectomy. Many adjuvant techniques have been introduced over recent years: imaging techniques are discussed in Chapter 6; radiology, aspiration/cytology and needle biopsy have established important roles; various forms of transillumination, thermography and duct injection have not proved sufficiently useful to warrant routine usage. Until recently, ultrasound has fallen into the same category, but improving technology is changing the situation, especially in association with localization to facilitate aspiration cytology. While radiology has improved on the diagnostic accuracy of clinical techniques alone, skilled clinical examination and needle exploration can still provide a high degree of diagnostic accuracy and are especially important in centres where ancillary aids are not readily available.

In the past, there has been a tendency to biopsy all breast lumps irrespective of their characteristics. This can result in a large number of biopsies. In one series[1], 75% of benign biopsies showed tissues which can be regarded as normal. Benign lumps need just as careful assessment as malignant ones – in an effort to avoid unnecessary biopsies and, in particular, repeated unnecessary biopsies.

Clinical Assessment of a Breast Lump

History

The history is important in the assessment of breast lumps, particularly in relation to duration of the mass, fluctuation in size with the menstrual cycle and associated pain. Each must be considered in association with the overall clinical picture – no one feature should be allowed to dominate clinical thinking. In the past, it has been widely thought that a painful lump is not malignant but this is not so[2]. However, the pain indicative of cancer differs in characteristics from that of cyclical mastalgia (Chapter 8).

Inspection

Detailed and systematic examination is of great importance, particularly in elucidating signs of malignancy. These are well known, but two of these, skin attachment and nipple retraction, can sometimes be caused by benign conditions.

Cancer is the likely diagnosis when nipple retraction is associated with a lump, but two benign lumps may also cause nipple retraction. A chronic abscess associated with periductal mastitis may cause retraction by a combination of shortening of ducts and areola oedema. A large cyst or fibroadenoma arising centrally among the major ducts can cause relative shortening by displacement and so give rise to apparent nipple retraction (Figure 5.1).

The same mechanism can operate with skin attachment. Haagensen[3] calls this false retraction. Large cysts or fibroadenomas can displace Cooper's ligaments and give rise to apparent skin fixity and distortion, while a chronic abscess associated with periductal mastitis will lead to actual skin attachment, oedema and sometimes *peau d'orange*. Hence the necessity to obtain histological confirmation in all cases of suspected malignancy.

Palpation

Consistency, surface characteristics and mobility in relation to surrounding tissues are each important in diagnosing benign lesions. A fibroadenoma has a characteristic rubbery consistency, a smooth or smoothly lobulated surface and a degree of mobility within the breast which can only be described as extraordinary – this combination of characteristics provides an unequivocal clinical diagnosis. This classic pattern is usual in young girls, but is often obscured in older women by incarceration of the fibroadenoma in a background of involutional changes such that the fibroadenoma is robbed of its classic discrete, smooth surface and mobility and the diagnosis comes as a histological surprise after excision of a solitary lump.

While palpation of a moderately tense cyst is equally characteristic, the clinical findings vary greatly depending on the degree of intracystic

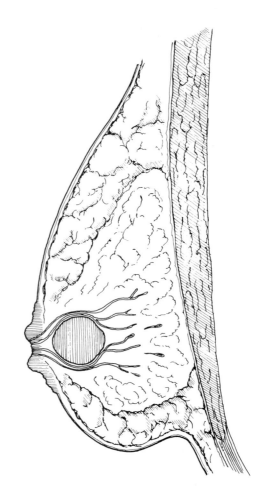

5.1 *A large benign cyst may stretch and distort main ducts or Cooper's ligaments, leading to 'pseudoretraction' of skin or nipple.*

tension, which may vary from normal tissue tension to a hardness which exceeds that of cancer. Thus cysts are commonly misdiagnosed. They may be missed completely because they are soft; in other cases cancer is confidently diagnosed because the cyst is so hard. This alone justifies the passage of a fine needle in every breast lump because the finding of unexpected fluid will save the patient much distress and unnecessary surgery. The surface of a cyst is usually smooth, but a large cyst may be lobulated and occasionally, a group of small cysts will feel nodular so as to simulate a fibroadenoma.

Assessment of the mobility of a breast lump within the surrounding tissue provides diagnostic information (Figure 5.2); there are three degrees of mobility of a lump in relation to the surrounding breast tissue.

Because a fibroadenoma has no attachment to surrounding capsule except for a single stalk, its mobility is extreme. The wall of a cyst is confluent with the fibrous breast stroma, hence the surrounding parenchyma can be felt to move with the cyst giving it an intermediate degree of mobility. At the other extreme, an infiltrating cancer fixes the surrounding breast tissue so that the affected quadrant of the breast moves with the

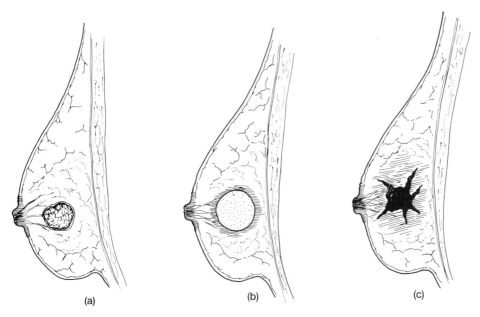

5.2 *Mobility of breast lumps in relation to surrounding breast tissue. (a) Fibroadenoma; (b) cyst; (c) cancer. The shaded area indicates the amount of breast tissue 'moving' with the lump.*

mass. But, occasionally, a very large cyst or benign tumour will have a similar effect by stretch-fixation of Cooper's ligaments so that the quadrant of the breast moves with the lump.

Palpation is even more important for ill-defined lumps – by far the commonest problem in breast assessment is to decide whether an area which feels abnormal to the patient is truly abnormal, or whether it is part of general nodularity of the breast. This arises particularly when a woman's attention is drawn to the upper outer quadrant of the breast by premenstrual pain or tenderness. Careful assessment to determine the pattern of nodularity in both breasts is essential. In doubtful cases it is useful to stand behind the patient and palpate both breasts simultaneously (Figure 5.3). In this way it is surprising how often an apparent single mass is found to be bilateral and symmetrical when the mirror image sections of the breast are examined together. Where it is still uncertain whether or not an area of nodularity is discrete, a cytology specimen can be taken and the patient re-examined in early or mid-cycle when normal nodularity will be minimal.

Fixity to skin and deep structures is unusual with benign conditions except those associated with chronic inflammation.

A complete physical examination, including axillary and supraclavicular palpation is important in all breast disease, but rarely provides discriminatory information with benign conditions.

Assessment using Ancillary Investigations

Aspiration Cytology

In the past, the classic teaching for clinical diagnosis of a lump was to follow the sequence:

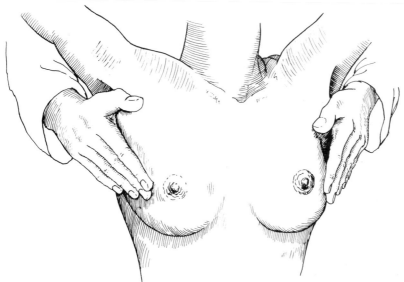

5.3 *Mirror image palpation of both breasts simultaneously helps assessment of doubtful lumps.*

inspect, palpate, percuss, auscultate. Today the sequence should be: inspect, palpate, percuss, auscultate, insert a needle. The last is a natural extension of clinical examination to give an added dimension to palpation.

It is sound policy to insert a needle into every breast lump for three purposes: to assess the consistency of the mass, to aspirate fluid if it proves to be a cyst, and to provide a cytological specimen if blood-stained fluid is obtained or the lesion proves to be solid. The rubbery feel to the needle point of a fibroadenoma or involutional nodularity is as characteristic as the softness and absence of resistance with fat, and the grittiness of cancer. Equally characteristic is the sudden sensation experienced when the needle tip traverses fibrous tissue to enter a cyst.

Technique is important in taking a specimen for cytological study (Chapter 18) and equipment to provide an optimal specimen should always be available. A specimen for examination is taken from any breast mass with two exceptions. A cytological examination of cyst fluid is unnecessary unless the fluid is blood stained, or a residual mass is palpated. It is also unnecessary for a *classic* fibroadenoma in a young woman under the age of 25 – when cytology may even be misleading.

Ultrasound

This has not proved of great use in breast diagnosis in the past, but the development of small, portable machines of high resolution is proving to be useful in guiding needle aspiration of small lumps or of impalpable masses detected by radiology or by ultrasound itself[4]. This is discussed further in Chapter 6.

Needle Biopsy (*see* Chapter 18)

The provision of histological material by a biopsy needle such as the Trucut is of particular value in the management of malignant masses of 2 cm or larger, because an adequate specimen gives a definitive diagnosis. Its usefulness is more limited in benign conditions, because adequate samples are notoriously difficult to obtain from the rubbery tissue typical of cyclical nodularity and fibroadenoma. Here aspiration cytology is more useful provided an experienced cytologist is available. In spite of these limitations, needle biopsy should be considered in all discrete breast lumps but a low yield of satisfactory specimens will have to be accepted in benign disease.

Mammography (*see* Chapter 6)

Clinical assessment, needle aspiration and cytology have lessened the role of mammography for a well-defined mass. Its greatest use is as a screening technique in detecting subclinical pathology and hence its routine use is best reserved for the older patient – 40 years or more. Here mammography is more accurate than in young women and screening in this age group has been shown to be worth while. Nevertheless, in any patient over the age of 25, mammography may provide helpful information where a lump presents a difficult diagnostic problem after clinical and cytological assessment. It is best used selectively in this way rather than routinely. We do not use mammography below the age of 25 – cancer is exceedingly rare, mammography often inaccurate, and the carcinogenic effect of radiation is likely to be greatest during the time of rapid glandular development.

Management of Nodularity

Normal Nodularity or Dominant Lump?

The commonest presenting lump in women during the reproductive period is the normal breast nodularity, or the cyclical nodularity of ANDI, seen in the upper outer quadrant and axillary tail of the breast.

To decide whether a mass is dominant or merely part of normal or cyclical nodularity is critical for an early carcinoma must not be missed; it is equally important that the surgeon does not embark on a series of biopsies of normal nodular breasts in young women, with increasing scarring and repeated worry every time an area of tenderness develops. Yet to avoid missing cancer in the 'at risk' age group (more than 25 years of age), discrete persisting lumps must be excised, irrespective of the results of ancillary investigations. Assessment is essentially clinical in young women, supplemented by cytology and/or mammography in older women where there is doubt as to whether or not a dominant mass is present.

To avoid unnecessary biopsy, a well-defined approach must be taken to determine whether a mass is dominant and persistent.

If a single examination is inconclusive, the following sequence is useful:

1. Examine both breasts simultaneously as described (*see* Figure 5.3).
2. Examine the patient during the first half of the menstrual cycle.

3. Use cytology, repeatedly if necessary.
4. Review the patient over a period of 2 months. If doubt persists, by then it should be obvious that one is dealing with normal nodularity, or biopsy should be undertaken.

Where full assessment shows nothing more than general nodularity, reassurance and explanation of the physiological basis of the nodularity is adequate treatment. Specific treatment is only required when pain is the major symptom and this is dealt with in the section on breast pain (Chapter 8).

However, particular notice should be taken of a patient who is certain that she can feel an abnormality in her breast, especially over the age of 40. A woman may feel an abnormality some time before her medical attendant is able to do so, and the older the patient, the more likely she is to be right. Such a patient should be observed for 6 months, even when no abnormality is found on examination or investigation.

Assessment of a Discrete or Dominant Mass

Having decided that a lump is not just part of normal nodularity, the physical characteristics should be carefully assessed to make a specific diagnosis. This is useful as a discipline in sharpening one's diagnostic acumen, but it is also important because some discrete lumps are due to normal structures. If the clinical features are definitely those of a normal structure and are confirmed by ancillary investigations, biopsy can be avoided but the emphasis must always be on biopsy where the slightest doubt persists regarding the diagnosis of any persisting dominant mass in a woman of cancer age group.

A further possible approach to this problem is to use an agent which reduces nodularity. This might not only cause regression of the nodularity which was causing diagnostic difficulty, but in so doing make any hidden cancer more obvious. Danazol is effective in reducing cyclical nodularity and we are exploring its use in this way. However, there is insufficient information available about the effect of danazol on discrete masses, including early cancer, to recommend its use at present in any way except investigational.

Features of Individual Lesions

Normal Sructures

Prominent Fat Lobule

Fat lobules are often easily palpable and one may become more prominent than its fellows. This is seen most frequently along the inferior margin of the breast or over the axillary tail, due perhaps in both cases to pressure from a brassière. The superficial nature of the lesion, its site, soft smooth consistency and softness to a needle point, will usually allow confident diagnosis.

Prominent Rib

It is not uncommon for a patient, usually young, to present with a 'breast lump' which appears to be normal breast tissue over a normal prominent rib. Sometimes the rib is asymmetrical – more often it is identical to the opposite side and it is difficult to know why the patient has suddenly become aware of the rib. Occasionally, radiology of the rib cage is necessary before reassuring the patient.

Intramammary Lymph Node

These are usually confined to the axillary tail of the breast and impalpable – because they are small and embedded in the breast stroma. Sometimes lymph nodes in the outer quadrant of the breast proper may enlarge sufficiently to be palpable. Although they feel cystic, they are slightly elongated and peripheral to the breast area where cysts are commonly found. They have a soft feel to a needle point. They have a characteristic appearance on mammography – a smooth ovoid lesion, sometimes with a notch along one margin. Lymphocytes are found on cytology. It is usually possible to make a diagnosis and avoid surgery.

Accessory Breasts

These occur under the anterior axillary fold, are usually bilateral and come to notice during pregnancy or if the patient gains weight. The condition is described more fully in Chapter 15.

Edge of a Previous Biopsy Wound

Patients may present complaining of a 'lump' at the site of a previous scar. It is due to the persistent defect in the breast which sometimes occurs if a biopsy wound is not closed by deep sutures. The most important aspect is awareness. It is discussed further on p. 47.

ANDI

Fibroadenoma

This tumour, in its classic form, is the most easily diagnosed breast lump. When it occurs in the age group of 15–25 years it is rubbery firm, smooth or lobulated and extremely mobile, clinical diagnosis is highly accurate and confirmation by ancillary tests is not necessary. Indeed, cytology is likely to be misleading unless a well-experienced cytologist is available, because the epithelial cells of fibroadenoma may simulate malignancy.

Fibroadenomas are also commonly seen in later life when the diagnosis is much more difficult. The patient has now reached the cancer age group, so definite exclusion of malignancy is mandatory. The fibroadenoma is caught up in the involutional fibrosis of the breast, so that it loses its characteristic smoothness and mobility; it requires full assessment as for any other dominant lump – by clinical assessment, mammography, cytology and biopsy if indicated.

The clinical and radiological similarities between fibroadenoma, cyst and some circumscribed cancers (especially medullary cancer) should be remembered. Where an otherwise typical fibroadenoma is softer than expected, a phyllodes tumour should be suspected (see Chapter 7).

Cyclical Nodularity ('Fibroadenosis'; 'Chronic Cystic Mastitis')

The problem of cyclical nodularity is that already discussed – the discrimination between general nodularity and a prominent mass in an individual patient. The problem becomes worse as normal nodularity moves across the spectrum to the more severe cyclical nodularity of ANDI.

Perhaps the most interesting aspect of this problem is why some patients with cyclical nodularity develop a dominant lump. In many cases, cyst formation or localized extravagant adenosis with or without fibrosis may underlie the mass, but in other cases, histological findings are no different to adjacent clinically unremarkable breast. Exaggerated local end-organ response to hormonal stimulation seems the most likely cause. The dominance of stroma over epithelial tissue in quantitative terms would point a finger at the stroma. With the large amount of specialized, hormonal-responsive stroma present in the lobule, a considerable increase in fibrocyte size or numbers, or stromal oedema, could occur without producing obvious changes on light microscopy – changes which could be significant overall when multiplied by the number of lobules in the area. This remains a major area of ignorance in breast pathophysiology. Attempts to demonstrate local oedema by physical methods have not been successful and further work is needed.

The term 'fibroadenosis' had been included in this section to allow discussion of this widely used term in a clinical context and to provide an opportunity for condemnation of the term 'fibroadenosis', together with the concepts and implications with which it has been associated by generations of surgeons and pathologists. The

major implication of the term – that it represents a specific clinical syndrome associated with a specific pathological process – has no basis in fact, and this problem has been discussed fully in Chapter 3.

The recognition of the basic normality of cyclical nodularity as a part of ANDI should be extended to histological assessment. Pathologists should be encouraged to drop the terms 'fibroadenosis' and 'chronic cystic mastitis' following the philosophy of Foot and Stewart[5] who wrote: 'Chronic cystic mastitis is so ingrained in the minds of some pathologists that this diagnosis of a locally excised portion of breast almost amounts to a surgico-pathologic reflex.'

Cysts

A cyst is the commonest discrete mass found in patients presenting to a breast clinic – a fact causing little surprise since it has been estimated that about 1 in 10 of all women will develop a symptomatic breast cyst during their reproductive life, and recurrent or multiple cysts are common.

Clinical diagnosis is surprisingly uncertain; variation in size, variation in shape due to lobularity or multiplicity, variation in consistency due to intracystic pressure mean that cysts can as easily be missed completely as confidently diagnosed as cancer. Fortunately, definite diagnosis is made certain by simple needle puncture; this alone provides the justification for inserting a needle into every suspected dominant breast lump. Aspiration is also the first step in management (Chapter 9).

Galactocele

This presents in the same way as a cyst, some time after parturition. It is managed in the same way as other cysts, and is discussed more fully in Chapter 9.

Sclerosing Adenosis

This presents most commonly as a radiological abnormality, a chance histological finding or as a cause of mastalgia. When it presents as a lump, it is dealt with as any dominant mass, and requires no specific treatment. It is dealt with in Chapter 10. The remaining lesions listed in Table 5.1 present in more specific fashion than the manifestations of ANDI and are dealt with in the appropriate sections of the book.

Follow-up after Assessment and/or Benign Breast Biopsy

This subject has been dealt with in Chapter 4 in relation to cancer risk. It is particularly important in busy breast clinics because routine follow-up of patients presenting with breast lumps can quickly swamp clinic facilities and interfere with the efficient care of new referrals. The following principles guide our own practice:

1. Young girls under the age of 25 should be discouraged from re-attendance.
2. A definite decision regarding biopsy should be made in older women by 2 months, and the lump biopsied or the patient discharged unless there are strong indications of increased cancer risk.
3. Patients aged 25–50 with significant cancer risk indicators as set out in Chapter 4 have annual checks and at least biennial mammography, although there is at present no clear evidence that this is beneficial.
4. Patients over the age of 50 should be entered into regular population breast screening programmes.

A number of studies are under way investigating various forms of maintenance therapy, e.g. danazol, evening primrose oil etc., as a means of preventing recurrent cysts and nodularity. None of these studies can yet be regarded as providing clear evidence of benefit, but further results are likely to be published in the next few years.

Management of Recurrent Lumps following Biopsy

Many breast lumps, such as fibroadenoma, cysts and nodularity, are prone to be multiple over a period of time. However, a new lump may be cancer so any new lump must be reassessed in the same way as the original lump.

A different situation arises when a lump appears in the region of a previous biopsy. It must also be reassessed completely but a number of additional factors need consideration.

Recurrent fibroadenoma may represent inadequate removal of the stalk or involvement of adjacent lobules. Excision biopsy of the recurrent lump rather than enucleation is indicated.

Recurrent cyst is common and requires no treatment other than re-aspiration provided the rules governing aspiration are adhered to (Chapter 9).

The breast parenchyma may fail to heal following a biopsy, leaving a palpable dip with prominent edge in the breast tissue. The prominent edge is frequently mistaken for a new mass.

A recurrent lump following biopsy of nodularity of ANDI may be due to:

1. The edge of the biopsy wound.
2. Scarring.

3. To pathology that was missed at the original biopsy.
4. To progression of the original lesion.
5. To a new lesion.

Such a lump must be carefully reassessed with a view to avoiding biopsy if (1) or (2) can be confirmed; (3) should always be considered if the interval is short and the operator relatively inexperienced; (4) is particularly important where the initial biopsy showed high grade epithelial dysplasia or carcinoma *in situ*, because progression is common in these conditions.

Breast Masses in Adolescence

A number of papers have reported studies of breast tumours in adolescence (Table 5.2). Stone *et al*[6] reported 143 masses between the ages of 10 and 20. The incidence increased steadily throughout the decade with a marked predominance from 16 to 20 years: 70% were fibroadenomas, 6% cysts and 12% 'hyperplasias' – presumably nodularity of ANDI. Other diagnoses were seen in only one or two cases.

Table 5.2 Summary of breast masses found during adolescence (10–20 years).

Male	Gynaecomastia[a]
Female	Premenarchal development of breast bud[a]
	Fibroadenoma[a]
	Cyst[c]
	Intraduct papilloma[b]
	Subareolar abscess[b] (periductal mastitis)
	Giant fibroadenoma[c]
	Adenocarcinoma[c]
	Nipple and areolar
	Retention cysts[b]
	Inversion[b]
	Molluscum contagiosum[c]
	Leiomyoma[c]

[a] Common; [b] uncommon; [c] rare.

A second study[7] of 40 cases gives a similar distribution although this paper includes virginal hypertrophy. These papers do not mention premenopausal asymmetrical development of the nipple bud. This is much the commonest swelling of the early part of adolescence. Recognition is vital, because ill-advised biopsy will lead to amastia. A further paper on the subject is that by Sandison and Walker[8]. Among 151 specimens were 114 fibroadenomas, 3 duct papillomas, 4 cysts and 4 cases of duct ectasia. This is a particularly helpful paper.

Much concern is often expressed that fibroadenoma in this age group must be removed because of the possibility of cancer. Although the few cases of cancer in this age group (it is exceedingly rare and none were seen in Sandison and Walker's series) have usually been misdiagnosed as fibroadenoma, review of case reports and our own experience shows that this diagnosis has been made because of the age group, not because of typical physical signs of fibroadenoma. Thus, masses with rapid growth, recent nipple retraction, surrounding tissue and lymph node involvement have been diagnosed as fibroadenoma. The risk of cancer can, for practical purposes, be ignored in an adolescent with a lump showing the *typical* features of the common fibroadenoma.

Lumps in the male breast in adolescence are less common – one series[6] reported 22 cases over a 15-year period. All were due to gynaecomastia. Unlike girls, there is a marked peak incidence at the age of 13/14. Gynaecomastia is much more common than this series would suggest but, like this series,

we have seen no other cause for breast mass in an adolescent male (*see* Chapter 16).

Breast Lumps in Older Women

The incidence and nature of benign breast lumps in older women (more than 55 years) differs from those of the reproductive period. In a comprehensive study, Devitt[9] reviewed 581 women in this age group presenting with benign breast disorders. The commonest presentation was with non-specific nodularity, 25% associated with pain. Eight per cent had simple cysts, most under the age of 60 and there was a significant relationship to postmenopausal hormone therapy. Eight patients had fibroadenomas, four calcified. Thus a similar range of benign breast lumps is seen in the older women, but characterized by a much lower incidence and a much lower frequency compared to cancer than that seen during reproductive life.

REFERENCES

1. Cox P. J., Li M. K. W. & Ellis H. Spectrum of breast disease in outpatient surgical practise. *Journal of the Royal Society of Medicine* 1982; **75**: 857–859.
2. Preece P. E., Baum M., Mansel R. E., Webster D. J. T., Fortt R. W., Gravelle I. H. & Hughes L. E. Importance of mastalgia in operable breast cancer. *British Medical Journal* 1982; **284**: 1299–1300.
3. Haagenson C. D. *Diseases of the Breast.* Philadelphia, 1986, W. B. Saunders, p 252.
4. Fornage B. D., Faroux M. J. & Simatos M. D. Breast masses – US guided fine-needle aspiration biopsy. *Radiology* 1987; **162**: 409–414.
5. Foote F. W. & Stewart F. W. Comparative studies of cancerous versus non-cancerous breasts. *Annals of Surgery* 1945; **121**: 6–53.
6. Stone A. M., Shenker R. I. & McCarthy K. Adolescent breast masses. *American Journal of Surgery* 1977; **134**: 275–277.
7. Bauer B. S., Jones K. M. & Talbot C. W. Mammary masses in the adolescent female. *Surgery, Gynecology and Obstetrics* 1987; **165**: 63–65.
8. Sandison A. T. & Walker J. C. Diseases of the adolescent female breast. A clinico-pathological study. *British Journal of Surgery* 1968; **55**: 443–448.
9. Devitt J. E. Benign disorders of the breast in older women. *Surgery, Gynecology and Obstetrics* 1986; **162**: 340–342.

6 Breast Imaging Methods

There are several techniques available for imaging the breast. These fall into two broad categories: the well-tried and dependable methods and those under current investigation or of doubtful use.

Techniques of Proven Value

Mammography

The most commonly used and most thoroughly investigated breast imaging modality is mammography – radiography of the breast. This radiographic technique has been in use for over 30 years and its value and accuracy in diagnosis has been demonstrated over the years. The main impact of this method, of course, has been on the diagnosis and management of breast cancer but it also has its place in the investigation, evaluation and management of benign breast disorders and benign disease of the breast.

Xeromammography

The basic mammographic technique may be a xeroradiographic method utilizing electrostatic imaging with dry, powder processing. The inherent advantages of the xeroradiographic method are the ability to penetrate dense breast tissue and so show lesions that might otherwise be obscured, and the highlighting of microcalcifications and the margins of breast lesions and structures due to the 'edge-enhancement effect' of the process.

Film-Screen Mammography

This method uses conventional, liquid chemical processing and, when used without grid facilities, has the advantage of a greatly reduced radiation dosage to the breast. However, it suffers from the great disadvantage of poor imaging of dense breasts. There is a failure of penetration of dense breast structures so that quite large lesions and microcalcifications also can be completely obscured. The more recent introduction of grid techniques with film-screen mammography has improved film imaging of dense breast tissue. The radiation dose to the breasts engendered by grid–film–screen mammography is similar to xeromammography.

Contrast Studies

Additional radiological investigative methods may be used. These are ductography, a positive contrast method of demonstrating ductal abnormalities, and pneumocystography, a negative contrast examination of breast cysts.

Ductography

This is useful in cases of nipple discharge of any type arising from one duct or, if from many ducts, then in the duct showing blood staining or different colouration. The causes of discharge include cysts, duct ectasia, granuloma, abscess, epithelial hyperplasia, papilloma, carcinoma and galactorrhoea due to prolactinoma.

The discharge should be examined cytologically and tested for blood. The nipple is cleaned with spirit and the selected duct cannulated. Diluted, bubble-free, radiographic water-soluble contrast medium is injected slowly until a feeling of fullness in the breast is experienced by the patient. The cannula is withdrawn and the nipple sealed with Micropore. Two mammographic views at right angles to one another are then taken.

The various types of discharge are not necessarily indicative of the underlying cause. It is important to realize that carcinoma or papilloma may be present with serous or watery discharge and not only with obvious blood-stained discharge. Connections with small cysts may be demonstrated (see Figure 12.2) and enlargement of ducts (Figure 6.1) and intraductal filling defects (Figure 6.2). A filling defect may be due to papilloma, carcinoma, granuloma or inspissated secretion. It may not be possible to differentiate these conditions but ductography demonstrates the location, nature and extent of the abnormality and helps towards a rational operative approach.

Contraindictions are the presence of mammary infection or infection of the nipple. A rare complication is the development of a localized or generalized mastitis as a result of sensitivity to the contrast medium. There are considerable variations in the extent to which ductography is used in different units. This is discussed further in Chapter 12.

Pneumocystography

This is used diagnostically when a blood-stained aspirate is obtained from a cyst. The cyst is punctured under sterile conditions and aspirated to dryness. An equal volume of air is then injected slowly and mammographic examination performed. The aspirated fluid should be cultured and examined cytologically. An intracystic mass is shown in cases of intracystic papilloma (*see* Figure 9.9) or carcinoma (Figure 6.3). It may not be possible to differentiate one from the other radiologically, although an extracystic extension and distortion of the cyst are suggestive of carcinoma. The situation and extent of the intracystic mass is shown preoperatively. It may be used therapeutically in recurring breast cysts. Approximately 60% of simple cysts do not refill after pneumocystography possibly due to an irritant effect on the cyst lining which causes adhesion following absorption of the air. In addition, the inner lining of the cyst in these cases is well demonstrated following air insufflation.

Contraindications include the presence of infection within the breast, the cyst or on the skin, and also blood dyscrasias. Breast abscess is a possible complication, but is usually due to activation of a covert abscess by leakage of infected contents into the breast stroma. Haematoma may occur in blood dyscrasias.

Ultrasound Examination

During the last 5 years or so, new ultrasound apparatus has become available enabling relatively sophisticated images of breast lesions to be obtained. It is often stated that ultrasound is the 'best' way of demonstrating a breast cyst. The method, of course, is unnecessary when the lesion is palpable as aspiration will confirm the clinical impression and also treat the patient. It is rarely necessary to know whether small impalpable cysts are present. This knowledge leads to the temptation of unnecessary aspiration under ultra-

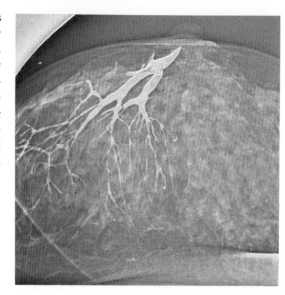

6.1 *Duct ectasia demonstrated on duct injection.*

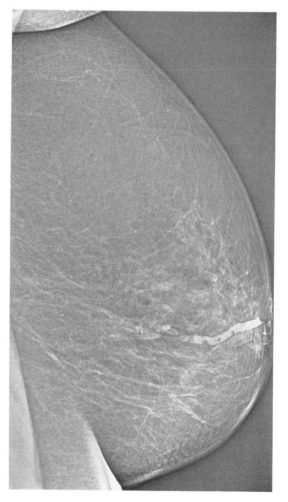

6.2 *Papilloma shown by duct injection. Same patient as in Figure 12.3.*

sonic guidance – a procedure carried out in some screening clinics. The modality can be used to demonstrate intracystic lesions and, in this

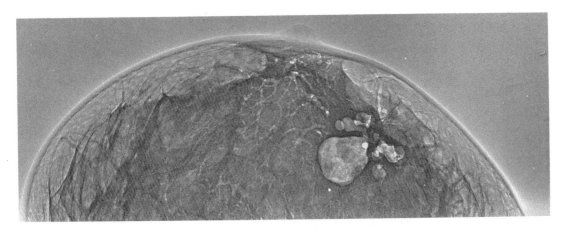

6.3 *Pneumocystography showing intracystic carcinoma.*

respect, is best used when a blood-stained aspirate has been obtained clinically. Duct ectasia may be demonstrated. Differentiation between solid and cystic lesions is possible, but this is not invariably accurate. It is possible in 'over 95% of cases'[1] (Figure 6.4).

The use of ultrasound has been advocated in the mammographically dense breast, because lesions may be obscured radiographically in such breasts[2]. This is true when an inadequate mammographic technique is employed, but is not often necessary when xerography or grid mammography are employed because penetration of dense breasts and differentiation between tissues and lesions is achieved with these techniques.

There are disadvantages to the ultrasonic method: fine microcalcifications may not be shown so that important evidence of breast disease is not available and, in addition, biopsy guidance to lesions identified by microcalcifications only is not possible. Coarse calcifications can be shown and, with large calcified lesions, a significant lesion could be obscured by the distal attenuation obtained in such cases. Spurious ultrasonic appearances of malignancy may be obtained with 'localized fibrocystic disease'[2]. Dense, generalized ANDI ('fibrocystic disease') could obscure a malignancy, i.e. in the very cases advocated as being suitable for ultrasonic examination. In addition, malignant lesions may give the ultrasonic features of benign disease. For complete examination, many images of each breast are required, the number depending on the size of the breast. Alternatively, video recordings may be

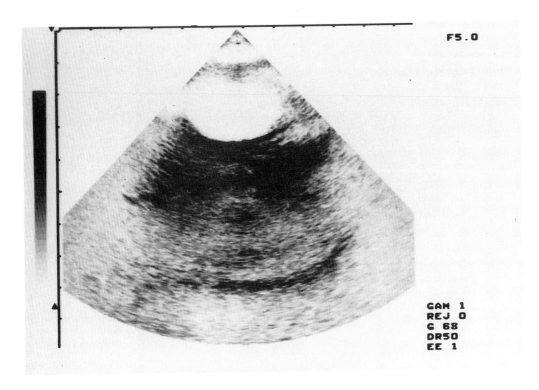

6.4 *A simple breast cyst demonstrated by ultrasonography.*

taken. In both cases, viewing is more tedious than with mammography.

Localization Techniques of Impalpable Lesions

The radiological features of some benign conditions, especially sclerosing adenosis, and subclinical malignancy can be identical. Thus, biopsy is necessary to exclude malignancy in these impalpable lesions; approximately 50% will prove to be benign. These suspicious mammographic appearances include distortion of breast architecture, lesions with irregular or ill-defined margins and the presence of a group of fine microcalcifications. The descriptive pinpointing of the abnormality of the lesion to a particular quadrant is inadequate because the patient is not in the same position for mammography as for surgery. Consequently, a localization method for these small lesions is necessary to ensure accurate surgical biopsy. Our method has been described and discussed by Preece et al[3]. Briefly, it involves the injection of 0.5 ml of a mixture of water-soluble, radiographic contrast medium and Patent Blue Violet dye directly into the breast by the radiologist to the site of the mammographic abnormality employing measurements from the nipple and overlying skin. The breast is then radiographed in two projections at right angles to one another. The contrast medium is demonstrated radiographically and its distance from the radiographic abnormality is measurable. Illustrations of this technique are given in Chapter 18 (Figures 18.11–18.14). The mammographic images and measurements accompany the patient to theatre and the biopsy is carried out. It is then mandatory to radiograph the specimen to confirm that the lesion has been excised. Histological examination of paraffin sections is recommended in this particular situation rather than frozen section examination.

Another technique employed is the use of a curved-end retractable wire, the curved end being released once the needle has been inserted into the appropriate position as checked by mammography. This is a popular technique, well described by Homer[4]. The released, curved end of the wire forms a 'hook' in or close to the impalpable lesion, its position having been checked radiographically before release. An external stabilizing device is then fixed to the wire to prevent inadvertent envelopment of the wire in the breast (Figure 6.5). The surgeon cuts down along the wire, palpates the hook and excises the hook and lesion. The specimen plus hook is then radiographed to ensure that the suspicious lesion has been excised (Figure 6.6). Because of the

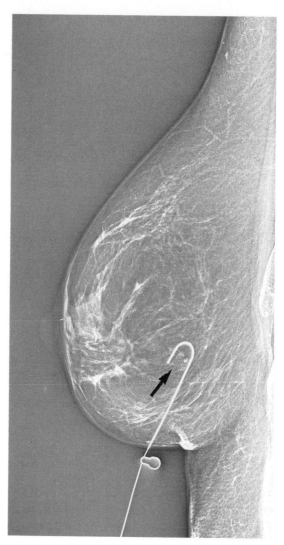

6.5 *A hooked needle fixed in situ. The lesion is arrowed.*

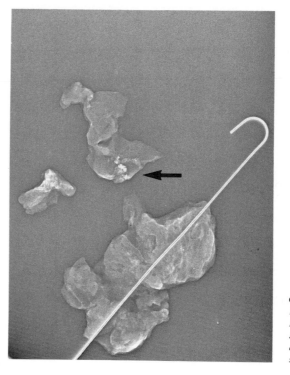

6.6 *Specimen radiography including the hooked needle. The lesion is arrowed – it has been dissected free to be sent separately for histology.*

relative flexibility of the wire, locating the tip within the breast at surgery is not always as easy as might be supposed – hence the continuing popularity of double dye biopsy in some centres.

When the impalpable, suspicious lesion is a small mass, ultrasound guidance may be used for fine needle aspiration cytology or to direct a hook needle or the needle for dye localization to the correct location. If only mammographic calcification is present, a radiographic technique will be necessary. Recently, a stereoscopic radiographic technique has become available enabling fine needle aspiration cytology or localization by hook needle or dye injection to be carried out very accurately.

The actual method used for localization biopsy is of little consequence as long as good localization is employed, the biopsy specimen is proved to contain the abnormality by specimen radiography and histological examination of paraffin, rather than frozen, sections is undertaken. However, with fine needle aspiration cytology a problem arises when benign cytology is obtained. One must ask whether needle aspiration of a small impalpable, mammographically detected lesion is sufficiently accurate to exclude malignancy. This depends greatly on the expertise of the clinician and cytologist and many would advocate excision biopsy in such a situation, because it is generally held that a negative cytology result should be regarded as a 'no result'.

Techniques of Uncertain Value

Other imaging modalities have been or are still being investigated. They are of uncertain value, especially the more recent introduced sophisticated methods of computerized tomography and magnetic resonance imaging which, at present, are of limited value but may, with technical development, become useful eventually. They are of course of great value in the management of distant metastases from breast carcinoma, but at present of little use in the evaluation of local breast disease, especially benign breast disorders.

Thermography

Thermography has been largely discarded as a non-specific technique with high false-positive and high false-negative rates in the diagnosis of breast cancer[5]. In a series of 110 women with histologically proven benign breast disease, 22% had abnormal thermograms, 15% equivocal thermograms and 63% normal thermograms.

Even in inflammatory conditions 8% had normal thermograms[6]. Moskowitz et al[7] maintain that it is not useful in identifying women with proliferative disorders. Thermography has little demonstrable value in the management of benign disease.

Diaphanography

Diaphanography or 'light-scanning', the modern application of transillumination, demonstrates cysts very well but is a slow method of examination and very operator dependent. Fibroadenoma may mimic carcinoma and microcalcifications are not shown. There is also difficulty in demonstrating lesions situated more than 2 cm beneath the skin surface[8].

Computerized Tomography and Magnetic Resonance Imaging

Both techniques show the same morphological features as mammography but can distinguish between fluid-containing lesions and solid lesions. However, they are far more expensive and time consuming and neither shows fine microcalcification – an important radiological feature of malignancy and also some benign breast diseases. At present, these methods are not indicated in the local investigation of breast disease.

Doppler Ultrasound Scanning

By using Doppler scanning, quantitative assessment of blood flow can be assessed transcutaneously. When used in combination with ultrasound sector scanning, the technique is known as 'duplex scanning'. The sector scan is used to define breast lesions and to differentiate cystic from solid lesions. Doppler flow studies may then give additional useful information in distinguishing between solid benign lesions and malignant lesions.

Most published work has concentrated on the detection of malignant lesions, but Boyd et al[9] report positive results with duplex scanning of benign lesions although the numbers are small.

Mammography in Benign Breast Disorders

Benign breast lesions in the majority of cases present fairly characteristic mammographic appearances. They are usually smooth in outline and rounded, ovoid or lobulated in shape. These lesions may occur singly but more often there are multiple lesions present (Figure 6.7) and usually bilaterally. There may be a surrounding 'halo' of compressed fat indicating that there is no infiltration. Breast structures such as ducts and trabeculae are displaced rather than disrupted. Duct ectasia may present as enlarged, dense or transradiant ducts converging on the nipple (*see* Figure 11.18). Difficulties in interpretation arise with irregular or ill-defined lesions such as abscess, plasma cell mastitis (*see* Figure 11.20) and fat necrosis. Lesions giving rise to distortion, e.g. sclerosing adenosis or previous biopsy scars (Figure 6.8), cause difficulties also.

Calcifications in benign disease are usually coarse and smooth and occur in characteristic forms in duct ectasia (*see* Figure 11.19) and fibroadenoma (Figure 6.9) but phyllodes tumour may simulate the latter. Fine microcalcifications occur in epithelial hyperplasia, sclerosing adenosis and papillomatosis and then may cause diagnostic difficulties.

Indications for Mammography in Benign Disorders

1. Confirmation of the clinical diagnosis: the diagnosis of benign disorder on mammography is usually possible. The accuracy of diagnosis was 97% in our unit[5]. The distinction between cyst and fibroadenoma is rarely possible unless characteristic calcification is present.

2. As an aid in clinically difficult or doubtful cases, e.g. in the common situation of nodular breasts, where multiple palpable lesions are present, and radiological evidence of malignancy might differentiate one lesion from the others.

3. Exclusion of malignancy in patients in the cancer age group in such situations as non-cyclical mastalgia or vague breast symptoms where no lesion is palpable. Fear of cancer is a major cause of morbidity in these cases, and

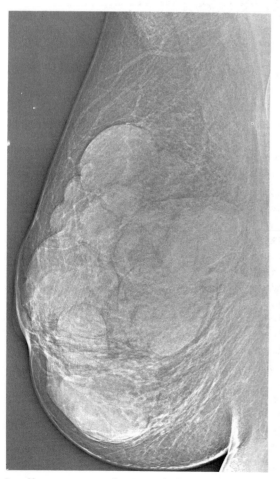

6.7 *Xeromammogram showing multiple rounded lesions – cysts.*

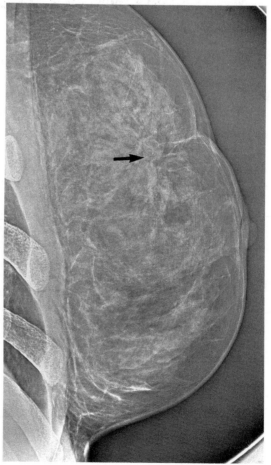

6.8 *Xeromammogram showing distortion due to a biopsy scar.*

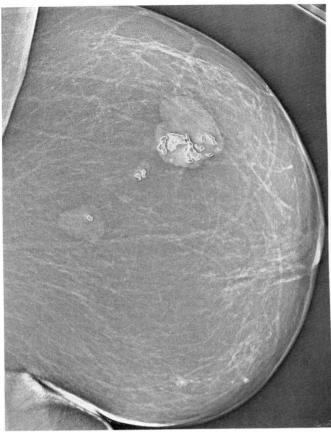

6.9 *Calcification in a fibroadenoma.*

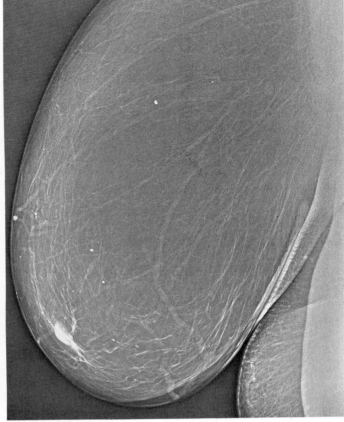

6.10 *N1 Wolfe pattern.*

negative mammograms will be very helpful in management.

4. In the clinical management of non-operative cases: the added reassurance of the presence of benign disease is valuable. Repeat mammographic examination in 6 weeks time for doubtful inflammatory conditions and in 6 months time for microcalcifications of doubtful significance can also be useful in these cases.

5. In the postbiopsy breast where the effects of scarring may make interpretation of palpatory findings difficult. It is advisable to carry out mammography 2–3 months following biopsy so that any distortion caused by the biopsy will be apparent. This mammogram will then be a base-line examination so that any later changes will be more easily detected.

Wolfe Parenchymal Patterns

Wolfe[10, 11] described four basic breast parenchymal patterns on mammography:

1. N1 – a parenchyma which is completely or mainly fatty (Figure 6.10).

2. P1 – the presence of prominent ducts occupying 25% or less of the breast (Figure 6.11).

3. P2 – prominent ducts occupying over 25% of the breast (Figure 6.12).

4. DY – the presence of a dense parenchyma, a 'dysplasia' (Figure 6.13).

Wolfe maintains that the risk of developing breast cancer can be predicted using these four basic radiographic patterns in women over 30 years of age. The N1 group has the lowest risk, P1 a low risk, P2 a high risk and DY the highest risk of developing breast cancer. In two studies, Wolfe found that the risk of developing cancer in the DY group was 21–37 times as great as in the N1 group. There are two groups at significant risk: the P2 and DY; and two groups at relatively low risk: N1 and P1.

Gravelle *et al*[12] have shown an association between these radiographic patterns and epidemiological risk factors. In particular, women with increased risk due to nulliparity or late age of first child showed a significant increase in the proportion of P2 and DY patterns. It was also shown that variables such as age and weight were related to the proportion of high-risk mammograms[13]. A further prospective study by Gravelle *et al* of parenchymal patterns showed that women

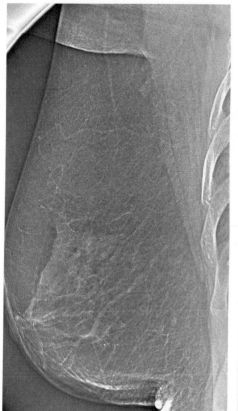 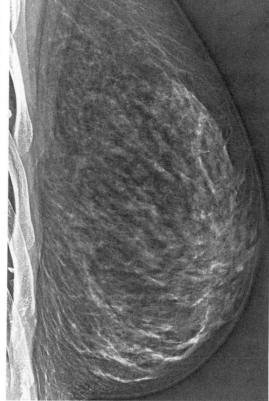 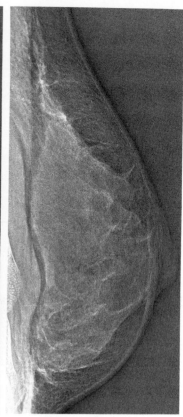

6.11   *P1 Wolfe pattern.*   6.12   *P2 Wolfe pattern.*   6.13   *DY Wolfe pattern.*

with DY and P2 patterns had nearly four times the risk of developing cancer compared with women having N1 or P1 patterns[14]. The combination of the 'high risk' patterns with age, weight, parity and age at birth of first child may identify groups at particularly high risk.

This has been discussed further in Chapter 4.

REFERENCES

1.   Dempsey P. J. & Wilson P. C. The use of automated sonography in total clinical breast evaluation. In: Leopold G. R. (ed.) *Clinics in Diagnostic Ultrasound*, Vol 12, Chap 4. London, Churchill Livingstone, 1984
2.   Guyer P. B. & Dewbury K. C. Ultrasound of the breast in the symptomatic and X-ray dense breast. *Clinical Radiology* 1985; 36: 69–76.
3.   Preece P. E., Gravelle I. H., Hughes L. E., Baum M., Fortt R. W. & Leopold J. G. The operative management of sub-clinical breast cancer. *Clinical Oncology* 1977; 3: 165–169.
4.   Homer M. J. Localisation of non-palpable breast lesions: Technical aspects and analysis of 80 cases. *American Journal of Roentgenology* 1983; 140: 807–811.
5.   Evans K. T. & Gravelle I. H. *Mammography, Thermography and Ultrasonography in Breast Disease*. London, Butterworths, 1973.
6.   Jones C. H., Greening W. P., Davey J. B., McKinna J. A. & Greeves W. J. Thermography of the female breast: a five year study in relation to the detection and prognosis of cancer. *British Journal of Radiology* 1975; 48: 532–538.
7.   Moskowitz M., Fox S. H., Brun del Re R. R., Milbrath J. R., Bassett L. W., Gold R. H. & Shaffer K. A. The potential value of liquid-crystal thermography in detecting significant mastopathy. *Radiology* 1981; 140: 659–662.
8.   Bartrum R. J. & Crow H. C. Transillumination light scanning to diagnose breast cancer. *American Journal of Roentgenology* 1984; 142: 409–414.

9. Boyd J., Jellins J., Reeve T. S. & Kossoff G. In: Jellins J. & Kobayashi T. (eds.) *Doppler Examination of the Breast.* Chichester, John Wiley & Sons Ltd, 1983.

10. Wolfe J. N. Risk for breast cancer development determined by mammographic parenchymal pattern. *Cancer* 1976; **37**: 2486–2492.

11. Wolfe J. N. Breast patterns as an index of risk of developing breast cancer. *American Journal of Roentgenology,* 1976; **126**: 1130–1139.

12. Gravelle I. H., Bulstrode J. C., Wang D. Y., Bulbrook R. D. & Hayward J. L. The relation between radiographic features and determinants of risk of breast cancer. *British Journal of Radiology* 1980; **53**: 107–113.

13. Gravelle I. H., Bulstrode J. C., Bulbrook R. D., Hayward J. L. & Wang D. Y. The relation between radiological patterns of the breast and body weight and height. *British Journal of Radiology* 1982; **55**: 23–25.

14. Gravelle I. H., Bulstrode J. C., Bulbrook R. D., Wang D. Y., Allen D. & Hayward J. L. A prospective study of mammographic parenchymal pattern and risk of breast cancer. *British Journal of Radiology* 1986; **59**: 487–491.

7 Fibroadenoma and Related Tumours

Terminology

A World Health Organisation party has simply defined a fibroadenoma as 'a discrete benign tumour showing evidence of connective tissue and epithelial proliferation'[1]. It has long been recorded and recognized as an entity and as a benign tumour – Sir Astley Cooper used the term 'chronic mammary tumour'. In its classic form it is one of the commonest, best recognized and most easily managed conditions, yet paradoxically fibroadenomas which are not entirely typical have given rise to more confusion than most breast conditions. This is due to the use of a plethora of terms to describe the more exuberant forms of tumour (in either a histological or clinical sense). Indeed, it is the confusion caused by clinical variants (those of large size or rapid growth) or histological variants (hypercellularity or atypia) which has been the root of the problem. More recently, there is a better understanding of the wide spectrum of histological appearance and disease behaviour with mixed epithelial and connective tissue proliferation, but the benefits of this better understanding can only be gained by insisting on precise terminology.

The fibrous stromal element of these tumours is the key to classification and behaviour, with any epithelial variant being treated as a secondary problem. Thus the term 'fibroadenoma' is used for all such tumours in which the fibrous stroma is of low cellularity and regular cytology. It covers tumours of all sizes, because their behaviour is basically similar, i.e. uniformly benign, whatever the size. The group of tumours where the stroma shows markedly increased cellularity and atypia is termed 'phyllodes tumour' (cystosarcoma phyllodes in older terminology). It is stressed that this diagnosis is made on histological grounds, not size. So while most phyllodes tumours are large, the term should also be applied to small tumours if they show the appropriate histological features. Most phyllodes tumours also behave in a benign fashion, although showing a tendency to local recurrence. But there is a spectrum of clinical behaviour, and an occasional case will be frankly malignant and may metastasize.

In summary, fibroadenoma is common, usually small but sometimes large, always benign. Phyllodes tumour is uncommon, usually large but sometimes small, usually benign but occasionally malignant. The two lesions cannot be distinguished clinically and not always on macroscopic section. Both occur throughout reproductive life, fibroadenoma predominantly in the first half, phyllodes tumour more commonly in the second.

Age is an added and important factor, for tumours of adolescence usually behave in benign fashion irrespective of histology. Tumours of the perimenopausal period occasionally recur and then behave in more serious fashion, even if histologically they look benign at the first presentation.

Fibroadenoma

This tumour appears usually in young women as a rubbery-firm, smooth, very mobile mass. These features – and in particular its striking mobility – are so characteristic that a confident diagnosis can be made in most cases in young women.

Age and Natural History

Clinically, the lesion is predominantly a tumour of young women. This would be expected from its lobular origin, for the time of greatest lobular development is the first years after the menarche. Yet studies have always shown the median age of diagnosis as about 30 years. This seems older than clinical experience suggests but is confirmed in our Cardiff series (Figure 7.1). The older patients are diagnosed in the pathology department, not in the clinic, and this can be explained on differing physical characteristics of fibroadenomas in different age groups. Lesions with classic physical signs (discrete, smooth, mobile) appear in the 16–25 year age group, being noticed accidently while bathing or dressing. In the later age group the classic clinical symptoms may be obscured by coexisting involutional changes and the histological diagnosis may come as a surprise following excision of a clinical dominant mass, which lacks the notable discreteness and mobility of fibroadenoma in the younger girl. Many fibroadenomas will not be felt in the young firm breast and, if left alone, will remain static or gradually increase in size until 1–3 cm in diameter, taking 1–5 years to do so. During the growth phase, the tumour doubles in size in 6–12 months[2] and is then likely to remain static for the rest of the patient's life or gradually decrease in size. They may become clinically apparent in the third or fourth decade as the tumour enlarges or the breast becomes softer or more pendulous after childbirth.

The paper by Kern and Clark[3] is frequently quoted as providing evidence that fibroadenomas may be observed to regress while under clinical observation. In fact, the paper is a histological study of mastectomy specimens and any relation to clinical regression is very circumstantial. Significant regression while under clinical observation must be very uncommon if it occurs at all, although it is accepted that fibroadenomas probably involute by the time of the menopause. Studies using ultrasound to monitor clinical impressions would be very interesting.

A few fibroadenomas first become obvious as discrete masses in the late years of reproductive life. These may show a remarkable propensity for growth, rapidly reaching a large size. They have the gross and histological features of a simple fibroadenoma and behave in a benign fashion (but see p. 69). It is interesting that similar rapid growth of a fibroadenoma is also seen in the 13 to 18-year age group, so that 'giant' fibroadenomas tend to have a bimodal distribution at the extremes of reproductive life (Figure 7.2). Four of the five fibroadenomas in the 11 to 15-year age group in this series were more than 4 cm in diameter, as were about 15% of those between 16 and 25 years. Large tumours are fewer in the next decade but reappear in smaller numbers around the menopause. Giant fibroadenomas in both adolescent and menopausal age groups are uncommon, but the giant tumours of adolescence

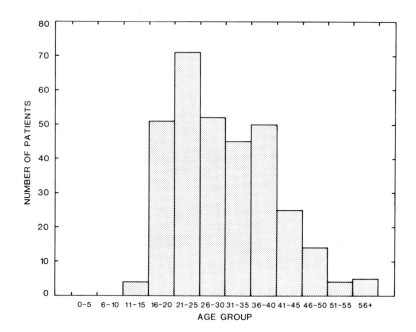

are more common than at the menopause. The infrequency of fibroadenoma after the menopause suggests that they involute with perimenopausal breast involution. During this process they may calcify. Devitt[4] reported a series of 4379 women over 55 years who presented with a breast complaint. Only eight had fibroadenomas, and four of these were calcified.

Very small superficial nodules of fibroadenomatous tissue, 3–4 mm in diameter are also noted clinically, and often remain unchanged for many years, suggesting that similar small static lesions deep in the breast are likely to be present much more frequently than clinically recognized. This has been borne out by histological study of whole breast sections. Cheatle[5] found small fibroadenomas in 25% of normal breasts.

Thus simple fibroadenomas fall into four main groups:

1. The small, static fibroadenoma of 3–4 mm palpable in the superficial breast.
2. The commonest type reaching a diameter of 1–3 cm before becoming static makes up 80%

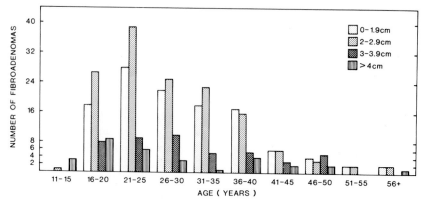

of all fibroadenomas and hence must be regarded as the 'norm'.
3. The very few giant fibroadenomas of adolescence and the perimenopausal age groups are discussed later.
4. This leaves about 10% in the 4–5 cm group which are distributed fairly evenly over the age range, but form a higher proportion in the perimenarchal and perimenopausal age groups.

Do these larger tumours constitute a different group in terms of histology or behaviour? Foster *et al*[6] have looked at this question by comparing the cellularity of fibroadenomas of different size groupings. Stromal cells were counted by grey level analysis from a computer-linked TV image. They found no relationship between stromal cellularity and size of fibroadenomas, but cellularity was related to the age of the patient. The mean cell count in patients younger than 20 years was almost double that of older patients, although there was a second lesser increase in stromal cellularity just before the menopause which might be explained by the stimulation of unopposed oestrogen at this time. Thus larger tumours did not appear to be related to cellularity and there is no obvious reason at present why some fibroadenomas should grow to a larger size than average. There is also no reason to treat these larger fibroadenomas differently, nor in our series did they have a particular tendency to recur or to be multiple.

Incidence

In most clinical series the frequency of fibroadenoma is about half that of cancer. In one series of 2005 consecutive outpatient consultations analysed in our unit, 360 patients had discrete lumps requiring excision; of these, 75 were fibroadenomas and 148 were cancers. The ratio in Haagensen's series[2] was 1.4, but this probably reflects the special nature of his cancer referral practice. However, only a minority of fibroadenomas are diagnosed clinically and small histological 'fibroadenomas' can be found in most breasts if looked for carefully enough (Chapter 3).

Fibroadenomas are more common in the left breast and predominate in the upper outer quadrants (Figure 7.3). This distribution reflects the amount of breast parenchyma in the different quadrants.

Pathology and Pathogenesis

We have already discussed in detail in Chapters 1 and 3 our reasons for regarding this condition

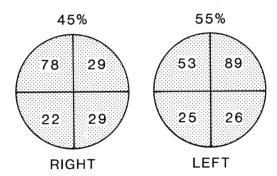

7.3 *Distribution of fibroadenomas in breast quadrants – Cardiff series.*

as part of ANDI – an aberration of normal lobular development rather than a tumour. There is good histological evidence that these tumours develop from the breast lobule – for instance, elastic tissue is present in ducts but not present in normal lobules, and elastic tissue is not seen in fibroadenomas[7]. The lobular origin explains many features of fibroadenoma, for instance, why most arise in young women at the time of maximal lobular development and why the stroma forms such a major element in fibroadenomas. This is derived from the hormone-dependent stroma of the lobule and not the simple fibrous stroma of the breast parenchyma. It also explains why most of the (very rare) cases of cancer arising in a fibroadenoma are of the more 'benign' type – lobular carcinoma *in situ*.

Steroid receptors have been studied in fibroadenoma[8]. Oestrogen and progesterone receptors can be demonstrated in relatively low concentrations in both cytoplasm and nucleus. These receptors are more easily demonstrated in fibroadenoma than other ANDI conditions.

The aetiology of fibroadenoma is not known, but the fact that lobular proliferation is a response to oestrogen stimulation suggests that it may arise as the result of a lobule becoming unusually responsive to oestrogen. It grows both by proliferation of the lobule and also involvement of adjacent lobules – a fact of relevance to the significant recurrence rate after removal.

The macroscopic appearance is of a sharply demarcated rounded or bosselated tumour with a white, glistening, bulging surface. The surface is irregular due to the epithelial lined clefts which break up the uniformity. If the surface is brownish, phyllodes tumour should be considered.

The histological appearance is very characteristic, a combination of loose pale stroma and duct-like structures lined by regular epithelial cells. There is a tendency for this to follow one of two broad patterns, to which Cheatle[5] gave the terms 'pericanalicular' and 'intracanalicular'. In the first the epithelial structures were abundant, wih the appearance of stroma surrounding circular ducts (Figure 7.4a). In the intracanalicular form (Figure 7.4b), the preponderance of stroma tends to push into elongated epithelial lined clefts, so that these now appear to surround islands of stroma. It is now recognized that both patterns are often seen in a single fibroadenoma, and there is no useful purpose in maintaining the differentiation.

The tissues of a fibroadenoma will respond to external influences in a manner similar to normal breast lobules. Thus they will undergo hyperplastic changes during pregnancy, secrete milk during lactation and involute at the menopause. The hyperplastic changes of pregnancy may outgrow the blood supply, leading to infarction.

It is important to recognize the wide variety of histological changes which may be seen in typical fibroadenomas compared to fewer variations in clinical behaviour. Such histological changes include apocrine and squamous metaplasia, neither of which is significant. Marked hyperplasia of epithelial elements is also common but does not reflect aggressive behaviour. However, such florid epithelial changes cause trouble to cytologists, and benign fibroadenoma is an important cause of false-positive diagnosis of cancer on cytology in all but the most experienced hands.

The widespread use of the contraceptive pill in young women makes it difficult to obtain accurate data on the role of the Pill in pathogenesis. There is no evidence that the use of the Pill increases the risk of developing fibroadenoma and the epidemiological data available suggest that it may be associated with a decreased incidence. This has been reviewed by Thomas[9]. Three of four studies show that the risk of developing fibroadenoma is more than halved among those taking the Pill, particularly long-term users. The epidemiological studies suggest that it is the progestogen element of the combined Pill which is protective.

In contrast, it has been suggested[10] that the incidence of multiple breast fibroadenomas is increasing and that this increase is associated with the use of the Pill. Multiplicity in Western populations is usually of the order of two to four lesions in one or both breasts. Our clinical experience regarding multiplicity and the Pill is similar to that quoted, although we have no data to support this impression. However, much higher numbers of fibroadenomas are sometimes reported in Negro and Oriental races. These tend to have a familial basis[2, 11] without an association with use of the Pill. We have seen as many as 40 fibroadenomas in a Chinese woman and much higher numbers have been reported.

An interesting negative association between current cigarette smoking (but not former smokers) and fibroadenoma has been reported[12].

Clinical Features

The clinical features are so characteristic in a young woman that the diagnosis can be made with a degree of confidence equalled only by that of a cyst after aspiration. The features are not so characteristic in older women, where the diagnosis should be made with care. One group[13] have reported a diagnostic accuracy of only 50%, but it is clear from their paper that they have not taken cognisance of the differing clinical signs of fibroadenoma in different age groups.

In the young woman, it is a smooth, round or lobulated, firm discrete swelling whose mobility has been quantified by the term 'breast mouse'. The degree of mobility is truly remarkable, and the diagnosis should be circumspect when a lesser degree of mobility can be demonstrated. One exception to this rule is a fibroadenoma arising behind the nipple, where the surrounding ducts will limit its mobility. (It is not always recognized that there is much lobular tissue behind the areola in many women, explaining the findings that cysts and fibroadenomas, both of lobular derivation, are sometimes found behind the nipple.) The extreme mobility of the tumour in young women is due to encapsulation (Figure 7.5) and to the softness and pliability of breast stroma in this age – in spite of the density of the young breast on mammogram. This also explains why fibroadenomas may appear on palpation to be much more superficial in the breast than their true position – a fact which has led many a surgeon to rue the decision to remove a fibroadenoma in a young girl under local anaesthetic.

The classic picture is not so obvious in older

7.4 *The histological patterns of pericanalicular (right) and intracanalicular (left) fibroadenomas.*

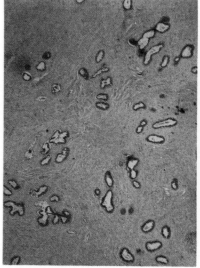
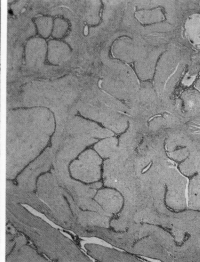

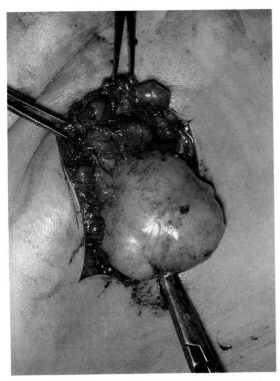

7.5 *The typical fibroadenoma of adolescent girls has a well-defined capsule, giving the tumour great mobility.*

the patients are not followed long term. Our own experience in Cardiff is similar. Seven percent of patients, had multiple tumours on presentation, and 7% had a further fibroadenoma either before or after the diagnosis for this survey[6]. One-third of the metachronous tumours occurred in the same quadrant as the first fibroadenoma, with an average time of 4 years to the second presentation. The mean age of patients with multiple tumours was 4 years less than those with single tumours. All these figures must be regarded as understatements, because complete follow-up of patients is very difficult in this age group and many tumours undoubtedly go unnoticed. It has been suggested that multiple fibroadenomas are more common in non-Caucasian populations, e.g. Chinese and Negroes. This has been our own experience in a small number of such cases and of our colleagues working in developing countries, but we can find no good data to substantiate this. However, reports of individual cases where one or both breasts are replaced by huge numbers of fibroadenomas have been made in Oriental or Negro races. The tumours vary greatly in size and growth potential.

Special Investigations

Mammography

Mammography is best avoided in younger women, both on grounds of poor diagnostic yield in the dense breast of this age, and radiation risk.

women where involutional fibrotic changes surrounding the tumour will decrease its mobility. In this age group, fibroadenoma often masquerades as a dominant mass of ANDI (fibroadenosis) and is removed as such, the fibroadenoma being revealed only after sectioning (Figure 7.6). The physical signs of cancer and fibroadenoma may then come much closer together and fibroadenoma should not be diagnosed clinically in this age group until cancer has been excluded unequivocally.

Fibroadenomas are sometimes discovered in the elderly, as a small, stony, hard, discrete mass, still moderately mobile. At this age the physical characteristics are again so precise that a clinical diagnosis can often be made with confidence. However it can readily be (and must be) confirmed by mammography that the stony-hard consistency is due to calcification (Chapter 6). It is a reasonable assumption that small fibroadenomas discovered in the late reproductive or postmenopausal periods arose many years earlier, remained static, and are then discovered only as a result of involutional changes allowing them to be palpated more readily.

Fibroadenomas are often multiple to the extent of three or even four developing concurrently or successively in both breasts. Haagensen[2] reported an incidence of multiple tumours of 16% among both Caucasions and Negroes in his series, and points out that this is a minimal figure because

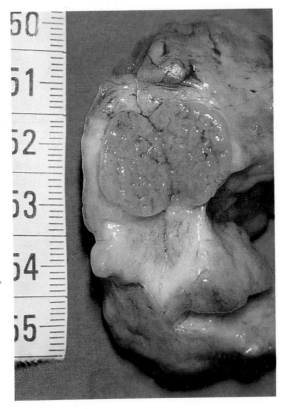

7.6 *A fibroadenoma in a 35-year-old patient. The typical clinical features were obscured by the involutional changes in the surrounding breast tissue.*

Certainly it is not necessary in the diagnosis of fibroadenoma under the age of 25.

In the older patient, a solitary smooth lesion is seen, of similar density to the surrounding breast tissue when small, and more dense when large. When small it may be difficult to detect, except as a smooth border outlined by the mammary fat. It may be surrounded by a halo of compressed fat, when the diagnosis is easier. The radiological appearance may be identical to that of a cyst, but needle aspiration will readily differentiate the two.

In the postmenopausal period, at least half of all fibroadenomas will show typical stippled calcification, similar to that seen in a uterine fibroid (see Chapter 6). Fibroadenolipoma of the breast is an uncommon hamartomatous lesion with distinctive radiological and pathological features[14]. It is described further in Chapter 17.

Ultrasonography

The ultrasonic features of fibroadenoma have been reviewed by Cole-Beuglet et al[15]. They include a round or oval sharp contour, weak internal echoes in a uniform distribution and intermediate attenuation.

MRI

Magnetic resonance imaging has been investigated[16] in 12 patients. It was concluded that the appearances were so variable that this technique is unlikely to be helpful in differentiating benign and malignant circumscribed tumours.

Cytology

A typical cytological appearance of fibroadenoma can be recognized by experienced cytologists, but, in less experienced hands, the hyperplastic epithelium typical of fibroadenoma may suggest a malign significance which is not justified by behaviour. Cytology is not indicated in a young girl with a typical fibroadenoma, but needle aspiration has a place where the features are not entirely typical, because cysts and galactoceles are occasionally seen in this age group. Cytology is of course indicated in older women.

Management

Most textbooks in the past have recommended removal of all fibroadenomas, irrespective of age or other considerations. Yet most fibroadenomas are self-limiting and many go undiagnosed. In practice, solitary fibroadenomas in young women are usually removed on diagnosis, to alleviate patient concern. However, it is not unreasonable to take a flexible attitude related to age group. In women under the age of 25, cancer is so rare that a typical fibroadenoma can be left with impunity. However, our own approach is to remove the tumour if the patient wishes to be rid of it, but to watch if for 6 months if she wishes to avoid operation. Occasionally such tumours are said to regress, but more commonly they remain static or increase in size under observation, in which case the patient will usually request removal. However, the high incidence of hypertrophic scars in young girls, particularly in the upper medial portion of the breast, should be explained to patients and will often result in agreement to conservative treatment of static lesions in this area.

We prefer this flexible approach in patients under the age of 25, and routine removal of all fibroadenomas over this age, to the alternative proposed by Wilkinson and Forrest[13]. They are undertaking a study where all fibroadenomas in patients under the age of 35 are observed, providing cytology is negative. This carries some risk of missing cancers, as they have found already in their preliminary study. More recently, Cant et al[17] have considered this question, and concluded with us that a conservative policy is safe in women under the age of 25 years, although they found that a majority would prefer excision. The operative detail of fibroadenoma excision is discussed in Chapter 18.

Hormonal Therapy

There has been a tendency on the European continent to treat fibroadenomas, along with other breast masses, by hormonal therapy, tamoxifen, danazol and progestogens among others (e.g. Cupceancu[18]). It is difficult to assess results because of the lack of histological diagnosis or long-term follow-up. We have not followed this practice because of the uncertain long-term effects of hormonal manipulation, especially with tamoxifen, in young women.

Recurrence after Surgery

New fibroadenomas which appear after removal of a previous tumour are often referred to as recurrent tumours, but this is a loose term and covers at least three groups.

1. Recurrence at the site of previous removal may represent incomplete removal, or adjacent lobules undergoing the same process. Some surgeons believe that removing the base of the 'stalk' lessens the risk of recurrence and this seems a reasonable step to take.

2. Newly noted tumours in the same or opposite breast represent the multiplicity of fibroadenomas often seen on careful histological examination of 'normal' breasts. Clinical experience suggests that multiple fibroadenomas may be occurring more frequently in recent years, although there are few firm data to support this.

3. It is not unknown for the original tumour to be missed and an adjacent area of nodularity excised, particularly if the operation is not carried out by the surgeon who examined the patient before operation. It is important that the surgeon familiarize himself with the site and characteristics of the lesion before the patient goes to theatre.

In the Cardiff series of 322 patients, 23 patients are known to have developed a further tumour during follow-up, with an interval of 1–6 years (mean 2.6 years), 16 in the same breast and 7 in the opposite. Of the 16 'recurrent' tumours in the same breast, 9 were at the same site and 7 elsewhere. Recurrence at the same site was not related to the size of the fibroadenoma, nor to use of the contraceptive pill. Two of these patients have developed a carcinoma during the follow-up period, neither at the site of the fibroadenoma. During the same period, 7 cases of phyllodes tumour were also treated – none of which had recurred at the time of the study, but one has recently recurred after an interval of 8 years.

Local recurrence of fibroadenoma should be excised because of the small risk of a more active tumour. New tumours elsewhere in the breast are best observed under the age of 25 in an attempt to avoid multiple scars, but excised over the age of 25 to obviate diagnostic error. Patients (usually Negro or Oriental) with very large numbers of fibroadenomas (40 or more) need to be managed on an individual basis. It is not realistic to keep removing them and a decision must be made between observation, selective removal of symptomatic or worrying lesions, and bilateral subcutaneous mastectomy. We know of no reports of the malignant potential of multiple familial fibroadenomas.

Variations in Histological Appearance of Fibroadenoma

Pregnancy

Fibroadenomas frequently show increase in size during pregnancy and secretory changes during lactation, and may show involution after parturition. Moran[19] described 10 cases removed during pregnancy. Azzopardi[7] describes cases showing similar secretory changes to those of lactation in patients receiving large doses of progestogens.

Infarction

Infarction is a complication most commonly seen during pregnancy and lactation. It is usually asymptomatic, but may lead to an increase in size, raising the spectre of lactational cancer. Unrecognized infarction may well be the cause of the calcified fibroadenomas characteristically seen in the elderly patient. Wilkinson and Green[20] report 10 cases of infarction of fibroadenomas but infarction of 'normal' breast tissue can also occur in pregnancy[21] and may be misdiagnosed as cancer.

Sclerosing Adenosis

This may occur in a fibroadenoma and present some difficulty in histological assessment, but has no other implications for clinical management.

Juvenile Fibroadenoma

Ashikari et al[22] studied 181 fibroadenomas in adolescent females and picked out 12 which they regarded as being floridly glandular and with a more cellular stroma. They gave these the name of 'juvenile fibroadenoma', but there is no uniformity of opinion among pathologists as to the specificity of this subgroup and it remains to be determined whether the histological picture they describe has a special clinical significance. The term is best avoided for the present. The clinical entity of giant fibroadenoma of adolescence is considered on p. 66.

Cancer in a Fibroadenoma

The common presence of epithelial hyperplasia in fibroadenomas, which is of no serious import, has lead to over diagnosis of cancer in the past. It is now recognized that exuberant hyperplasia can be ignored[6]. Cancer is rare and usually takes the form of lobular carcinoma in situ, as would be expected from the lobular origin of fibroadenoma. Haagensen[2] reports two cases treated conservatively, i.e. by local excision, without further trouble. If lobular carcinoma in situ (LCIS) is found in a fibroadenoma after enucleation, it would seem prudent to do a further local excision to determine whether the LCIS is present in the surrounding breast and then treat it accordingly.

Ductal carcinoma in association with fibroadenoma is much less common, and takes two forms: direct infiltration from an adjacent cancer and cancerization of the fibroadenoma by tumour growing along the duct into the epithelial clefts – a process analogous to the cancerization of lobules by duct cancer. In either case, the fibroadenoma should be ignored in deciding on a treatment policy for the cancer. The subject of cancer arising in fibroadenoma has recently been reviewed[23].

There is no strong evidence that the presence of a fibroadenoma is associated with an increased risk of subsequent cancer. In a follow-up of 322 fibroadenomas[6] only two cancers were found, neither related to the site of the fibroadenoma. But the question is an open one. Certainly any increased risk must be small. This question is considered more fully in Chapter 4.

Adenoma of the breast

There has long been argument as to whether or not a true adenoma of the breast exists – or whether these tumours just represent epithelial dominance in a fibroadenoma. Recently it has been established that adenoma is a distinct entity[24].

Giant Fibroadenoma – Definition

This is predominantly a condition of the extremes of reproductive life, the first 5 years after the menarche and a decade before the menopause, when a fibroadenoma keeps growing beyond the usual 1–3 cm diameter. Fibroadenoma is designated 'giant' on the basis of its clinical size alone. This is a matter of definition which has varied widely in the past, some authors suggesting a weight of 500 grams, some 5 cm and others 10 cm in diameter. In practice, most tumours are closer to 10 cm than 5 cm and sudden growth in size is a dominant feature of adolescent tumours. Since the great majority of common fibroadenomas reach only 2–3 cm in size, greater than 5 cm seems a reasonable definition to pick out this group, particularly when associated with rapid growth. Ashikari et al[22] combined cellularity of the stroma with size but this is confusing. Size and histology are better kept separate, because clinical behaviour in young girls does not parallel histological appearance. They should be considered in relation to age: adolescent or perimenopausal.

Nomenclature

Nomenclature and definition are often confused due to the loose employment of three terms: giant and/or juvenile fibroadenoma, cystosarcoma phyllodes and sarcoma. Haagensen[2] set out clearly the histological features of the main groups, showing that giant fibroadenoma, phyllodes tumor and sarcoma should be defined on histological features only. His classification has been endorsed by Azzopardi[7] with a significant modification – that the term 'cystosarcoma' be dropped because these tumours are so rarely malignant. This view is now achieving general acceptance with three terms used for breast tumours with a conspicuous stromal element: fibroadenoma; phyllodes tumour and sarcoma; and 'pure' sarcoma of the breast, as set out above. Phyllodes tumour carries a benign connotation, and phyllodes sarcoma is malignant – the differentiation being made on the degree of cytological aberration; both are tumours showing a combination of stromal and epithelial tissues. Pure sarcoma is a tumour of connective tissue only. It behaves in a much more malignant fashion than phyllodes sarcoma, and is outside the scope of this book.

The entity of 'juvenile fibroadenoma' is not easily defined. The term has usually been used to designate a fibroadenoma in adolescence which grows rapidly and often reaches a large size, but some authors, e.g. Ashikari et al[22], describe histological features which they feel are specific to a subgroup of fibroadenomas in this age group. However, as discussed above, this histological specificity is not generally accepted and there is at present no agreement that juvenile fibroadenoma is a distinct histological group. There is no advantage to the term over classification on the basis of size alone.

Giant Fibroadenoma of Adolescence

This is a rare but important condition where an unusually large fibroadenoma occurs at or within a few years of puberty. It may be defined more precisely as a fibroadenoma-like tumour greater than 5 cm in diameter and presenting between the ages of 11 and 20 years. The importance of the group lies in their presentation and management. At presentation the diagnostic problems range from failure to detect an abnormality, to confusion with malignancy or virginal hypertrophy. Management has been obscured by unnecessary confusion with other related clinicopathological entities, including phyllodes tumour, and particularly the fibroadenomatous tumours seen later in life. The subject has been reviewed recently[26].

Giant fibroadenomas in this age group may be associated with multiple fibroadenomas, but usually only one enlarges to a great degree.

Nambiar and Kannan-Kuty[25] regarded giant fibroadenoma as a more or less distinct clinicopathological variant, but our own studies show no great difference (apart from the size), in disease behaviour or cellularity when compared with smaller fibroadenomas[6]. It is important that this condition be recognized as benign and that it be separated from phyllodes tumour or phyllodes sarcoma. Nambiar and Kannan-Kuty[25] reported 25 cases and found a further 61 in the literature. They reported no recurrence or distant metastases but their own 25 patients were all Chinese, Malays or Indians. Haagensen reports seven cases, of which five were Negro and only two Caucasians. We have treated four patients aged 14–16 and one aged 18[26], all Caucasians.

Clinical Features

Although these are varied, there is a remarkable overall similarity in the features described in all publications on this subject. Onset at or soon after puberty, sudden growth, prominent veins and occasional skin ulceration due to pressure are typical. Patients frequently report cyclical changes in the affected breast with premenstrual pain and increased breast size and tension during menstruation. The growths are unilateral, but it is not uncommon for a fibroadenoma of conventional size to present at the same time or later in the opposite breast.

It might be thought that a giant tumour would be diagnosed without difficulty, but this is not always the case. It often occurs at the time of rapid breast development and the mass is obscured by this development. If the consistency of the mass is similar to that of normal breast it may be regarded merely as asymmetry of the breasts (Figure 7.7). In other cases it may be clear that there is a well-defined mass, firmer than the rest of the breast. In the third group, malignancy is simulated by such rapid growth that there are large dilated veins present over the mass (Figure 7.8). Pressure necrosis of the overlying skin may occur, so that carcinoma or sarcoma is diagnosed.

Pathology

A wide spectrum of changes in both epithelial and connective tissue elements is found in these tumours. The epithelial element may show varying degrees of hyperplasia, while the stroma varies from fibrous to cellular, with or without mitotic activity, and thus may embrace the spectrum of phyllodes tumour. However, significant cellular atypia is not a feature, and this is important. In our experience, a number of cases have been

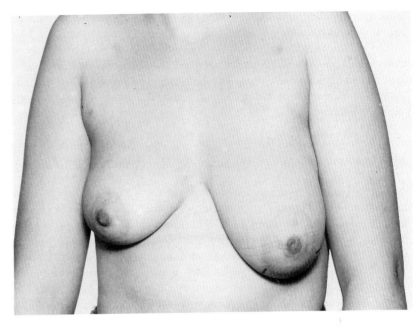

referred with cytology or histology reports where the pathologist has considered the appearance as sufficiently worrying to recommend wider excision or mastectomy. Where such a report is given in an adolescent patient, further opinions should be sought from pathologists of great experience as these tumours act in a clinically benign fashion, even though clinical and histological features at first sight may suggest malignancy[27].

Race

A review of the literature suggests that these tumours are more common in Negroes and Oriental races, and discussion with surgeons working in countries with these populations would suggest that this is true. It is significant that any reports

7.7 *Eighteen-year-old patient presenting with recent breast asymmetry. She was unaware of the presence of a large discrete mass in the left breast.*

7.8 *Benign giant fibroadenoma of adolescence. Rapid growth, vascularity and pressure skin necrosis raised the question of malignancy.*

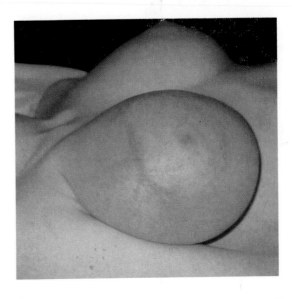

of malignancy in tumours in this age group have been in Negroid or Oriental races, so the tumours should be treated more cautiously in these groups than need be the case in Caucasians. However, it would still appear that the vast majority of adolescent tumours in all races are benign in their clinical behaviour.

Management

Age is of great importance in assessing giant breast tumours – for practical purposes these lesions in adolescence are always benign. Our small series of six cases[26] showed no recurrence, and the literature supports the view that discrete giant tumours in Caucasian adolescents, which contain both epithelial and connective tissue elements, even though they may have a wide spectrum of histological appearances, have a uniformly benign clinical behaviour[27]. Some of our tumours had a typical fibroadenoma appearance on histology, others had an appearance indistinguishable from benign phyllodes tumour. We are not aware of any report of local recurrence or malignancy in such tumours in Caucasians of this age group, and age takes precedence over histological assessment in adolescence. It is

reasonable to treat these lesions, on the basis of clinical diagnosis, by enucleation. Mammography and biopsy do not influence the treatment but may even lead to a false diagnosis of malignancy and consideration of unnecessarily radical treatment. Clearly a different attitude will be taken to tumours in patients over the age of 20, and perhaps young patients of non-Caucasian race.

Giant fibroadenomas tend to be deeper in the breast than is clinically apparent and, for this reason, are best approached from behind through a submammary incision, the Gaillard–Thomas approach (*see* Chapter 18). With large tumours, the remaining breast exists only as a compressed rim around the periphery, but this may be expected to expand and lead to a breast of roughly normal size and contour (Figures 7.9 and 7.10). We believe that more radical surgery is not indicated in this age group, irrespective of histological findings, because recurrence is a clinical curiosity in Caucasians, even when histological features cause concern. Nambiar and Kannan-Kutty recommend excision with a margin of normal tissue, similar to that which many authors, including ourselves, would advocate for phyllodes tumour in older patients. They recommend this in contradistinction to enucleation, which they advise against. However, it is not clear how local excision is achieved. With larger tumours the normal breast exists as a thin compressed rim around the tumour and excision would be tantamount to a simple mastectomy, the operation which is necessary for large phyllodes tumours in older women.

Simple mastectomy as recommended and practised in the case reported by Holbrook and Ramsay[28] is certainly to be condemned. Complex reconstructive procedures, such as the insertion of a de-epithelialized flap and silicone prosthesis as recommended by Hoffman[29] are also inappropriate. Such an approach ignores the fact that the

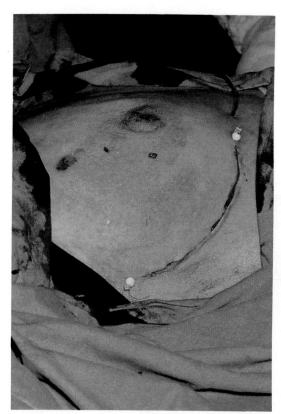

7.9 *The tumour has been enucleated via a submammary (Gaillard–Thomas) approach, leaving only a thin rim of compressed breast tissue.*

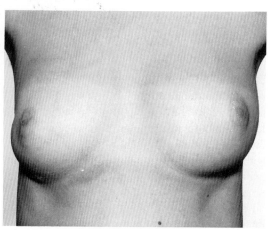

7.10 *One year later, the breast has regained almost normal size.*

breast remnant rapidly returns to normal after removal of the fibroadenoma (Figure 7.10), a process which might well be inhibited by an implant. Even closure of the cavities by sutures is unnecessary and may lead to breast distortion.

Giant Breast Tumours of the Perimenopausal Period

Giant tumours of the breast show a second peak of incidence in the pre- and perimenopausal period. Such tumours need careful clinical and histological assessment to put them in one of five categories:

1. Giant fibroadenoma.
2. Recurrent and progressive fibroadenoma.
3. Phyllodes tumour and phyllodes sarcoma.
4. Pure sarcoma.
5. Carcinoma.

The last two are outside the scope of this book.

Giant Fibroadenoma

A large tumour which clearly has the histological features of a benign fibroadenoma will usually behave in a benign fashion. It may be treated as a fibroadenoma of normal type in younger age groups, although it may not enucleate, because of associated involutional fibrosis in the surrounding breast.

Recurrent and Progressive Fibroadenoma

This is a rare but important variant characterized by multicentricity and recurrence after surgical excision. In reported cases, there has been a tendency to increasing histological activity on succeeding biopsies. One case under our care is typical of cases reported in the literature.

A female patient, born 1935, presented in 1964 with a 3 × 2 cm nodule, which was excised and reported on histology as a benign fibroadenoma. In 1967 she presented again with gross nodularity of the breast. Most of the tissue of the right breast was involved in a nodular process, which was treated by removal of three-quarters of the breast tissue. Histologically it was found to consist of 'fibroadenosis' mixed with nodules of benign fibroadenoma up to 5 cm in diameter. In 1973 the breast was back to its original size (Figure 7.11) and gross nodularity led to removal of one-quarter of the breast mass. The macroscopic description was 'tough fibroadenosis' but the

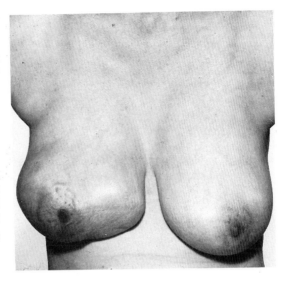

7.11 *Recurrent giant fibroadenoma of the perimenopausal period. See text for details.*

histology again showed benign fibroadenomatous tissue.

In 1978 the patient was seen in our unit. Further gross nodularity of the breast and marked discomfort lead to a biopsy of the largest (5 cm) mass which showed a fibroadenoma in which 'the spindle cell fibrous stroma differs from previous biopsies and now had undoubted hallmarks of malignancy'. Simple mastectomy was performed and the whole breast was found to be replaced by a huge fibroadenomatous mass.

In 1987 the patient was well with no evidence of local or distant recurrence. These very rare cases probably represent a progression of benign fibroadenoma to malignancy that constitutes the exception rather than the rule. Even so, the degree of malignancy is low, unlike that of primary sarcoma of the breast.

Phyllodes Tumour and Phyllodes Sarcoma (Cystosarcoma Phyllodes)

Although we are dealing with phyllodes tumour and phyllodes sarcoma under the heading of giant tumours of the perimenopausal period, this is only because they are seen most commonly in this form and at this stage of life. Small tumours of only a centimetre or so occur, and in any age group. The pathology and management of these smaller tumours are similar to the more classic presentation discussed here. This is a tumour with a dramatic clinical picture and aggressive histological features, so it is not surprising that it has received attention beyond any it deserves in view of its predominantly benign behaviour. It was Johann Muller who first gave it this name in 1838[30], because it is often cystic and classically has leaf-like projections into it. While these were accurately descriptive, the term 'sarcoma' is not justified in a majority of cases, and hence the suggestion that the term 'phyllodes tumour' be substituted, with the term 'phyllodes sarcoma' restricted to the small proportion which justifies this designation on histological grounds or by clinical behaviour. This is another condition where confusion reigns, and much of the blame must again be directed against imprecise terminology. Since the tumour may be neither cystic nor sarcomatous, 'cystosarcoma' should be abandoned in favour of phyllodes tumour or phyllodes sarcoma. This case is well argued by Azzopardi[7].

The tumour is distinct from giant fibroadenoma, macroscopically as well as histologically, but it must be reiterated that the diagnosis is a histological one which may apply to any size tumour. The histological features may be seen in small as well as large tumours. Likewise, it is the pathologist who should decide (on histological grounds) whether the term 'sarcoma' is justified. To diagnose the tumour, both epithelial and fibrous stromal elements must be present, with the stroma showing cellularity, irregularity, hyperchromatism and significant mitosis. Stromal changes are patchy, so many sections need to be studied in the assessment of a large tumour.

An excellent description of the histological details assessed by the pathologist is provided by Azzopardi[7]. The macroscopic and microscopic appearance of giant fibroadenoma and phyllodes tumour are contrasted in Figures 7.12–7.15.

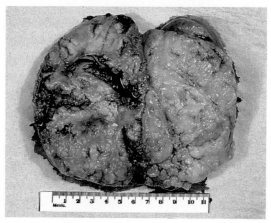

7.13 *Giant fibroadenoma – macroscopic, uniform, whitish appearance of fibrous tissue.*

Aetiology

The tumour is clearly related to fibroadenoma in some cases, because patients may develop both lesions and histological features of both lesions may be seen in the same tumour. However, whether phyllodes tumour develops from a fibroadenoma or both develop simultaneously, or phyllodes tumour may arise *de novo*, is not clear. What is important is that it should not be confused with pure sarcoma (without any epithelial element), for these have a greater degree of malignancy and lumping the two together can obscure the essentially benign nature of many phyllodes tumours.

Clinical Features

Haagensen[2] reports approximately 1 phyllodes tumour to every 40 fibroadenomas. Our own hospital experience is similar; 7 phyllodes tumours were diagnosed during a period when 332 fibroadenomas were treated. The age distribution is broad – from 10 to 90 in Haagensen's series of 84 patients, but with a majority between 35 and 55 years. Bilateral tumours are very rare. Phyllodes tumour is rare in patients before the age of 20, when it appears to behave in a particularly benign fashion, regardless of the histological features.

Most tumours grow rapidly to a large size before the patient presents, but the tumours are not fixed in the sense of a large carcinoma. This is because they are not particularly invasive – the bulk of the tumour may occupy the whole breast, and produce pressure ulceration of the skin, but still show some mobility on the chest wall. The tumours are usually softer than fibroadenomas, grossly bosselated and the skin over them shows large dilated veins. The axillary lymph nodes are

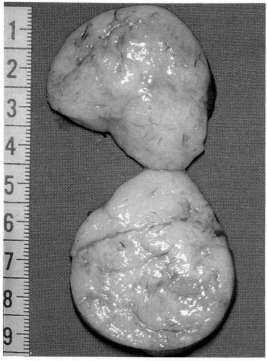

7.12 *Giant phyllodes tumour – macroscopic, brown, irregular, cellular, leaf-like masses, necrosis and haemorrhage. Note similarities and contrasts to Figure 7.6.*

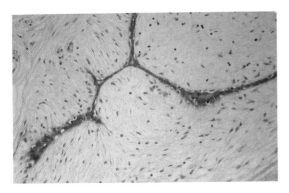

7.14 *Giant fibroadenoma – microscopic, hypocellular stroma.*

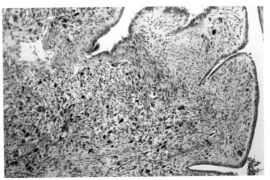

7.15 *Phyllodes tumour (sarcoma) microscopic. Cellular stroma with marked pleomorphism.*

not usually involved – a reasonable estimate of the incidence in the malignant subgroup is 10%, so overall the figure is very low.

On section, the tumour is well defined, but histologically may show limited invasion of the pseudocapsule of compressed breast tissue – accounting for the tendency to local recurrence. On cut surface, they have a moist, necrotic, characteristically brownish appearance (*see* Figure 7.13), sometimes with obvious mucoid, haemorrhagic or necrotic areas, and a softer consistency than a fibroadenoma. The brown colour is notable even with smaller tumours (Figure 7.16) and should alert the surgeon to this diagnosis.

Behaviour

While phyllodes tumour shows a distinct tendency to recur locally if excised by a close margin, local or distant metastasis is uncommon. In fact those tumours assessed as benign after comprehensive histological study can be expected to have an excellent prognosis. Those which are histologically malignant (phyllodes sarcoma) are unpredictable in behaviour.

In Treves and Sunderland's study[31] of 77 cases, 50% of those classified as malignant metastasized. A number of workers[31-33] have tried to assess the malignant potential. It is generally felt that mitotic rate is the best guide, although far from uniformly predictive. A mitotic rate less than 4 per 10 high power fields (HPF) carried an excellent prognosis, 5–9/10 HPF is intermediate and more than 10/10 HPF carries a worse prognosis. Small tumours (less than 4 cm diameter) also have an excellent prognosis. Rhodes *et al*[34] have recently reviewed the histological assessment of malignancy.

The overall favourable prognosis is shown by Haagensen's series – only 4 out of the 84 patients are known to have metastasized[2]. While we have seen local recurrence in patients, none has as yet metastasized.

Treatment

Age is important in the management of these lesions. Under the age of 20, all should be treated by enucleation, because they behave in a benign manner.

The situation is less clear-cut in older patients. Few surgeons have sufficient experience to be dogmatic about management. Haagensen reports one of the largest series, and recommends wide local excision as the primary approach to treatment of benign phyllodes tumours. He has a local recurrence rate of 28% among 43 patients treated by local excision, with a minimum 10-year follow-up. But only three of the recurrences required secondary mastectomy, and none has died from the tumour. Only 1 in 21 patients treated by mastectomy – simple or radical – developed local recurrence, a phyllodes sarcoma which rapidly produced both local and systematic metastases.

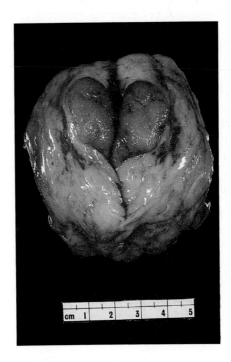

7.16 *Small benign phyllodes tumour. Note similarity to Figure 7.6, but distinct brownish colour.*

For small lesions where the diagnosis is suggested by the macroscopic appearance we would excise the tumour with a 1 cm margin of normal breast tissue. If histology is benign, this would be sufficient treatment, with a quadrantic excision for intermediate lesions. Where the diagnosis is first recognized on histological examination of an excision biopsy specimen, we recommend quadrantic excision of the scar, as a means of ensuring adequate local clearance. For large lesions and recurrent lesions, a good clearance inevitably involves near total mastectomy and we prefer simple mastectomy, with immediate reconstruction should the patient wish it. We feel that mastectomy is a small price to pay for

freedom from local recurrence, and that reconstruction can readily lessen the price. We are reinforced in this policy by the fact that the stroma sometimes shows increased malignancy with recurrence.

The histological association of carcinoma with phyllodes tumour is similar to that discussed under fibroadenoma (see p. 65) – a predominance of lobular carcinoma in situ, and occasionally involvement of the lesion from adjacent cancer. Unlike fibroadenoma, there is some evidence for an increased incidence of related carcinoma, simultaneous or subsequent – in patients with phyllodes tumour[35] and is an added reason for careful long-term follow-up of such patients.

REFERENCES

1. World Health Organisation. *Histological Typing of Breast Tumours*, 2nd ed., 1981.
2. Haagensen C. D. *Diseases of the Breast*, 3rd ed. Philadelphia, W. B. Saunders, 1986.
3. Kern W. H. & Clark R. W. Retrogression of fibroadenoma of the breast. *American Journal of Surgery* 1973; 126: 59–62.
4. Devitt J. E. Benign disorders of the breast in older women. *Surgery, Gynecology and Obstetrics* 1986; 162: 340–342.
5. Cheatle G. L. Hyperplasia of epithelial and connective tissues in the breast: its relation to fibroadenoma. *British Journal of Surgery* 1923; 10: 436–455.
6. Foster M. E., Garrahan N. & Williams S. Fibroadenoma of the breast – a clinical and pathological study. *Journal of the Royal College of Surgeons (Edinburgh)* 1987; (in press).
7. Azzopardi J. G. *Problems in Breast Pathology.* London, W. B. Saunders, 1979.
8. Nardelli G. B., Lamaina V. & Siliotti F. Steroid receptors in benign breast disease, Gross cystic disease and fibroadenoma. *Clinical and Experimental Obstetrics and Gynecology* 1987; 14: 10–15.
9. Thomas D. B. Role of exogenous female hormones in altering the risk of benign and malignant neoplasms in humans. *Cancer Research* 1978; 38: 3991–4000.
10. Weigenstein L., Tank R. & Gould R. E. Multiple breast fibroadenomas in women on hormonal contraceptives. *New England Journal of Medicine* 1971; 284: 676.
11. Naraynsingh V. & Raju G. C. Familial bilateral multiple fibroadenomas of the breast. *Postgraduate Medical Journal* 1985; 61: 439–440.
12. Berkowitz G. S., Canny P. F., Vivolsi V. A. et al. Cigarette smoking and benign breast disease. *Journal of Epidemiology and Community Health* 1985; 39: 308–313.
13. Wilkinson S. & Forrest A. P. M. Fibroadenoma of the breast. *British Journal of Surgery* 1985; 72: 838–840.
14. Crothers J. G., Butler N. F., Fortt R. W. & Gravelle I. H. Fibroadenolipoma of the breast. *British Journal of Radiology* 1985; 58: 191–202.
15. Cole-Beuglet C., Soriano R. Z., Kurtz A. B. & Goldberg B. B. Fibroadenoma of the breast. Sonomammography correlated with pathology in 122 patients. *American Journal of Radiology* 1983; 140: 369–375.
16. Stelling C. B., Powell D. E. & Mattingly S. S. Fibroadenomas: histopathologic and M. R. imaging features. *Radiology* 1987; 162: 399–407.
17. Cant P. J., Madden M. V., Close P. M. et al. Case for conservative management of selected fibroadenomas of the breast. *British Journal of Surgery* 1987; 74: 857–859.
18. Cupceancu B. Short term tamoxifen treatment in benign breast diseases. *Endocrinologie* 1985; 23: 169–177.
19. Moran C. S. Fibroadenoma of the breast during pregnancy and lactation. *Archives of Surgery* 1935; 31: 688.
20. Wilkinson L. & Green W. O. Jr. Infarction of breast lesions during pregnancy and lactation. *Cancer* 1964; 17: 1567–1572.
21. Hasson J. & Pope C. H. Mammary infarcts associated with pregnancy presenting as breast tumours. *Surgery* 1961; 49: 313–316.
22. Ashikari R., Farrow J. H. & O'Hara J. Fibroadenomas in the breast of juveniles. *Surgery, Gynecology and Obstetrics* 1971; 132: 259–262.
23. Yoshida Y., Takaoka M. & Fukumoto M. Carcinoma arising in fibroadenoma. Case report and review of world literature. *Journal of Surgical Oncology* 1985; 29: 132–140.
24. Hertel B. F., Zaloudek C. & Kempson R. L. Breast adenomas. *Cancer* 1976; 37: 2891–2905.
25. Nambiar R. & Kannan-Kutty M. Giant fibroadenoma (cystosarcoma phyllodes) in adolescent females. A clinico-pathological study. *British Journal of Surgery* 1974; 61: 113–117.
26. Raganoonan C., Fairbairn J. K., Williams S. & Hughes L. E. Giant breast tumours of adolescence. *Australia and New Zeland Journal of Surgery* 1987; 57: 243–247.
27. Mies C. & Rosen P. P. Juvenile Fibroadenoma with atypical epithelial hyperplasia. *American Journal of Surgical Pathology* 1987; 11: 184–190.
28. Holbrook W. A. & Ramsay J. H. Giant fibroadenoma of the breast. *Bulletin of the School of Medicine of the University of Maryland* 1956; 41: 58–63.

29. Hoffman S. H. Giant fibroadenoma of the breast: immediate reconstruction following excision. *British Journal of Plastic Surgery* 1978; 31: 170–172.

30. Muller J. *Uber den Feinern Bau and die formen der krankhaften geschwulste.* Berlin, G. Reimer, 1838.

31. Treves N. & Sunderland D. Cystosarcoma of the breast – a malignant and a benign tumour. A clinico-pathological study of 77 cases. *Cancer* 1951; 4: 1286–1332.

32. Lester J. & Stout A. P. Cystosarcoma phyllodes. *Cancer* 1954; 7: 335–353.

33. Norris H. J. & Taylor H. B. Relationship of histological features to behaviour of cystosarcoma phyllodes. Analysis of 94 cases. *Cancer* 1967; 20: 2090–2099.

34. Rhodes R. H., Frankel K. A., Davis L. & Tatter D. Metastatic cystosarcoma phyllodes. *Cancer* 1978; 41: 1179–1187.

35. Rosen P. P. & Urban J. A. Coexistent mammary carcinoma and cystosarcoma phyllodes. *Breast* 1975; i: 9–15.

8   Breast Pain and Nodularity

Mastalgia is one of the commonest symptoms in patients attending a breast clinic and is also the most frequent reason for breast-related consultation in general practice[1, 2]. Many alternative terms have been used to describe mastalgia in the past, including the term 'mastodynia' introduced by Heineke in 1821 and 'mazodynia' used by Birkett in 1850. The mixing of pathological with clinical terms noted in Chapter 3 has caused confusion in the past and it is better to use mastalgia to denote the *symptom* of pain in the breast without any specific pathological connotation being implied.

Historical Note

The literature amply demonstrates that breast pain is the commonest presenting symptom of breast conditions and it would be natural to assume that it was a well-documented subject with clear definitions and guidelines for management. Unfortunately, this is not the case; the literature devoted to mastalgia is poor in both quality and clarity. Most of the problem is due to attempts to relate poorly defined clinical presentations with pathological terms as previously discussed in Chapter 3. Birkett in 1850 in his textbook of breast diseases[3] described breast pain as 'mazodynia' and noted two subtypes: with induration (nodularity) or without induration. He noted premenstrual exacerbation of tenderness in the nodular group and suggested aperients and tonics as treatment. Cheatle and Cutler[4] in 1931 used the term 'mazoplasia' to describe bilateral painful nodular breasts, and suggested it was present to some degree in all women's breasts. Later authors used the all-embracing term 'chronic mastitis' to denote painful nodular breasts[5, 6], with some attempting to define degrees of severity[7]. Carl Semb described various degrees of painful nodularity in his exhaustive study of 1928[8], but also mixed symptomatic terms with pathological descriptions.

Geschickter wrote a whole chapter in his 1945 book on the subject of mastodynia (painful breasts) and described many of the clinical features of mastalgia[7], but as had others before him, concluded that mastodynia progressed into the various forms of chronic cystic mastitis.

Thus, despite a small number of exhaustive studies by these eminent clinicians and pathologists, there is no clear account of mastalgia as a *symptom*. In 1971, a special research clinic was set up within the Cardiff Breast Clinic in order to answer some of the questions regarding mastalgia and benign breast disease. The findings of this mastalgia clinic, which has continued to study this problem to the present, form the substance of this chapter.

Frequency of Breast Pain

The frequency of breast pain as a presenting symptom of breast disorders in various clinics is shown in Table 8.1. The exact frequency is difficult to ascertain as many studies do not state the population from which the study group is drawn. An example is Geschickter's detailed account which described 375 cases of mastodynia seen in Baltimore over a period of 50 years, but the incidence of other breast conditions is not stated[7].

Table 8.1   Frequency of breast pain as a presenting symptom in benign and malignant breast disease.

Study	Percentage of patients attending complaining of mastalgia
Semb[8]	85
Southampton Breast Clinic[9]	50
Cardiff Breast Clinic	45
General Practice[1,2]	47–52
Working Population (M&S–Cardiff Study)	66
Screening Clinic[10]	70

In general, it can be seen that breast pain is present in about 50% of patients presenting to surgical clinics with breast problems but higher levels of around 65–70% were volunteered by women interviewed at a screening clinic and at screening carried out on site in a group of working women at a large retail chain store (Table 8.1).

Mastalgia in Breast Cancer

Although this book does not deal with cancer, the role of breast pain in the diagnosis of early breast cancer is often thought to be of great importance. Several papers make the point that, although breast pain is an uncommon symptom in breast cancer, it does not exclude the diagnosis. Preece[11] noted that mastalgia due to cancer has no specific diagnostic features. However, it differed from cyclical premenstrual mastalgia in that it was unilateral, persistent and constant in position. Of 17 patients who presented with mastalgia alone out of a population of 240 operable breast cancers, he found 5 were T0 tumours and 5 T1 tumours, suggesting that mastalgia as a *sole* presenting symptom is associated with smaller tumours. The literature on this topic is generally consistent as Table 8.2 demonstrates.

Table 8.2 Frequency of breast pain as a presenting symptom of operable breast cancer.

Study	Percentage of cancers presenting with pain
Preece[11]	7
River[12]	24
Haagensen[13]	5
Smallwood[9]	18
Yorkshire Group[14]	5

Classification

The previous attempts at classification based on pathological terms did not give any practical help in the understanding or management of mastalgia. A pressing need was to classify accurately the symptom of mastalgia and this was initially done by drawing up a protocol in the Mastalgia Clinic describing several features of the symptom (Table 8.3).

In addition, a comprehensive gynaecological history was taken and careful physical examination performed. All the patients studied in the Mastalgia Clinic had already been examined clinically by an experienced breast surgeon and by mammography (when indicated) to exclude carcinoma of the breast. These patients thus presented with painful breasts with or without

Table 8.3 Contents of the Cardiff Mastalgia Protocol.

Feature	Examples
Descriptive terms	Tenderness/heaviness/burning
Periodicity	Continuous, intermittent
Duration	
Distribution in breast	
Radiation	
Aggravating factors	Physical contact
Relieving factors	Analgesics/drugs/well-fitted brassière
Diurnal pattern	
Disturbance of lifestyle	Sleep loss/marital problem/can't hug children
Dominant hand	

Table 8.4 Frequency of patterns in 232 prospectively documented mastalgia patients.

Pattern/diagnosis	No. (%)
Cyclical pronounced	93 (40)
Non-cyclical	62 (27)
Tietze's syndrome	25 (11)
Trauma (post-biopsy)	19 (8)
Sclerosing adenosis	11 (4.5)
Cancer	1 (0.5)
Miscellaneous/non-breast	21 (9)

From Preece *et al*[15].

nodularity. Cases with a discrete lump were managed as detailed in Chapter 5.

Analysis of the initial 232 patients studied with this protocol defined certain patterns of mastalgia[15]. The frequency of each type is shown in Table 8.4.

Cyclical Pronounced Pattern

The commonest pattern was the cyclical pronounced pattern which is so named because it shows a definite relationship to the menstrual cycle, almost always premenstrual with a duration varying from 1 week up to 4 weeks (Figure 8.1). This group probably represents the 'mastodynia' group of previous reports, although some authors state that associated nodularity excludes 'mastodynia'. The cyclical pronounced patient almost invariably has nodularity of a varying degree which is maximal in the upper outer quadrant, and shows similar cyclicity to the pain. Obviously, many women experience 2 or 3 days premenstrual breast tenderness or heaviness and this should be regarded as normal (Figure 8.2). Fine nodularity which begins a short time before menstruation and regresses postmenstrually is equally normal; the difficult problem is deciding where normality ends and disease begins.

The cyclical group has been given the adjective 'pronounced' to denote the increased intensity of the symptom defined either by duration (> 1 week per cycle), or by severity documented using a pain chart (Figure 8.3). Severity is necessarily a subjective assessment, as is all assessment of pain in clinical practice, but obtrusive features in the lifestyle, such as sleep loss, work disturbance or interrupted sexual activity, can give some guide.

Other characteristics of the cyclical pronounced group are shown in Figure 8.4 and it is worth noting that the terms 'heaviness' and 'tenderness to touch' are used frequently to describe symptoms of the pattern. Bilateral pain and nodularity are also common. The pain often radiates to the axilla and down the medial aspect of the upper arm, presumably as a referred pain via the intercostobrachial nerve. A well-taken history will often reveal the temporal association with the menstrual cycle, but we have found a simple pain chart to be extremely useful in displaying this pattern (*see* Figure 8.3). It is readily completed by most patients and has the added advantage of giving a simple quantitation to the symptom (days of pain) which is useful for assessing effectiveness of therapy. Mammography has proved unhelpful in the cyclical pronounced pattern, as the non-specific changes of radiological density ascribed to fibroadenosis have been the main feature, and no specific radiological appearance correlates with the site or side of pain.

Non-cyclical Pain

The second largest group (27%), the non-cyclical pattern, is distinguished principally by its lack of relationship with events in the menstrual cycle and again this is well shown by the simple pain chart (Figure 8.5). This pattern occurs in both pre- and postmenopausal women in contradistinction to the cyclical pattern and for this reason the mean age of these patients is 43 years compared to 34 for the cyclical group. The non-cyclical pattern differs in several other respects from the cyclical (Figure 8.6). The pain tends to be well localized in the breast and is more frequently subareolar or inner quadrant. Simultaneous bilateral pain is less frequent and the descriptive terms of 'burning, drawing or abscess-like' are different. Other terms indicative of a transient sharp quality, such as pricking or stabbing, have also been commonly used and may last for minutes or days at a time. When the pattern was assessed quantitively using a linear analogue scale (*see* later), it was scored by the patients at a lower intensity than the cyclical pattern. Nodularity is less prominent than in the cyclical group and there may be no palpable abnormality at the site of pain.

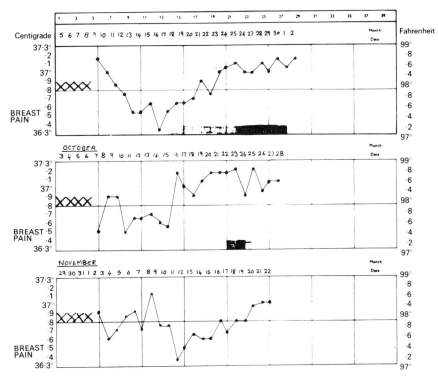

8.1 *Basal body temperature chart recorded by a patient with mastalgia. The first two cycles show a biphasic ovulatory pattern and breast pain occurred for about 2 weeks premenstrually in the first cycle (top level) and for about 4 days in the second cycle. No pain occurred in the third cycle (lower panel) which appears to have a non-ovulatory temperature pattern. This chart demonstrates the association of mastalgia with ovulation and the variation in one woman from cycle to cycle. XXX = menstrual period.*

| Record the amount of breast pain you experience each day by shading in each box as illustrated. | ■ Severe pain ◪ Mild pain ● No pain | For example:– If you get severe breast pain on the fifth of the month then shade in completely the square under 5. Please note the day your period starts each month with the letter 'P'. | Please bring this card with you on each visit. |

8.2 *Breast pain chart showing daily recording of breast pain. The chart shows 3–4 days of mild premenstrual pain per cycle which would be regarded as normal. P = period.*

Mammography has been of some interest in the non-cyclical group, as the radiological changes of coarse calcification and ductal dilatation attributed to duct ectasia or periductal mastitis have been commonly seen in this group. Of the 62 patients documented, no less than 42 showed radiological evidence of duct ectasia somewhere in the painful breast and of these 20 showed calcification of secretory disease at the site of complaint. These findings led us initially to describe the non-cyclical pattern as the 'periductal mastitis' pattern, but we prefer to use the former term as first it conforms to our previously stated principle of not mixing symptomatic with pathological terms, and secondly there is no histological evidence that non-cyclical pain is due to the pathological changes of duct ectasia. A further term, 'the trigger spot', for this pattern or at least a subgroup of it, has been introduced[16], and is claimed to have the special feature that pressure by palpation at the indicated site of pain will reproduce the patient's pain. However, in our experience, while this picture is seen in some patients, it does not describe the overall group and there is no correlation with any histological picture at the site of complaint[17].

Tietze's Syndrome

Tietze's syndrome[18] or painful costochondral junction syndrome is not a true breast pain but the pain is often felt in the region of the breast as the breast overlies the costal cartilages, which are the source of the pain (Figure 8.7). It has a characteristically chronic time course and, on examination, one or several costal cartilages are tender and feel enlarged. Typically the pain is felt within the medial quadrants of the breast and increased pain occurs on pressure over the affected cartilage. Radiological examination of these patients reveals no abnormality in the costal cartilages or specific features in the breast.

Trauma and Sclerosing Adenosis

The trauma group, 8% of the total, complained of a persistent non-cyclical type pain localized to a previous benign biopsy scar. There were no specific findings apart from the presence of the scar, but on enquiry it was revealed that several of the biopsies had been complicated by infection or haematoma. In addition, some of the painful scars had been made across Langer's lines of tension and this may be an important factor.

Eleven patients had pain at the site of sclerosing adenosis (seven proved histologically and four shown on mammography), but there were no clear diagnostic features to the descriptive terms used by the patients. Cancer was an uncommon cause of pain as these cases were generally filtered out in the general breast clinic and only one case was seen of a cancer developing during observation in the Mastalgia Clinic. This patient had a well localized pain with no lump at presentation and negative mammography, but the pain persisted for 1 year and a repeat mammogram showed an impalpable cancer. Cancer usually shows a non-cyclical pain chart, as illustrated

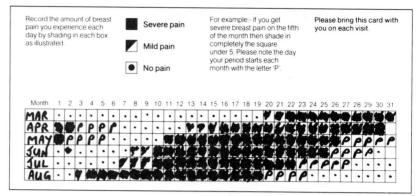

8.3 *Pain chart of a patient with cyclical pronounced mastalgia showing 2–3 weeks of severe to mild mastalgia per cycle over 6 months.*

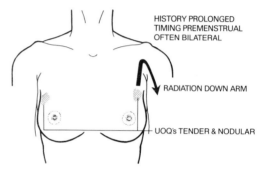

8.4 *Diagram showing the clinical features of cyclical mastalgia. It is premenopausal; mean age = 34 years. Descriptive terms are 'heaviness' and 'tenderness to touch'; relieved by menstruation and menopause.*

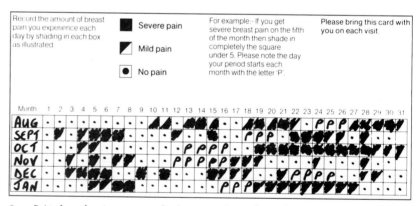

8.5 *Pain chart showing a non-cyclical pattern of mastalgia. There is no demonstrable relationship to any phase of the menstrual cycle.*

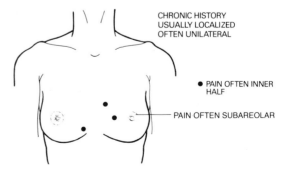

8.6 *Diagram showing the clinical features of non-cyclical mastalgia. It is pre- or postmenopausal; mean age = 43 years. Descriptive terms are 'drawing' and 'burning'; not relieved by reproductive events.*

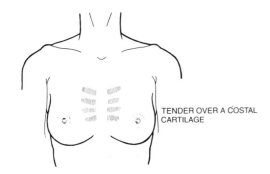

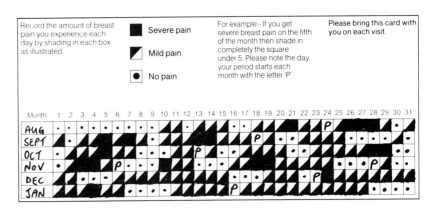

8.7 *Diagram showing the clinical features of Tietze's syndrome. It is often unilateral; any age; no time pattern; no palpable abnormality; chronic course.*

8.8 *Pain chart of a patient who subsequently developed a small palpable cancer at the site of pain. The chart shows a typical non-cyclical but persistent pattern.*

in Figure 8.8 of a patient who was found to have a cancer in a small lump which developed at the site of the pain. The miscellaneous group consisted of patients who were unclassifiable into the preceding groups or were shown to have pain due to a non-breast cause, such as gallstones or angina. About 10–13% of patients presenting with breast pain will be found to have a cause outside the breast, particularly of musculoskeletal origin, such as cervical spondylosis[19].

Other general findings for the whole group of patients were that mastalgia is commoner in the left breast and half of the patients had experienced pain for over 1 year prior to consultation. Thus mastalgia is often prolonged and seems to have a predeliction for the left breast as does cancer. In summary, there are three major pain patterns: the cyclical pronounced, non-cyclical and Tietze's syndrome and only these three will be considered further in the discussion of therapy.

Aetiology of Mastalgia and Nodularity

History

Many of the surgeons who wrote about the clinical description of mastalgia also speculated on the cause of the condition, but modern hormone estimations were unavailable and most of the conclusions remained pure speculation. Several workers suggested that some ovarian influence was responsible for the cyclical pattern of mastalgia as they had noted the association with the menstrual cycle and also the absence of the problem after the menopause[6, 7]. Perhaps we should not be too critical of these scientists because aetiological terms coined by them have a very familar ring today and hormones were undiscovered at the time. Cutler proposed a luteal abnormality and Geshickter described a relative hyperoestrogenism.

Other theories were those of excessive water retention or, more importantly, neuroticism. Astley Cooper began the trend of describing mastalgia patients as 'being of a nervous disposition' but also added that this was a personal impression[20]. Unfortunately this trend continued, without any rational scientific basis, and was brought up-to-date almost a century and a half later by a leading gynaecologist with the comment in a major gynaecology textbook that mastalgia patients were 'frustrated, unhappy nulliparae'[21]. Even such an authority as Haagensen wrote that women with severe breast pain were 'in general, unstable and hypochondriacal although they are not frankly psychotic'. These impressions and hypotheses have now been examined scientifically.

Studies of Aetiology

Water Retention

Oedema due to water retention has been suggested as a cause of both mastalgia and the premenstrual tension syndrome because women had reported weight gain and breast and ankle swelling in late cycle.

As a result treatment with diuretics was proposed[22]. There was, however, no study in the literature showing that general oedema was associated with mastalgia. We therefore carried out estimations of total body water using tritiated water in mastalgia patients and asymptomatic normal women[23]. This study clearly showed that there were no significant differences in water gain between the fifth and twenty-fifth days of the cycle when mastalgia patients were compared with normal controls and this was true even for the cyclical group who displayed the typical premenstrual increase in breast pain. Therefore, simple retention of body water does not seem to be correlated with mastalgia, although it might be argued that intramammary oedema is more important. As mentioned previously, breast swelling is common in the luteal phase when assessed volumetrically[24, 25], but there is no way currently of measuring which component of breast tissue is responsible for the swelling.

Psychoneurosis

We next turned our attention to the hypothesis that mastalgia patients were more neurotic than other patients as suggested by Astley Cooper. Using the well-validated Middlesex Hospital Questionnaire (MHQ), specifically designed as a rapid screening test for differentiating between 'normals' and psychiatric cases[26], we tested the psychoneurotic profiles of 300 patients presenting to hospital with mastalgia (cyclical and non-cyclical) and 156 patients presenting with varicose veins[27]. The scores of the varicose vein and mastalgia patients were significantly lower than those of psychiatric outpatients, which had been published by the MHQ designers (Table 8.5). Moreover, the only differences between mastalgia cases and varicose vein patients were in favour of the former. This study showed conclusively that there is no scientific foundation for the impressions of those who believed mastalgia patients to be psychoneurotic.

Table 8.5 Neuroticism scores of mastalgia patients compared with patients with varicose veins (mean ± s.d.).

	Mastalgia (n = 300)	Varicose veins (n = 156)	Psychiatric outpatients (n = 173)
Anxiety	7.6 ± 0.23	7.8 ± 0.30	11.0 ± 0.26[a]
Depression	4.2 ± 0.16	5.1 ± 0.21	7.6 ± 0.29[a]
Phobia	5.0 ± 0.16	5.7 ± 0.22	6.8 ± 0.29[a]

[a] Significantly greater than mastalgia or varicose vein groups. High scores imply abnormality (MHQ questionnaire).

Endocrine Abnormalities

The advent of accurate radio-immunoassays for estimation of blood hormones and the discovery of human prolactin as a separate entity from growth hormone, caused a rapid upsurge in interest in the 'hormonal imbalance' hypotheses previously discussed. From previous work, three main theories emerged regarding the aetiology of painful nodular breasts:

1. Increased oestrogen secretion from the ovary.
2. Deficient progesterone production ('relative hyperoestrogenism').
3. Hyperprolactinaemia.

Early studies failed to support the first two theories, as steroid levels were no different in patients or controls[28-30], but a French group in 1979 showed a significantly depressed level of luteal progesterone[31], thus supporting the second theory. Further, the same group obtained symptomatic relief by correcting the depressed progesterone level with an exogenous progestogen. Unfortunately, no other group has been able to find a definite defect in luteal phase progesterone and in all British and American studies there was no significant difference between mastalgia patients and controls[29, 32]. Our experience is similar and, in a study of 50 mastalgia patients and 18 controls, we failed to show any difference in luteal phase progesterone between the two groups[33]. Further studies of the free fraction of progesterone measured daily in the saliva failed to reveal any differences between controls and mastalgia patients in Wales or Scotland[34, 35]. The case for a luteal defect therefore remains unproven and the therapeutic value of progestogens is also debatable (see later). A recent review concludes that there are no significant differences in basal levels of ovarian steroids and gonadotrophins in women with benign breast conditions compared with controls[36].

Prolactin was only accepted as a separate hormone from 1970 onwards, and a specific radio-immunoassay became available a year later, but since then, a great deal of attention has been focused on the hormone. As the major lactogenic hormone, there are prima facie reasons for believing that it may play a role in a condition which is thought to be due to overstimulation of a normal physiological process. However, several studies of random basal prolactin levels showed no significant differences between normals and patients with benign breast disorder (BBD) (review by Wang and Fentiman)[36], but analysis of prolactin secretion in normal women showed that the hormone is secreted in a pulsatile manner and has a diurnal variation[37]. Both these factors suggest that random sampling of basal prolactin is inappropriate. In order to avoid these problems, Malarkey measured 24-hour profiles, but again failed to find any differences between controls or biopsied benign disease cases at any time of the day or night[30]. However, a further study of daily sampling at a fixed time throughout the menstrual cycle revealed a small but statistically significant difference between women with cystic disease and controls.[38].

The above studies were performed on random or 24-hour basal prolactin levels, but a more recent approach is the examination of the dynamics of the pituitary release of prolactin.

Prolactin is almost unique in that its secretion is tonically inhibited by dopamine (Figure 8.9),

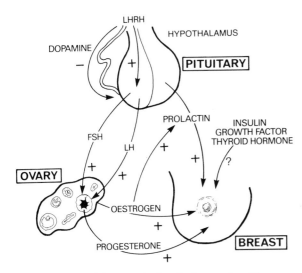

8.9 *Diagram of the control of prolactin secretion. The principal control is the tonic inhibitory effect of dopamine, but note that oestrogen acts to elevate prolactin levels. In practice, the relationships are more complicated than depicted in this simple diagram.*

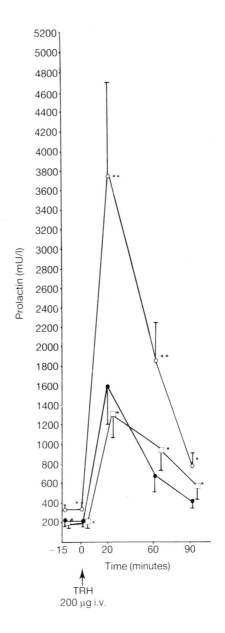

8.10 *Thyrotrophin-releasing hormone (TRH) test in women with cyclical and non-cyclical pain and controls. The cyclical mastalgia patients (O, n = 17) show a significantly increased peak release of prolactin at 20 minutes. The non-cyclical patients (□, n = 7) have a similar response to controls (●, n = 11). Values given are the mean ± 1 s.e.m. Mann–Whitney U test: ★p = non significant; ★★p < 0.05. (From Kumar et al[41], with permission of Cancer.)*

but recent work suggests that neural control of prolactin is extremely complex[39]. However, prolactin secretion by the pituitary can be stimulated by the use of thyrotrophin-releasing hormone (TRH) and domperidone. Both agents produce an immediate rise in serum prolactin in normals and test different sections of the control system, as TRH is directly stimulatory to the lactotrophs while domperidone antagonizes the inhibitory action of dopamine on prolactin secretion. Peters examined the stimulated prolactin response to TRH in a mixed group of benign disease patients and found the patients with mastodynia had a significantly greater rise in prolactin compared with controls[40]. We also examined the pituitary control of prolactin secretion in 17 patients with cyclical mastalgia compared with 11 controls and confirmed Peter's findings that the TRH-induced rise of prolactin is significantly greater at 20 minutes (Figure 8.10) and is maintained up to 60 minutes post-injection[41]. The basal prolactin levels were not significantly different between the groups. The enhanced prolactin response is also seen after domperidone administration (Figure 8.11), whereas the TSH response to TRH is not different between mastalgia patients and controls. These studies strongly suggest that there is a disturbance of hypothalamic control in women with cyclical mastalgia and this 'fine tuning' defect may be the primary problem in painful nodular breast disease. It is of interest that a similar defect has been demonstrated in the cyclical oedema syndrome, which has many similarities to cyclical mastalgia although they are distinct conditions[42].

Other Aetiological Theories

Other theories that have been put forward include the over-stimulation of breast cells due to interference with ATP degradation by methylxanthines consequent on high caffeine intake[43]. There is some biochemical evidence to support this contention, but caffeine intake appears to be much lower in British women and may not be relevant in the UK.

A recent hypothesis proposes an abnormality of prostaglandin synthesis secondary to deficient essential fatty acid (EFA) intake in the diet[44]. This is supported by circumstantial evidence that other stigmata of EFA deficiency such as increased sebum secretion are commoner in BBD patients[45]. The end result of EFA deficiency is postulated to be amplification of prolactin effects on breast

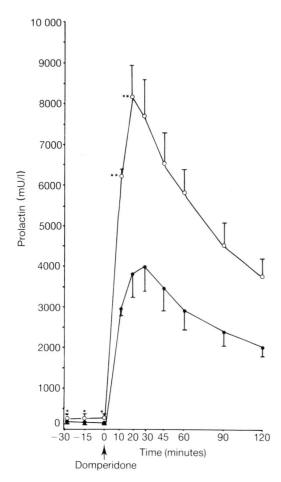

8.11 *Domperidone test in women with cyclical mastalgia (n = 12) compared with controls (n = 11). Domperidone 10 mg i.v. (bolus) gives a typical high peak of prolactin secretion but the cyclical mastalgia patients show a significantly higher peak prolactin release at 20 minutes. Values given are the mean ± 1 s.e.m. Mann–Whitney U test: *p = non-significant; **p < 0.002. (From Kumar et al[41], with permission of* Cancer.*)*

cells because of deficient production of prostaglandin E_1.

In summary, it is clear that the cherished and widely accepted hypotheses of neuroticism and general water retention have found little support in experimental results and modern work suggests that control mechanisms of pulsatile secretion of gonadotrophins and/or prolactin are abnormal in patients with painful nodular breasts. The possibility of an end-organ abnormality remains to be investigated in detail.

Management of Patients with Mastalgia and Nodularity of the Breast

The first consideration in management is the taking of a careful history and examination of the breast. If a dominant or discrete lump is present, management is as detailed in Chapter 5.

We are then left with the patients with mastalgia and nodularity and those with diffusely nodular breasts that are painless. The latter group requires no active treatment and can be discharged if there are no other indications for follow-up. The next section on therapy deals with patients with mastalgia and nodularity and the term 'mastalgia' is used to denote pain with or without nodularity.

Reassurance

For patients with mastalgia of whatever pattern, the first and most successful treatment is reassurance that their symptoms are not due to cancer. Geschickter stated that 'cancer should be excluded; rule out infection, reassure and give support' and Billroth emphasized that 'friendly advice, reassurance and the banishment of suspicion and fear of dread disease is of great importance'. These quotations have been emphasized because the manner of delivery and conviction of the reassurance is very important, as it is certainly true that many women consult surgeons about their mastalgia because they fear there is cancer in their breasts. Reassurance of these patients does not cure their breast pain but alters their attitude to the pain, so that it is no longer a serious problem. One of the difficulties with active reassurance is that many surgeons dislike using the term 'cancer' in the patient's presence (even when discussing the absence of the condition), and so resort to various euphemisms, which are open to misinterpretation. For example, the following statement of reassurance was actually made to a patient with painful nodularity: 'You have something in your breast; don't worry about it and as there is nothing I can do about it, there's no point in me seeing you again.'

Most clinicians can translate the phrase to: 'You have fibroadenosis (ANDI); it is harmless and the cause is unknown, but as I don't know of any useful treatment for the pain, I don't think you need to come to Outpatient's for a repeat visit.' However, the patient's translation was: 'I have cancer; it is incurable and the surgeon is abandoning me!'

These points are made to underline that sympathetic, detailed reassurance is required and in our Mastalgia Clinic we have successfully treated 85% of 600 mastalgia patients by simple reassurance.

Some clinicians agree with Geshickter's recommendation of support for the painful breast. We generally find that our patients with persistent mastalgia have already fitted themselves with the most comfortable brassière they could find. However, there is a report of the therapeutic value of a well-fitting brassière[46], although the placebo effect of fitting a specially designed brassière in the hospital must have played a considerable part in the good results obtained.

The next step in management is concerned with those patients who have been reassured, but still find that mastalgia is a considerable interference to their lives. This group, in our experience, is about 5% of the new patient referrals to a breast clinic and the mastalgia in this group may be so severe as to cause marital friction because the husband is unable to touch his wife's breasts for 3 weeks every month or children to hug their mother for similar reasons. Since there is no clear-cut diagnostic pathophysiology in mastalgia, hormonal investigations have little place in management apart from a routine prolactin level in cases with galactorrhoea or amenorrhoea, to exclude a prolactinoma. It should also be remembered that a common presentation of both mastalgia and amenorrhoea is pregnancy, but this should have been excluded by an accurate history.

The Contraceptive Pill and Mastalgia

The role of the 'Pill' in the epidemiology of breast cancer is hotly debated and, due to the long lag between hormonal events and breast cancer occurrence, the matter remains unresolved. However, in terms of BBD, most reports have indicated a *protective* effect[47, 48]. We have recorded the type of 'Pill' taken by our mastalgia patients but on analysis there are no correlations between pain patterns and brands. Some women may experience mastalgia for the first time on starting a new oral contraceptive but most mastalgia then tends to disappear or is minimal. If a patient has severe mastalgia that starts for the first time on commencing oral contraception, it is worth advising either a change to a lower dose or if already on a 30 μg Pill, a change to a different brand. Little is known of the exact effects of exogenous 'balanced' mixtures of oestrogens and progestogens as the recent controversy regarding the 'potency factors' of different progestogens has shown[49, 50]. If mastalgia remains a major problem, then occasionally a change to mechanical methods of contraception may be helpful, but there is no guarantee of response and the risks of an unwanted pregnancy are increased. In our experience, the severity of the mastalgia dictates whether the patient will readily agree to stop taking the Pill.

Postmenopausal replacement therapy using oestrogens is a well-known cause of mastalgia and is treatable by withdrawal of the offending hormone or substitution by a low dose combined preparation which will prevent unopposed oestrogen effects on the breast.

Drug Therapy for Mastalgia

The many different hypotheses of aetiology of BBD discussed in the previous section have given rise to a number of specific therapies which are perhaps more logical than the previous empirical treatments (Table 8.6). However, it is important to clearly distinguish between controlled and uncontrolled studies because there is a powerful placebo effect in subjective symptoms such as pain. Our benchmark for studies is the double-blind, placebo-controlled trial and we have used this technique in nearly all of our therapeutic studies.

Table 8.6 Mastalgia: aetiological hypotheses and treatments.

Hyperoestrogenism	Androgens/anti-oestrogens (tamoxifen)
Luteal insufficiency	Progesterone/progestogens
Hyperprolactinaemia	Bromocriptine (dopamine agonist)
Increased gonadotrophin	Danazol (antigonadotrophin)
Dietary methylxanthines	Caffeine restriction
Dietary essential fatty acids (EFA) deficiency	Evening primrose oil (EFA supplement)
Local inflammation or fibrosis	Local steroid injection
Miscellaneous	Pyridoxine/thyroid hormones/Vitamin A/hormone replacement therapy

Diuretics

One of the popular treatments, certainly among general practitioners, is the administration of diuretics. These have no rational basis as was demonstrated by the lack of correlation of retention of body water with symptoms[23] and, as no placebo-controlled trial has shown any beneficial effect, it is likely that their 'efficacy' in general practice is due to the placebo effect. Pain is the subjective symptom *par excellence*, and for this reason all studies in mastalgia should be at least placebo controlled and preferably randomized between the active and placebo therapies.

Progestogens

The luteal deficiency hypothesis, recently championed by Mauvais-Jarvis and his colleagues[31] had also been considered by earlier workers and attempts were made to correct the progesterone deficiency by administration of luteal extracts with varying success. The apparent demonstration by the Paris group of a definite progesterone deficiency in BBD did give rise to hopes that simple correction by progestogens would be useful. Indeed, it was reported by a Belgian group that this was the case[51], but this double-blind study only showed improvement in thermographic appearances and not in clinical findings. Also, as previously mentioned, other groups had failed to find a progesterone deficiency. The efficacy of progestogens thus remains an open question, and awaits a properly controlled trial of therapy, but progestogens have been compared with placebo in the premenstrual syndrome and failed to show any benefit greater than the placebo effect[52].

Bromocriptine

The discovery of a small elevation of basal prolactin in BBD[38] and the availability of a specific prolactin-lowering agent, bromocriptine, suggested that the first truly specific treatment for mastalgia was attainable. In fact, a report of the effectiveness of bromocriptine had already appeared describing a good response in 10 or 15 patients in an open study[53]. Soon afterwards a controlled study showed that the drug was effective in relieving breast swelling in patients with the premenstrual syndrome[54].

These encouraging results were tested in the Cardiff Mastalgia Clinic in a double-blind, placebo-controlled trial carried out on 53 patients using a bromocriptine dosage of 2.5 mg twice daily[55]. Assessment of response, which had been sketchy with the previous two bromocriptine trials, was improved by using a simple scale for the clinician's assessment, and a subjective, self-rating visual linear analogue scale (VLA) for the patient's response (Figure 8.12). The VLA scales were completed independently of the clinician's assessment. Unlike the previous studies, the patients were randomized into their respective pain patterns to see if any pattern responded preferentially. The results of this trial showed that the cyclical pattern of pain was significantly reduced by bromocriptine compared with placebo but the non-cyclical pattern failed to respond (Figure 8.13). This trial demonstrated for the first time that patients classified according to a simple symptomatic classification responded differentially to a precise manipulation of the pituitary output of prolactin. Blood sampling during the trial confirmed the depression of prolactin levels on bromocriptine to subnormal levels as these patients were initially normoprolactinaemic as expected.

It is currently not understood how lowering of prolactin levels produces amelioration of mastalgia, but the mechanism is presumed to be due to a reduction in the overall stimulation of breast cells by prolactin, because it is known that bromocriptine does not lower sex steroid levels. When the data on serum prolactin levels were analysed to see if there was a correlation between amount of depression and symptom improve-

ment, no correlation could be found. This suggests that the effects may be more complicated than was first thought. As bromocriptine is a dopamine agonist, it is possible that there is a direct effect on breast tissue, independent of prolactin effects, if breast cells have dopamine receptors similar to those found on pituitary cells. However, recent studies in our laboratories have failed to detect dopamine receptors on human breast cells grown in monolayer culture.

Confirmation of the Cardiff results has come from other controlled trials[56-59], and it is clear from review of the literature that this drug is consistently effective in reducing the symptoms of mastalgia[60]. The problem with bromocriptine is that some women experience severe side-effects, the commonest being nausea, vomiting and dizziness, which have caused a 20% drop-out rate in many trials. The severity of side-effects can be reduced by introducing the drug slowly in an incremental scheme and avoiding doses higher than 2.5 mg twice daily (Table 8.7). The incidence of side-effects is variable and some women have no problems even at high dosage.

Danazol

Danazol was introduced in 1971 by Greenblatt who suggested it may have a role in mastalgia[61]. This agent, like bromocriptine, is unique in its

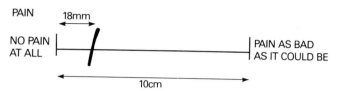

8.12 *A typical visual linear analogue (VLA) scale. The patient has made a mark 18 mm from the 'no pain' end and so a reading of 18 is obtained. This scale is sometimes known as an LAS scale (linear analogue scale).*

8.13 *VLA results of the Cardiff controlled trial of bromocriptine in mastalgia. Note the placebo response in both cyclical and non-cyclical patients, but the significantly lower scores, i.e. improvement, on bromocriptine in the cyclical patients. (From Mansel et al[55], with permission of the British Journal of Surgery.)*

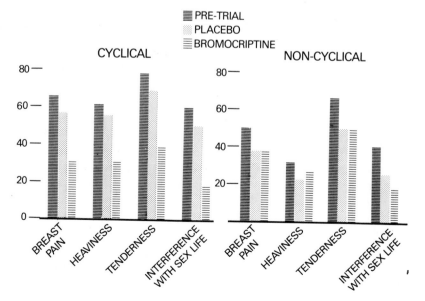

Table 8.7 Recommended incremental dosage scheme for bromocriptine therapy.

Days	Dose
1–3	1.25 mg at night with food
4–7	2.5 mg at night with food
8–11	1.25 mg in the morning and 2.5 mg at night (with food)
12 onwards	2.5 mg in the morning and 2.5 mg at night (with food)

action on the pituitary–ovarian axis. It was originally described as an impeded androgen and in monkeys it was shown to act as an antigonadotrophin, as it depressed serum FSH and LH and prevented ovulation. Its action in humans is not so clearly defined because it only interferes with FSH and LH levels at high dosage. It may have a local tissue effect as it has been shown to bind to both progesterone and androgen receptors but not to oestrogen receptors.

Greenblatt's group initially used the drug for treating endometriosis but a number of papers soon followed from the same group showing the usefulness of danazol in painful nodular breast disease[62, 63]. All these reports were of uncontrolled studies and appeared to be cumulative, and were thus open to the criticisms of lack of placebo control. We therefore carried out a double-blind placebo study in the Cardiff Mastalgia Clinic on 28 patients with cyclical mastalgia, using a detailed protocol similar to that described earlier[64]. This study showed that danazol was clearly beneficial in cyclical mastalgia producing both relief of symptoms and reduction in nodularity and these effects could be obtained with doses as low as 200 mg. The lower dose gave much lower side-effects and only a 10% drop-out rate was recorded in the trial. The hormonal effects of danazol treatment were a low luteal progesterone (suggesting anovulation) and an unchanged prolactin, so it appears the drug is working on the ovary or pituitary although only 30% of these patients were amenorrhoeic on the drug. The side-effects are mainly amenorrhoea, the incidence of which increases with dose up to 100% at 600–800 mg and various mild androgenic effects such as weight gain, acne and hirsutism. All of these effects are dose related and can be minimized by low dose therapy. Our current practice is to start at 200 mg daily and then use a maintenance dose of 100 mg daily on alternate days. A recently reported side-effect has been a lowering of the voice pitch which has been permanent in a small number of cases, but our experience is that only 5% of patients notice this symptom and it is generally reversible on stopping the drug. Danazol currently appears to be the best agent for severe

breast pain and nodularity with an overall improvement rate of 70% in our total group of 291 treated patients. Another double-blind, controlled study from Nottingham reported that danazol was superior to bromocriptine for cyclical breast pain[65].

Evening Primrose Oil

The fatty acid deficiency hypothesis has led to the testing of treatment by supplementing the diet with an essential fatty acid (EFA). One promising preparation is the oil of evening primrose (EPO) which is unique in containing 7% γ-linolenic acid and 72% linoleic acid and represents the richest natural source of EFAs known (Figure 8.14). A two-centre trial on 100 patients has suggested the compound may be useful for treating mild cases of cyclical mastalgia[66]. This agent is potentially useful in mild to moderate cases as it has virtually no side-effects. Patient acceptance is high as it is viewed as a 'natural substance' rather than a hormone or drug. Interestingly, the EPO trial also showed that non-cyclical pain was unresponsive to this therapy, as had been found in the bromocriptine trial. Further EPO trials to confirm these findings are currently underway.

Tamoxifen

The anti-oestrogen, tamoxifen was reported to be helpful in mastalgia in an Italian study[67], but this drug is currently only licensed for the treatment of breast cancer in the UK. A recent double-blind study of tamoxifen in Guy's Hospital showed that tamoxifen 10 mg daily significantly improved mastalgia. Side-effects were reported to be 'minimal', but in this study about 15% of the patients dropped out on therapy[68]. A potential problem of tamoxifen therapy in premenopausal women is an elevation of serum oestradiol on tamoxifen, although this was not found by Ricciardi and Ianniruberto[67]. A further problem has been raised by a recent toxicology study which showed that a small number of rats developed

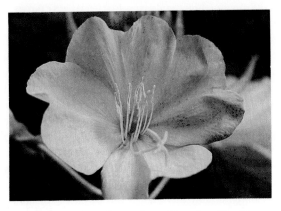

8.14 *The evening primrose flower (Oenothara biennis).*

liver tumours on high dose tamoxifen. The current recommendation of both the manufacturers and the Committee of Safety of Medicines is that tamoxifen should only be used in patients with malignant disease.

Other Therapeutic Approaches

The evidence for many other varied therapeutic approaches is generally poor and it is likely that the results reported are due to the placebo effect. The caffeine/methylxanthine theory suggests that withdrawal of dietary coffee, cola and chocolate would help the symptoms of BBD and this has been found in an open study by Minton et al[69]. The methylxanthine intake varies between different cultures and a proper trial of withdrawal of a dietary substance is difficult to control so these results need further study. However, if a patient was found to be drinking in excess of 10 cups of coffee each day, it would be worth changing to decaffeinated coffee, but this level of consumption in the UK is uncommon. The caffeine methylxanthine hypothesis has been challenged by several different investigators. Two case control studies, one of histologically diagnosed benign breast disease and one of fibrocystic disease, both failed to show any association with coffee consumption[70, 71]. A randomized trial of caffeine reduction with non-blind assessment showed some reduction in breast nodularity in the coffee abstaining group, but the changes were minor and there was no correlation of palpable nodularity at entry to the study with coffee consumption at that time[72].

A small number of studies have suggested that pyridoxine (vitamin B_6) may be useful in treating mastalgia on the basis that pyridoxine will enhance the decarboxylation of dopa to dopamine and so inhibit prolactin levels. Most studies have been uncontrolled and further it has been shown that pyridoxine treatment does not lower serum prolactin in patients with the amenorrhoea–galactorrhoea syndrome[73]. In contradistinction, a recent study has shown that pyridoxine lowers exercise-induced prolacin secretion[74]. A recent double-blind study using pyridoxine at a dose of 200 mg daily in cyclical mastalgia found that the vitamin did not significantly improve breast pain compared with placebo[75].

Other studies of vitamin A administration and treatment with thyroid hormone[76] have been reported to show improvement of mastalgia, but the studies were open and involved a small number of heterogeneous patients and are thus difficult to interpret.

Treatment of Non-cyclical Mastalgia

All the above treatments have been directed at the cyclical group of patients whether the authors have realized this or not, but our studies suggest that the cyclical group appears to have an endocrine basis and, in turn, appears to respond to endocrine-directed therapy. It also seems that the non-cyclical group appears to be unresponsive to manipulation of the endocrine system but this may be due to the aetiology of non-cyclical pain being an inflammatory process rather than an endocrine imbalance, a concept which is also supported by the pre- and postmenopausal distribution of cases.

In view of this, attempts have been made to treat the non-cyclical group with non-steroidal anti-inflammatory agents but there is no published evidence of their efficacy. Our experience of non-steroidal anti-inflammatory drugs is similarly disappointing. As an extension of this approach, Crile suggested that a local injection of lignocaine and prednisolone may be effective in relieving the localized non-cyclical pain[77]. His description corresponds to the 'trigger spot' subgroup mentioned previously and he found the steroid/local anaesthetic injection gave initial relief in two-thirds of the patients with continued relief in about one half of the patients followed. Our recent experience has shown better results; we have obtained a 70% response rate. We have also considered excision for this group of patients even where no obvious palpable abnormality was present at the site of complaint, which is the usual situation. We have chosen our cases for excision after at least three repeat visits to the clinic have revealed the site of the complaint to be constant and pressure on the indicated area mimics the pain. Excision of these 'trigger spots' has again given relief in 50% of patients. Histology of the excised breast has not shown any specific histological changes.

Surgical excision

More extensive surgical excision for mastalgia as a symptom is uncommon but prophylactic excision for premalignant disease has been performed more commonly and is considered in Chapter 4. For most types of mastalgia, except the trigger spot mentioned above, the symptom is so widespread that segmental resection is insufficient. Thus most surgeons have used subcutaneous mastectomy, or total mastectomy in earlier times. Most of these operations are carried out for 'prophylaxis' of breast cancer by plastic surgeons and documentation of the numbers and results of operations performed solely for mastalgia is very poor, although nearly all authors list mastalgia as an indication for the operation. In the Nottingham Breast Clinic, only four patients underwent subcutaneous mastectomies for mastalgia in 12 years but only two patients obtained relief of their symptoms and a further patient developed a fibrous capsule requiring removal of the prosthesis[17]. Our experience of a small number of cases is that the operation rarely cures mastalgia and this impression is confirmed by discussion with colleagues. In addition, we are reluctant to perform this operation because previous papers have understated the complications of the procedure, which are in fact numerous both in the early postoperative period and in the long term. Particularly troublesome is the fibrous contraction that occurs around implants, especially if they are placed subcutaneously (Figure 8.15). Additionally, nipple or areolar necrosis and infection of the prosthesis are not uncommon. Our view is that this operation is rarely indicated for breast pain because it has a low chance of therapeutic success and a high incidence of complications. A review of the detailed results of this operation performed for mastalgia is urgently needed but perhaps the paucity of published figures reflects other surgeons disquiet about this operation for this indication.

Natural History of Mastalgia

One of the problems of therapeutic trials in mastalgia is that the natural history of the condition is poorly documented. Because spontaneous remissions can occur, these may give a false impression of treatment benefit. Geschickter briefly described some features of the natural history of his mastodynia cases and noted that the majority found relief of pain at the menopause.

In an effort to correct this lack of knowledge, we undertook a review of all our mastalgia cases documented between 1973 and 1976 in the Cardiff Mastalgia Clinic[78]. There were a total of 258 patients and a follow-up of 66% was obtained by direct interview or postal questionnaire. Details regarding the duration of pain and spontaneous remission were obtained. The results showed that cyclical pain was most commonly relieved by hormonal events such as pregnancy and the menopause but this was not the case with non-cyclical pain. It also appeared that patients with cyclical pain who started having symptoms at an early age (< 20 years), tended to have persistent pain often throughout reproductive life, whereas a late age of onset was associated with a shorter overall duration of pain. This implies that younger patients may require treatment for prolonged periods as we had previously found that post-treatment recurrence of pain is common. In view of these findings, we aim to treat young patients with sèvere mastalgia in short intermittent bursts rather than continuous periods. However, patients near the menopause may be treated for longer periods in the expectation that their pain will be naturally resolved in the near future by their menopause.

It should be noted that patients investigated in the Mastalgia Clinic were by definition severe cases of long duration, so these findings do not apply to the many women who develop mild to moderate mastalgia in the fourth and fifth decades. In many of these patients, natural remission occurs within a few months.

Recommended Management

Our detailed management protocol and experience of treatment in nearly 300 mastalgia patients has been published recently[79]. The important points are shown in Table 8.8. The first priority is exclusion of cancer by appropriate tests and firm reassurance of the patient. This will be adequate treatment for around 85% of patients with mastalgia presenting to hospital and probably higher in general practice.

The 15% of mastalgia patients with severe mastalgia who are not helped by reassurance should then be assessed initially by a pain chart to define the pain pattern to give a base-line

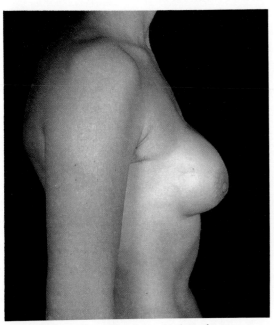

8.15 *Patient with a subcutaneous implant after subcutaneous mastectomy for benign breast disease. The breast is hard to palpation and projects rigidly from the chest wall.*

Table 8.8 Principles of mastalgia treatment.

1. Exclude cancer
2. Reassurance
3. Define pattern (pain chart or history)
4. Cyclical mastalgia (overall response 80%)
   (a) Evening primrose oil 6 capsules daily
   (b) Danazol 100–300 mg daily then reduce
   (c) Bromocriptine 1.25 mg increasing to 3.75–5 mg daily
5. Non-cyclical mastalgia (overall response 45%)
   (a) Danazol
   (b) Evening primrose oil
   (c) Bromocriptine
   (d) Lignocaine/steroid injection to trigger spots and Tietze's syndrome

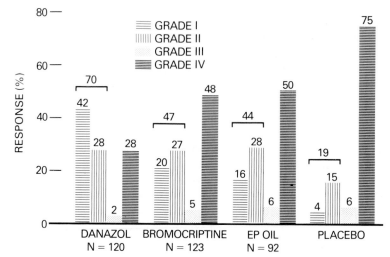

measurement of the number of days pain per cycle. Patients who are still troubled by their mastalgia after 2–3 months of charting (to allow for spontaneous remission) should be treated by one of the three main agents.

Cyclical Pain

Our current first choice is evening primrose oil as it has a reasonable response and is almost free of side-effects. In addition it does not interfere with the menstrual cycle – however, a major disadvantage is that it currently is not available on prescription and the patient will have to purchase her own supply. The next drug which we use is danazol which clearly has the best response rate overall (around 80%) but has definite side-effects (Table 8.9), especially on the menstrual cycle. However, low dose maintenance regimens of danazol using 25 or 50 mg per day have much lower side-effects. The next agent we use is bromocriptine which has an efficacy midway between danazol and evening primrose oil (Figure 8.16), but also gives side-effects in some 20% of patients (Table 8.9), principally nausea and dizziness. The drug does not disturb the menstrual

cycle and this is a positive advantage to some patients. Our review of treatment has shown that failure of response to one drug does not predict subsequent failure on another drug, so it is worth trying all three drugs in turn in an individual before concluding that the mastalgia is unresponsive.

Non-cyclical Pain

The overall response to the three principal drug therapies is much lower in non-cyclical patients at around 45%. The order of efficacy of the agents is still danazol, bromocriptine and evening primrose oil (Figure 8.17); because the response rates are so much lower, we would recommend using danazol first as this appears to offer the best chance of response. Again it is worth trying the other agents in turn, but the evidence from the controlled studies shows that both bromocriptine and evening primrose oil effects are equivalent to placebo in non-cyclical patients.

8.16 *The overall response rates of the Cardiff Mastalgia Clinic for treatment of cyclical mastalgia with danazol, bromocriptine, evening primrose oil and placebo. Grade I = no symptoms; grade II = substantial improvement in symptoms but some residual pain; grade III = poor response with substantial residual pain; grade IV = no response. The figures above each histogram are percentages.*

8.17 *The overall response rates of the Cardiff Mastalgia Clinic for treatment of non-cyclical pain with danazol, bromocriptine, evening primrose oil and placebo. Grades are as in Figure 8.16.*

Table 8.9 Side-effects of the principal therapies.

Therapy	Common side-effects	Incidence(%)
Danazol 100–400 mg	Weight gain Acne Amenorrhoea Hirsutism Reduction in breast size Voice change	25
Bromocriptine 2.5 mg twice daily	Nausea Dizziness Headache	20
Evening primrose oil 6 capsules daily	Mild nausea	<2

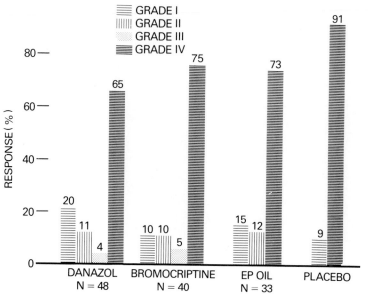

The use of local anaesthetic and steroid injection in non-cyclical mastalgia is well worth while if a persistent localized painful area can be demonstrated on repeat visits to the clinic. We use Depo-Medrone with Lidocaine injection (Upjohn) which contains methylprednisolone 40 mg and lignocaine (lidocaine) hydrochloride 10 mg/ml. The localized tender area is marked and 1 ml of the injection is carefully infiltrated at the level of the pectoral fascia. (The injection should not be subcutaneous as this will cause skin atrophy.) The only side-effect is mild local discomfort but this is quickly relieved by the local anaesthetic. Care should be exercised to make sure the injection is not too deep as we have seen one small pneumothorax following an injection into the axillary tail.

Choice of Drug with Regard to Side-effects

The choice of drug should be generally as recommended in Table 8.8 but the attitude of the patient may indicate the final choice. Patients who are fertile must take mechanical precautions against pregnancy if taking bromocriptine or danazol as both of these agents are potentially teratogenic and may interfere with concomitant oral contraception pills. Thus, a patient who is unable or refuses to use barrier contraception should be treated with evening primrose oil, which can be taken with the oral contraceptive. If patients dislike the idea of drug-induced amenorrhoea, the choice of agents will be between evening primrose oil or bromocriptine, neither of which alters the menstrual cycle. These choices are illustrated in the flow diagram in Figure 8.18.

Length of Drug Treatment

It appears from our studies that the good response obtained with most of the endocrine treatments was short lived, as might be expected if the postulated endocrine defect is long term. In the danazol trial, recurrence of symptoms was appearing after 3 months placebo treatment (Figure 8.19). We have found that about one-half of the patients have recurrent mastalgia at 6 months but some of these had milder pain than before. Other authors have similar experience[80]. Our current policy is to treat for 3 months initially and then discontinue the drug to see if symptoms recur. Of the 50% that do recur, some will not require further therapy as the pain is milder but the severe recurrences can be put back onto the original therapy if there had been a previous good

8.18 *A flow diagram of the management of mastalgia.*

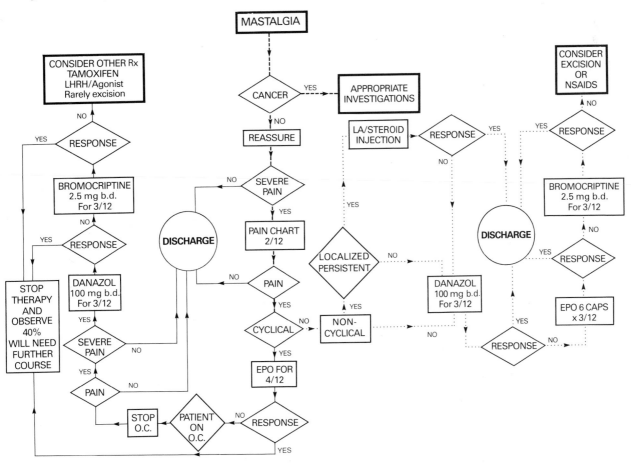

response, or on to an alternative if the initial response had been poor[79]. (This change of therapy often had occurred already, if the response had been poor.) These short treatment bursts limit drug costs and may be less suppressive to the pituitary–ovarian axis than continuous treatment, although studies of long-term usage and high dosage in both bromocriptine and danazol have not indicated any permanent suppression.

Conclusions

The series of detailed studies in the Cardiff Mastalgia Clinic have shown that the cyclical patients, defined by simple criteria, are different fom the non-cyclical on pituitary function testing and in response to two different endocrine drug treatments involving prolactin modulation. These studies provide powerful circumstantial evidence that prolactin is implicated in the genesis of

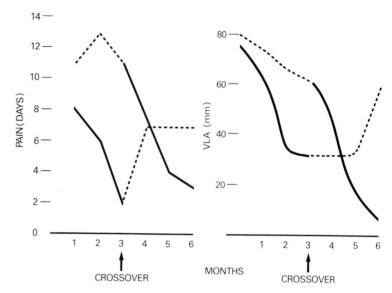

8.19 *The results of the Cardiff danazol trial for days of pain and VLA scores for tenderness. Note that symptoms return after 1–3 months when the patients took placebo (----) after a course of danazol (——).*

human breast pain and nodularity. The non-cyclical group remains enigmatic and difficult to treat effectively.

REFERENCES

1. Nichols S., Waters W. E. & Wheeler M. J. Management of female breast disease by Southampton General Practitioners. *British Medical Journal* 1980; **281**: 1450–1453.

2. Roberts M. M., Elton R. A., Robinson S. E. & French K. Consultations for breast disease in general practice and hospital referral patterns. *British Journal of Surgery* 1987; **74**: 1020–1022.

3. Birkett J. *The Diseases of the Breast and their Treatment.* London, Longman, Brown, Green and Longmans, 1850, p 164.

4. Cheatle G. L. & Cutler M. *Tumours of the Breast.* London, Edward Arnold and Co., 1931.

5. Atkins H. J. B. Chronic mastitis. *Lancet* 1938; **i**: 707–712.

6. Patey D. H. Two common non-malignant conditions of the breast. *British Medical Journal,* 1949; **i**: 96–99.

7. Geschickter C. F. Mastodynia (painful breasts). In: *Diseases of the Breast,* 2nd edn. Philadelphia, J. B. Lippincott Co. 1945, p 183.

8. Semb C. Pathologico-anatomical and clinical investigations of fibro-adenomatosis cystica mammae and its relation to other pathological conditions in mamma, especially cancer. *Acta Chirurgica Scandinavia* 1928; **64** (suppl. 10): 1–484.

9. Smallwood J. A., Kye D. A. & Taylor I. Mastalgia: is this commonly associated with operable breast cancer? *Annals of the Royal College of Surgeons* 1986; **68**: 262.

10. Leinster S. J., Whitehouse G. H. & Walsh P. V. Cyclical mastalgia: clinical and mammographic observations in a screened population. *British Journal of Surgery* 1987; **74**: 220–222.

11. Preece P. E., Baum M., Mansel R. E. *et al.* The importance of mastalgia in operable breast cancer. *British Medical Journal* 1982; **284**: 1299–1300.

12. River L., Silverstein J., Grout J. *et al.* Carcinoma of the breast: the diagnostic significance of pain. *American Journal of Surgery* 1951; **82**: 733–735.

13. Haagensen C. D. *Diseases of the Breast,* 3rd edn. London, W. B. Saunders, 1986, p 502.

14. The Yorkshire Breast Cancer Group. Symptoms and signs of operable breast cancer. *British Journal of Surgery* 1983; **70**: 350.

15. Preece P. E., Hughes L. E., Mansel R. E., Baum M., Bolton P. M. & Gravelle I. H. Clinical syndromes of mastalgia. *Lancet* 1976; **ii**: 670–673.

16. Bishop H. M. & Blamey R. W. A suggested classification of breast pain. *Postgraduate Medical Journal* 1979; **55**: 59–60.

17. Dowle C. S. Breast pain: classification, aetiology and management. *Australia and New Zealand Journal of Surgery* 1987; **57**: 423–428.

18. Tietze A. A peculiar accumulation of cases with dystrophy of the cartilages of the ribs. *Berliner Klinische Wochenschrift* 1921; **30**: 829–831.

19. La Ban M. M., Meerschaert R. & Taylor S. Breast pain: a symptom of cervical radioculopathy. *Archives of Physical and Medical Rehabilitation* 1979; **60**: 315.

20. Cooper A. *Illustrations of the Diseases of the Breast.* Part 1. London: Longman, Rees, Orme, Brown and Green, 1829, p 76.

21. Jeffcoate N. *Principles of Gynaecology,* 4th edn. London, Butterworths, 1975, p 550.

22. Israel S. L. *Menstrual Disorders and Sterility,* 5th edn. New York, Harper and Row, 1967, p 160.

23. Preece P. E., Richards A. R., Owen G. M. & Hughes L. E. Mastalgia and total body water. *British Medical Journal* 1975; **iv**: 498–500.

24. Ingelby H. & Gershon-Cohen J. (Eds.) *Comparative Anatomy, Pathology and Roentgenology of the Breast.* Philadelphia, University of Pennsylvania Press, 1960.

25. Milligan D., Drife J. O. & Short R. V. Changes in breast volume during normal menstrual cycle and after oral contraceptives. *British Medical Journal* 1976; iv: 494–496.

26. Crown S. & Crisp A. H. A short clinical diagnostic self-rating scale for psychoneurotic patients: the Middlesex Hospital questionnaire (MHQ). *Journal of Psychology* 1966; 112: 917–923.

27. Preece P. E., Mansel R. E. & Hughes L. E. Mastalgia: psychoneurosis or organic disease? *British Medical Journal* 1978; i: 29–30.

28. Swain M. C., Hayward J. L. & Bulbrook R. D. Plasma oestradiol and progesterone in benign breast disease. *European Journal of Cancer* 1973; 9: 553–556.

29. England P. C., Skinner L. G., Cottrell K. M. & Sellwood R. A. Serum oestradiol-17β in women with benign and malignant breast disease. *British Journal of Cancer* 1974; 30: 571–576.

30. Malarkey W. B., Schroeder L. L., Stevens V. C., James A. G. & Lanese R. R. Twenty four hour preoperative endocrine profiles in women with benign and malignant breast disease. *Cancer Research* 1977; 37: 4655–4659.

31. Sitruk-Ware R., Sterkers N. & Mauvais-Jarvis P. Benign breast disease. I: Hormonal investigation. *Obstetrics and Gynecology* 1979; 53: 457–460.

32. Walsh P. V., Bulbrook R. D., Stell P. M., Wang D. Y., McDicken I. W. & George W. D. Serum progesterone concentration during the luteal phase in women with benign breast disease. *European Journal of Cancer and Clinical Oncology* 1984; 20: 1339–1343.

33. Preece P. E. A study of the aetiology, clinical patterns and treatment of mastalgia. MD Thesis, University of Wales, 1982, pp 94–124.

34. Kumar S., Mansel R. E., Wilson D. W., Read G. F., Truran P. L., Hughes L. E. & Griffiths K. Daily salivary progesterone levels in cyclical mastalgia patients and their controls. *British Journal of Surgery* 1986; 73: 260–263.

35. Read G. F., Bradley J. A., Wilson D. W., George W. D. & Griffiths K. Evaluation of luteal-phase salivary progesterone levels in women with benign breast disease or primary breast cancer. *European Journal of Clinical Oncology* 1985; 21: 9–17.

36. Wang D. Y. & Fentiman I. S. Epidemiology and endocrinology of benign breast disease. *Breast Cancer Research and Treatment* 1985; 6: 5–36.

37. Nokin J., Vekemans M. & L'Hermite M. Circadian periodicity of serum prolactin concentration in Man. *British Medical Journal* 1972; 3: 561–562.

38. Cole E. N., Sellwood R. A., England P. C. & Griffiths K. Serum prolactin concentrations in benign breast disease throughout the menstrual cycle. *European Journal of Cancer* 1977; 13: 597–603.

39. Lancranjan I. & Friesen H. G. The neural regulation of prolactin secretion. In: Veale W. L. & Lederis K. (eds) *Current Studies of Hypothalamic Function*, Vol 1. Basel, S. Karger, 1978, p 131.

40. Peters F., Pickardt C. R., Zimmerman G. & Breckwoldt M. PRL, TSH and thyroid hormones in benign breast disease. *Klinische Wochenschrift* 1981; 59: 403–407.

41. Kumar S., Mansel R. E., Hughes L. E., Woodhead J. S., Edwards C. A., Scanlon M. F. & Newcombe R. G. Prolactin response to thyrotropin-releasing hormone stimulation and dopaminergic inhibition in benign breast disease. *Cancer* 1984; 53: 1311–1315.

42. Young J. B., Brownjohn A. M., Chapman C. & Lee M. R. Evidence for a hypothalamic disturbance in cyclical oedema. *British Medical Journal* 1983; 286: 1691–1693.

43. Minton J. P., Abou-Issa H., Reiches N. & Roseman J. M. Clinical and biochemical studies in methylxanthine-related fibrocystic breast disease. *Surgery* 1981; 90: 299–304.

44. Horrobin D. F. Cellular basis of prolactin action: Involvement of cyclical nucleotides polyamines, prostaglandins, steroids, thyroid hormones, Na/K ATPases and calcium: relevance to breast cancer and the menstrual cycle. *Medical Hypotheses* 1979; 5: 599–614.

45. Goolmali S. K, & Shuster S. A sebotrophic stimulus in benign and malignant breast disease. *Lancet* 1975; i: 428.

46. Wilson M. C. & Sellwood R. A. Therapeutic value of a supporting brassiere in mastodynia. *British Medical Journal* 1976; ii: 90.

47. Ory H., Cole P. & MacMahon B. Oral contraceptives and reduced risk of benign breast diseases. *New England Journal of Medicine* 1976; 294: 419–422.

48. Royal College of General Practitioners Study. *British Medical Journal* 1981; 282: 2089–2093.

49. Pike M. C., Henderson B. E., Krilo M. D. *et al.* Breast cancer in young women and use of oral contraceptives: Possible modifying effect of formulation and age at use. *Lancet* 1983; ii: 926–929.

50. Anderson T. J. Mitotic and apoptotic response of breast tissue to oral contraceptives. *Lancet* 1984; i: 99–100.

51. Colin C., Gaspard U. & Lambotte R. Relationships of mastodynia with its endocrine environment and treatment in a double blind trial with lynestrenol. *Archiv für Gynaekologie* 1978; 225: 7–13.

52. Day J. B. Clinical Trials in the premenstrual syndrome. *Current Medical Research and Opinion* 1979; 6 (Suppl 5): 40–45.

53. Schulz K. D., Del Pozo E., Lose K. H., Kunzig H. J. & Geiger W. Successful treatment of mastodynia with the prolactin inhibitor bromocriptine (CB 154). *Archiv für Gynaekologie* 1975; 220: 83–87.

54. Bendek-Jaszmann L. J. & Hearn-Sturtevant M. D. Premenstrual tension and functional infertility. *Lancet* 1976; i: 1095–1098.

55. Mansel R. E., Preece P. E. & Hughes L. E. A double blind trial of the prolactin inhibitor bromocriptine in painful benign breast disease. *British Journal of Surgery* 1978; 65: 724–727.

56. Blichert-Toft M., Anderson A. N., Henriksen O. B. & Mygind T. Treatment of mastalgia with bromocriptine. A double blind crossover study. *British Medical Journal* 1979; 1: 237.

57. Montgomery A. C. V., Palmer B. V., Biswas S. & Monteiro J. C. M. P. Treatment of severe cyclical mastalgia. *Journal of the Royal Society*

of Medicine 1979; **72**: 489.

58. Durning P. & Sellwood R. A. Bromocriptine in severe cyclical breast pain. *British Journal of Surgery* 1982; **69**: 248–249.

59. Mussa A. & Dogliotti L. Treatment of benign breast disease with bromocriptine. *Journal of Endocrinology* Invest 1979; **2**: 87–91.

60. Mansel R. E. A review of the role of bromocriptine in symptomatic benign breast disease. *Research Clinical Forum* 1981; **3**: 61–65.

61. Greenblatt R. B., Dmowski W. P., Mahesh V. B., Scholer H. F. L. Clinical studies with an antigonadotrophin–Danazol. *Fertility and Sterility* 1971; **22**: 102–112.

62. Asch R. H. & Greenblatt R. B. The use of an impeded androgen-Danazol in the management of benign breast disorders. *American Journal of Obstetrics and Gynecology* 1977; **127**: 130–134.

63. Greenblatt R. B., Nezhat C. & Ben-Nun I. The treatment of benign breast disease with danazol. *Fertility and Sterility* 1980; **34**: 242–245.

64. Mansel R. E., Wisbey J. R. & Hughes L. E. Controlled trial of the antigonadotrophin danazol in painful nodular benign breast disease. *Lancet* 1982; **i**: 928–931.

65. Hinton C. P., Bishop H. M., Holliday H. W., Doyle P. J. & Blamey R. W. A double blind controlled trial of danazol and bromocriptine in the management of severe cyclical breast pain. *British Journal of Clinical Practice* 1986; **40**: 326–330.

66. Pashby N. L., Mansel R. E., Hughes L. E., Hanslip J. & Preece P. E. A clinical trial of evening primrose oil in mastalgia. *British Journal of Surgery* 1981; **68**: 801.

67. Ricciardi I. & Ianniruberto A. Tamoxifen induced regression of benign breast lesions. *Obstetrics and Gynecology* 1979; **54**: 80–84.

68. Fentiman I. S., Caleffi M., Brame K., Chaudary M. A. & Hayward J. L. Double blind controlled trial of tamoxifen therapy for mastalgia. *Lancet* 1986; **i**: 287–288.

69. Minton J. P., Foecking M. K., Webster D. J. T. & Mathews R. H. Response of fibrocystic disease to caffeine withdrawal and correlation of cyclic nucleotides with breast disease. *American Journal of Obstetrics and Gynecology* 1979; **135**: 157–158.

70. Lubin F., Ron E., Wax Y., Black M., Furano M. & Skitrit A. A case control study of caffeine and methylaxanthines in benign breast disease. *Journal of the American Medical Association* 1985; **253**: 2388–2392.

71. Heyden S. & Fodor J. G. Coffee consumption and fibrocystic breasts: an unlikely association. *Canadian Journal of Surgery* 1986; **29**: 208–211.

72. Ernster V. L., Mason L., Goodson W. H. *et al.* Effects of caffeine-free diet on benign breast disease: a randomised trial. *Surgery* 1982; **91**: 263–267.

73. Lehtovirta P., Ranta T. & Seppala M. Pyridoxine treatment of galactorrhoea–amenorrhoea syndromes. *Acta Endocrinologica* 1978; **87**: 682–686.

74. Moretti C., Fabri A., Gressi L., Bonifacio V., Fracoli A. & Isidori A. Pyridoxine (B6) suppresses the rise in prolactin and increases the rise in growth hormone induced by exercise. *New England Journal of Medicine* 1982; **307**: 444.

75. Smallwood J., A-Kye D. & Taylor I. Vitamin B6 in the treatment of premenstrual mastalgia. *British Journal of Clinical Practice* 1986; **40**: 532–533.

76. Estes N. C. Mastodynia due to fibrocystic disease of the breast controlled with thyroid hormone. *American Journal of Surgery* 1981; **142**: 764–766.

77. Crile G. Injection of steroids in painful breasts. *American Journal of Surgery* 1977; **133**: 705.

78. Wisbey J. R., Kumar S., Mansel R. E., Preece P. E., Pye J. K. & Hughes L. E. Natural history of breast pain. *Lancet* 1983; **ii**: 672–674.

79. Pye J. K., Mansel R. E. & Hughes L. E. Clinical experience of drug treatments for mastalgia. *Lancet* 1985; **ii**: 373–377.

80. Rasmussen T., Doberl A., Rannevik G. & Tobiassen T. The Hjorring project on fibrocystic breast disease. In: Baum M., George W. D. & Hughes L. E. (eds) *Benign Breast Disease.* London, Royal Society of Medicine Symposium Series, 1984, p 135.

9　Cysts of the Breast

Cysts are the commonest abnormality found in patients presenting to a breast clinic – a fact of little surprise since it has been estimated that 7% of all women will develop a symptomatic breast cyst during their reproductive life.

Like many other breast lesions, cysts were described by Sir Astley Cooper in 1831[1]. The French surgeon, Reclus, provided a comprehensive account in 1883[2] – an account so accurate that the disease is still known by his name among French surgeons. Bloodgood[3] has achieved surgical immortality more easily than most with his attention-catching description of the 'blue-domed cysts' which bear his name.

A very large majority of breast cysts are a manifestation of ANDI – an aberration of normal lobular involution as described in Chapters 1 and 3. Unless otherwise specified, this chapter refers to these lesions. Less common forms of cysts are shown in Table 9.1.

The reasons for regarding this as an aberration of normal involution, and therefore part of the spectrum of ANDI, have been set out in Chapter 3. Haagensen[4] uses the term 'cystic disease' to include other elements of ANDI such as mastalgia and cyclical nodularity, but this can further confuse the issue, and it is preferable to consider each aspect separately. The management of macroscopic cysts is specific to that clinical presentation and unrelated to the other elements of ANDI.

Pathology

The pathology of breast cysts was only too familiar to surgeons when biopsy excision was the standard management of all cysts. Now the surgical trainee brought up on needle aspiration will see only the small cysts encountered by chance during breast surgery. These vary in size from those just visible to the naked eye to others up to 4–5 mm in diameter. They often occur in a cluster over an area 2–3 cm in diameter. These are the 'blue-domed' cysts (Figure 9.1) which have classically been considered to denote benign disease. These smaller cysts have no intrinsic significance except the potential to form larger cysts in due course.

Larger cysts are thin walled and of a brownish

Table 9.1　Breast cysts.

True breast cysts

1. ANDI (aberrations of normal lobular involution)
   Microcysts
   Apocrine macrocysts
   Non-apocrine macrocysts
2. Juvenile cysts
3. Galactocele
4. Oil cysts of fat necrosis
5. Papillary cystadenoma

Conditions which require differentiation from breast cysts

1. Dilated ducts/chronic abscess associated with duct ectasia/periductal mastitis
2. Cysts of the dermis and areola
3. Cysts associated with tumour necrosis
   Phyllodes tumour – benign and malignant
   Necrotic carcinoma
4. Hydatid cysts

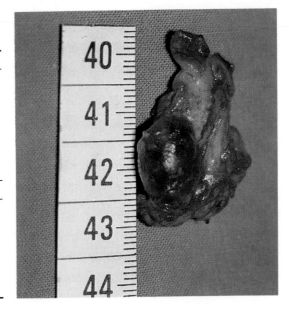

9.1　*A typical 'blue-domed cyst of Bloodgood' discovered by chance at biopsy for dominant nodularity. It should have been found by a needle point!*

colour, from the brown opalescent fluid within them. They usually present as an individual cyst but the single palpable cyst is likely to be the overt presentation of multiple, bilateral cysts, the majority of which are impalpable (Figure 9.2). The cysts may be uni- or multilocular but, even in unilocular cysts, constricting fibrous bands provide evidence of their origin from a single lobule or group of lobules (*see* Chapter 3). The fluid content of the cysts shows a wide range of appearances from clear to heavily turbid, and from light brown, through grey, to almost black (Figure 9.3). They do not contain blood unless there is an associated neoplasm. Crystal clear watery fluid is not seen in the common cysts of ANDI.

Multiple cysts are frequently impalpable due to the laxity of the cyst, allowing it to merge into surrounding breast tissue of similar consistency. But a very small increase in volume has a disproportionate effect on the intracystic pressure, explaining how a small increase in fluid can cause a large cyst to become tense and clinically apparent in a few days. This concept also explains the surprising fact that most cysts do not recur after aspiration. In fact, many do not disappear after aspiration but merely revert to their lax, impalpable state, as is readily shown by repeat mammography. Both increase and decrease in size may be seen on serial mammograms over a short period, suggesting that the balance between secretion and reabsorption or duct obstruction must be variable – so obstruction of the ductule draining the cyst is not a complete or irreversible process. Little is known of the dynamics of secretion and reabsorption of fluid by the cyst epithelium or through the cyst wall.

There is a rapidly expanding literature on the biochemistry of cyst fluid. It contains many steroid hormones[5, 6], beta human chorionic gonadotrophin (BHCG)[7] and relaxin[8], tumour markers such as fetoprotein and carcinoembryonic antigen (CEA)[9] and 'gross cystic disease proteins'[10], many of which are found in much higher concentrations than in blood, suggesting an active secretory process.

Incidence

There are surprisingly few satisfactory data on incidence of cysts in the general population. One autopsy study[11] of 225 women without overt clinical breast disease showed a 19% incidence of macroscopic cysts – 1–2 mm or more – and, in half, the cysts were bilateral. Foote and Stewart[12] reported 27% incidental cysts in 300 breasts

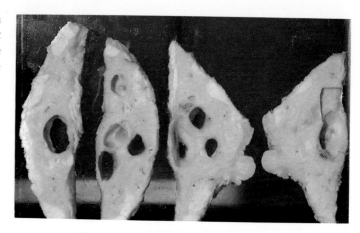

9.2 *A breast at autopsy – asymptomatic during life. It demonstrates the multiplicity of macroscopic cysts, and the diffuse nature of the involutional stromal changes of ANDI.*

removed for cancer. Haagensen[4] estimates that 7% of Western women will develop a palpable cyst, because this is the incidence of cancer, and in his practice cyst and cancer are seen with equal frequency. This must be a very rough approximation.

Pathogenesis

Many early workers and some recent writers have regarded cysts as dilated ducts. However, the clinical course and complications of duct ectasia and involutional cysts are very different, as is the underlying pathology of the two conditions. They should not be linked in any way, although they frequently coexist as different aberrations of involution.

Sir Alan Parks was one of the first workers to shed light on the problem when he described the process of cystic lobular involution (Hayward and Parks[13]). In this process, lobules develop microcysts during their involution, while maintaining some of the specialized lobular stroma around the epithelial acini. As long as this

9.3 *The range of colours of cyst fluid. The first specimen of opalescent fluid is common – the blood-stained fluid uncommon, and requiring further investigation.*

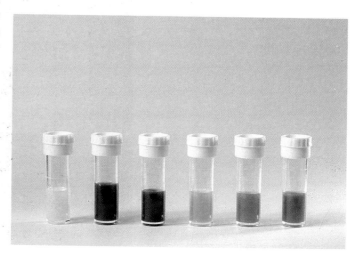

remains, the lobule may go on to complete involution – but if the specialized stroma is replaced by fibrous tissue before the small cysts have regressed, the cystic change is likely to persist. With time, the many small cysts representing the acini of the lobule will coalesce to form a smaller number of larger cysts (*see* Chapter 3). The lobular origin of macroscopic cysts is described by Azzopardi[14] who shows the value of elastic stains in demonstrating that each cyst derives from a lobule, enormously distended in the case of large macrocysts.

Many workers have noticed the presence of apocrine metaplastic epithelium in small cysts, and it has been believed that obstruction of the outflow from the lobule leads to distension, and conversion of the columnar apocrine cells to a flat cuboidal epithelium – or little epithelium at all.

Recent work has cast doubt on this simplistic approach from a number of directions, but there is still much uncertainty about detailed mechanisms. Studies from Bradlow's unit[15] have shown that cysts fall into two main groups, dependent on the ratio of Na^+ and K^+ in the cyst fluid. One group of cysts has a high ratio, similar to plasma, the other has a low Na^+ and high K^+ resembling intracellular fluid. Estimation of the Na^+/K^+ ratio in our own series of 725 patients shows a similar bimodal distribution (Figure 9.4). Measurement of pH has been reported as distinguishing between the two types of cyst, high K^+ cysts having a higher pH. Dixon and co-workers[16] regard a pH of 7.4 as the cut-off point, whereas Bradlow's group[17] recommend a pH of 7.0. Androgen conjugates are also found to be high in some cyst fluids, and low in others[18]. These findings, now confirmed by other workers, suggest that there may be at least two populations of cysts, possibly corresponding to those lined with apocrine epithelium (Figure 9.5) which is actively secreting in the high K^+ group, while in the others the flat epithelium (or no epithelium lining at all) acts more as a passive membrane (Figure 9.6).

This would suggest that the progression from micro- to macrocyst is dependent on the balance between secretion and outflow or reabsorption, and this balance might be upset in two ways. In one, obstruction of the ductule draining the original lobule would lead to back pressure and dilatation. A number of possible obstructing mechanisms have been suggested, including benign epithelial hyperplasia and fibrous obliteration of the lumen. But in many cases, the normal involutional fibrosis around the ductule, perhaps augmented by kinking, may alone be sufficient. In the second group, apocrine secretion in excess

of the reabsorptive capacity of the cyst may be important. It is these cysts with apocrine lining, particularly when this lining is papillary, which Haagensen[4] has suggested have a small but definite increase in malignancy associated with macroscopic cyst disease. However, larger careful studies have not confirmed an increased risk with any type of cyst – *see* Chapter 4. Patients with apocrine lined cysts are more likely to have multiple cysts and develop further cysts[19].

However, the diversion of cysts along the two paths of high or low Na^+/K^+ ratio occurs during macrocyst development, and not from the beginning. Dixon and his co-workers[20] have studied 40 microcysts, and found that all had high concentrations of androgen conjugates and a high K^+/Na^+

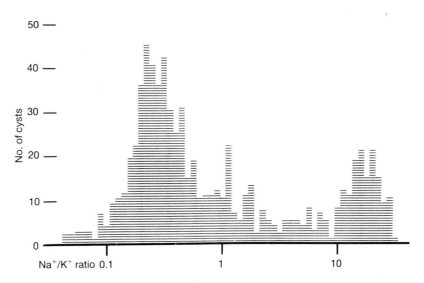

9.4 The bimodal distribution of breast cysts when characterized by Na^+/K^+ ratio of cyst fluid – Cardiff series

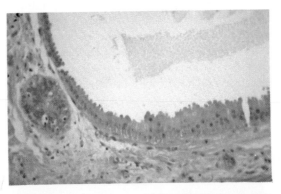

9.5 Wall of apocrine cyst – lined by tall pink columnar epithelium.

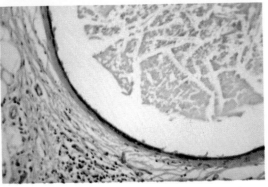

9.6 Cyst lined by flattened epithelium (sometimes the epithelial lining of the cyst wall is lost completely).

ratio. They have shown that microcysts form a single population lined by apocrine secretory epithelium -- the two types of macrocysts thus appear to develop from a single, apocrine type of microcyst.

Aetiology

Cyst formation can be regarded as a minor aberration of normal lobular involution; but the specific aetiological factors responsible for this aberration are unknown. There is some indirect evidence to implicate hyperoestrogenism, either absolute or relative. A number of cases seem to be related to oestrogen therapy, particularly in postmenopausal patients. Haagensen[4] regards the administration of oestrogen for menopausal symptoms as a potent cause of cysts in women over the age of 50, although Fechner[21] was unable to confirm this. Oestrogen also produces cysts in some rodents but since there are great differences between individual strains of mice, it hardly seems logical to transpose the findings to humans, although the fact that oestrogens also produce cysts in primates[22] is more convincing.

There is also some direct evidence in that England et al[23] demonstrated raised mean levels of serum oestradiol-17β in 13 women with cysts, although among these patients 7 had high levels, 4 normals and 2 reduced. Cole et al[24] also showed significantly elevated prolactin levels in cyst patients compared with controls or other patients with benign disease. At present, a hormonal basis for involutional cysts remains unproven. The cause of this condition is undetermined, and there is no conclusive evidence to support hormonal treatment of cysts – although it is reasonable to withdraw oestrogen supplements in such patients if it otherwise seems appropriate.

Clinical Features

Macroscopic cysts are frequently asymptomatic, the patient noting the mass accidentally when touching the breast. In other cases, sudden pain draws the attention of the patient to a large cyst, probably due to leakage of fluid into the surrounding tissue, giving chemical irritation. Pain may also be associated with disappearance of the cyst, which has presumably ruptured or discharged its contents into a duct. Pain is not usually related to the menstrual cycle, nor is variation in the size of the cyst. Nipple discharge is uncommon but does occur and duct injection has sometimes demonstrated communication with

a cyst in such a case. The discharge will then be typical of cyst fluid.

Fifty-five per cent of cysts are found in the left breast and 45% in the right – a ratio identical to that for fibroadenoma. Two-thirds occur in the upper outer quadrant, with the upper inner quadrant being next most common. Cysts are uncommon in the lower half of the breast. On examination, the physical characteristics vary widely according to a number of factors: size, intracystic pressure, depth and situation in the breast, and the characteristics of surrounding breast tissue.

Large cysts are frequently visible when the patient lies down (Figure 9.7). Generally the cyst is felt as a smooth, tense structure, readily palpable against the chest wall, and to some extent attached to breast tissue (see Chapter 5). Large cysts may be palpably multilocular. Lax cysts are palpated only with difficulty or not at all. Very tense cysts are so hard that carcinoma may be simulated closely. A large cyst may displace surrounding Cooper's ligaments, producing apparent skin attachment or even retraction (false retraction of Haagensen[4]). The diagnostic problem is fortunately solved readily by routine use of needle aspiration for *all* lumps.

A deep cyst may feel much more superficial in a youngish patient with pliable breast tissue and be missed entirely by timorous needling. Likewise, only the foremost loculus of a lobulated cyst may be felt from the surface, so that needling produces a suprisingly greater amount of fluid than expected. Conversely, needling of one of a cluster of cysts will produce less fluid than expected.

There is a strong clinical impression that multiple cysts are seen most commonly in buxom women, but no habitus is exempt – and single cysts are common in patients with small, dense breasts. There seems to be no relationship between age and multiplicity or recurrence.

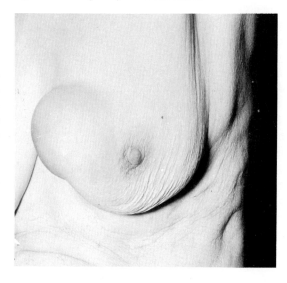

9.7 *A large visible cyst. This is an extreme example, but smaller cysts may also produce an eccentric contour when the patient lies down.*

Age

Cysts are predominantly a disease of the middle and late reproductive period, increasing in frequency from 35 years to a maximal incidence between 40 and 50 years. They are rarely seen before the age of 30, although we have seen a 5-cm cyst behind the areola in a 16-year-old girl, which did not recur after a single aspiration. Perhaps the pathogenesis differs in such juvenile cysts, although the clinical features were typical in this case. Cysts disappear rapidly after the menopause, unless the patient is taking hormone preparations. Of Haagensen's 2511 patients, 78% presented between 35 and 50 years, only 2.3% before the age of 30[4]. The rare cysts seen in the elderly tend to be large, and associated with a papillary tumour (p. 100), when the fluid will be blood stained. It seems likely that the even rarer cysts in the elderly not associated with tumour have a different aetiology to the premenopausal cyst – although little has been written about large non-neoplastic cysts in the elderly. Devitt[25] found that only 6% of symptomatic women over the age of 60 had breast cysts, compared with 15% of those less than 55 years presenting to a breast clinic. Furthermore, a majority of the older patients with cysts were taking hormone supplements.

Natural History

The natural history can be presented no better than through the results of Haagensen's[4] unique study, in which he has followed 2511 patients, 2235 for 5–30 years. Seventeen were multiple at first presentation on clinical examination (mammography and surgery would show much higher figures), 40% developed new cysts, the interval to a further cyst being progressively shorter with age – from an average of 10 years in the third decade to 2 years in the sixth. As would be expected, the greater the number of cysts, the shorter the interval to recurrence. With a minimum 5-year follow-up, 30% had only one cyst, 30% had 2–5 cysts, and the remainder had 6 or more. Fifty or more cysts over a prolonged period is not excessively rare. A further excellent paper is that of Jones and Bradbeer, who followed 322 cases for a minimum of 5 years, and obtained similar results[26].

Investigation (*see also* Chapter 6)

Radiological examination is not strictly necessary for cysts, but we utilize mammography for all cyst patients over the age of 30 years as a form of screening, to exclude an incidental cancer. Mammography will usually show cysts to be multiple and bilateral with numbers in excess of those detected clinically. Cysts are rounded, ovoid or lobulated with characteristics so similar to fibroadenoma as to make radiological differentiation impossible. Pneumocystography is useful if cyst aspiration reveals blood-stained fluid. In this case, a minimal amount of fluid should be removed so that the radiologist can easily locate the cyst. Irregularity of the surrounding tissues at one edge suggest infiltration in the rare cystic carcinoma. Such information is not essential because all cysts with blood-stained fluid should be excised but it gives useful information for preoperative assessment and planning. (The bright red, partial blood staining of a traumatic tap should be easily differentiated from the uniform, old blood of a cystic tumour.)

Ultrasound will readily diagnose a cyst, but is hardly necessary when the same information can be obtained so easily by needle aspiration. It may have a place in localizing small deep impalpable lesions – which may be cystic or solid – for needling.

Differential Diagnosis

Cysts are readily differentiated from solid lesions by needling. Three other cystic conditions need to be considered: the cystic form of fat necrosis (p. 175), galactocele (p. 99) and cystic papillary tumours, adenoma and carcinoma (p. 100). It cannot be stressed too often that a tense cyst can closely simulate cancer on palpation. The question of cancer should never be raised with a patient before a needle has been inserted into a breast lump.

Management

The last 40 years has seen the management of cysts pass from mandatory excision, through selective aspiration with cytological examination to routine (and if necessary repeated) aspiration alone. Patey and Nurick[27] had an early influence in the UK in managing cysts conservatively. The development of a conservative regimen for managing breast cysts has been one of the truly major advances in breast surgery. Like penicillin, it needs no controlled trial to prove its efficacy, and it is unfortunate that some conservative surgeons still deny patients its obvious benefit. Nevertheless, no aspect of breast disease management is without pitfalls and strict rules must be followed to avoid an occasional disaster.

Aspiration

The first investigation of every lump in the breast should be the insertion of a needle, and if this is practised cysts will be diagnosed at first consultation. A 21-gauge needle with a syringe of appropriate size to the estimated cyst volume is plunged directly into the cyst, fixed by two fingers of the opposite hand (Figure 9.8). No anaesthetic is necessary. The average cyst volume is 5–10 ml, but varies from less than a millilitre to 75 ml or more. A 10 ml or 20 ml syringe is usually convenient. Tong[28] has argued strongly in favour of the use of evacuated glass tubes ('Vacutainer'), but the benefit is probably marginal – particularly with large cysts. (Cysts are often more easily palpated with the patient sitting up – in such cases, the lump is localized and held while the patient lies down for aspiration.) If the mass proves to be solid, a cytological specimen is obtained, and this is facilitated if a syringe holder designed for obtaining cytology specimens is used. If the fluid is not blood stained, the cyst is aspirated to dryness, the needle removed and the fluid discarded. Cytological examination of cyst fluid is not useful or cost effective unless the fluid is blood stained. Many early workers advocated cytological examination of all cyst fluid[27, 28], but most large units have now abandoned it except when blood stained[29, 30]. The breast is carefully

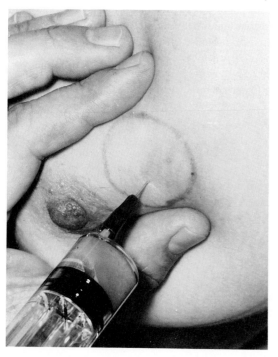

9.8 *Technique of aspirating a cyst – the cyst is immobilized by fingers of the left hand.*

palpated to exclude a residual mass – if one exists, it is re-needled for cytology (and to exclude a further cyst) prior to arrangements being made for excision biopsy.

If the fluid is blood stained, 1–2 ml only of fluid is taken for cytology and the patient referred for pneumocystography. The presence of blood is usually obvious, but in cysts with black fluid (usually not due to blood), any doubt should be eliminated by examining the fluid for blood by microscopy or a chemical occult blood test. Blood must be regarded as synonymous with tumour (usually benign, but sometimes malignant). Malignancy is more likely to be found in the elderly but even then the prognosis is favourable.

Mammography is best deferred for a week after aspiration as the trauma may cause diagnostic difficulty.

To summarize, there are two cardinal rules for safe cyst aspiration and these must always be observed:

1. The mass must disappear completely after aspiration. If not, it must be treated as any other persistent mass, with re-needling, cytology, mammography, needle biopsy and open biopsy as indicated by individual circumstances.

2. The fluid must not be blood stained. If it is, cytology and pneumocystography as outlined above may be helpful but we believe open biopsy should be undertaken in all such cases. Many workers have recommended that all cysts should be excised if the cyst refills after aspiration. This is not necessary or desirable if the above two rules are met, although it should be regarded as a further indication for mammography if this is not used routinely in cyst patients. We have seen no carcinoma associated solely with refilling of a cyst without blood-stained fluid, except as an incidental finding adjacent to the cyst.

Recurrent Cysts

Early recurrence is not rare but less common than might be expected. Because aspiration might not be expected to influence the natural history, one might anticipate universal recurrence. In fact, only about 10% of cysts refill to become palpable, although almost one half of patients will develop another cyst elsewhere in the breast – about one-third will develop more than one. We treat a recurrent cyst by repeated aspiration, and are not particularly concerned at the number of aspirations required. Fortunately cysts rarely refill after two or three aspirations. Recurrence is an indication for mammography but not for excision. Because recurrence usually occurs in patients with multiple cysts, excision is not appropriate treatment. A persistent mass, or blood-stained fluid, remain the only indications for excision. If recurrence becomes tedious for the patient, we will consider pneumocystography – for this seems to have a clinical benefit in lessening recurrence. Dixon and co-workers[19] have found that apocrine lined cysts, characterized by a high K^+/Na^+ ratio, are more prone to be multiple and to recur than non-apocrine cysts. Bundred (NJ, 1987, personal communication) studied 82 women to determine the best predictive factors for cyst recurrence within 2 years of aspiration. A high K^+ level, a K^+/Na^+ ratio greater than 3, and a low Cl^- level in the cyst fluid were all predictive of recurrence. The greater the number of cysts requiring aspiration at the first visit, the greater the chance of recurrence.

Follow-up

Although Haagensen[4] has given evidence that macroscopic cysts are associated with a definite – but quite small – increase in cancer risk, other workers have not confirmed this. Certainly we do not believe this to be an indication for regular follow-up unless other major risk factors are present. We instruct patients in self-examination and see them as necessary. We regard this policy as satisfactory until the risk factors associated with cysts are more precisely defined. This problem is discussed further in Chapter 4.

Hormone Therapy

The hormonal background to cysts is not defined sufficiently precisely to justify any form of hormone therapy unless part of a controlled study. One study of patients with recurrent cysts has reported a remarkable reduction (75%) in the number of cysts requiring aspiration after a course of danazol, 100 mg three times per day for 3 months[31]. Benefit was even greater at 6 months, i.e. 3 months after cessation of therapy. This was a small study and requires confirmation. Another trial of evening primrose oil is in progress and the results of further studies are awaited.

Mastectomy

Some surgeons recommend subcutaneous mastectomy, with silicone implant for extensive or recurrent cystic disease, either on the basis of reduction of cancer risk or for the physical and psychological benefit of the patient. We believe this practice should be condemned except in the most exceptional circumstances. Although cysts are a nuisance, they cause the patient no great harm – a different state of affairs to many patients who have complications after bilateral subcutaneous mastectomy with silicone implants. Until reconstructive techniques improve, it is difficult to justify on grounds of benefit to the patients.

Galactocele

A galactocele is an uncommon lesion in which a cyst filled with milky material develops after a period of lactation. There is a surprising paucity of information about this condition, compared with other aspects of breast pathology. Such literature as exists is often obscured by a tendency to confuse galactocele with duct ectasia and recurrent subareolar abscess. The confusion extends down to some of the most recent papers, particularly those which state that galactoceles are prone to lead to chronic sinuses. The first use of the term 'galactocele' has been attributed to Campbell who defined it in 1845 as a 'form of tumour which springs from one of the milk ducts, forming a cyst'.

The term is best confined to a specific clinical syndrome in which a woman develops a painless swelling of the breast from a few weeks to some months after ceasing lactation. The swelling is smooth and mobile and in fact has the exact physical characteristics of the usual breast cyst. Aspiration produces what is clearly milk, instead of one of the variety of fluids commonly found in breast cysts. The lesion disappears completely and is usually cured by a single aspiration, but like ordinary cysts, will occasionally require two or three aspirations. It may be found anywhere in the breast, but commonly towards the areola.

The aetiology and pathology are obscure. Lactation is an essential antecedent in the typical case (although the condition has been described in male infants!). It is usually stated to follow abrupt artificial cessation of lactation.

A simple explanation of the pathogenesis is that a pre-existing cyst which connects with the duct system fills with milk, either by secretion or retrograde filling, but the ductule draining the cyst becomes blocked, trapping the milk. This may become slightly thicker by absorption of water, but retains the obvious characteristics of milk. Since some cysts can be demonstrated to connect with the duct system, the surprising fact is that galactocele is not more common given the frequency of cysts in the breasts. Presumably the

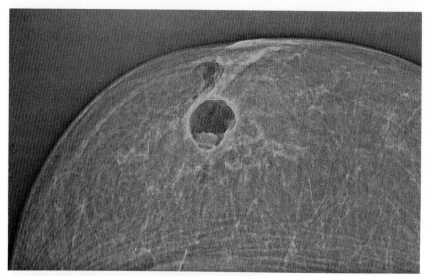

9.9 *Pneumocystogram for a cyst containing blood-stained fluid, demonstrating an intracystic papilloma.*

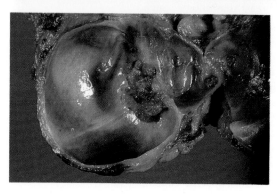

9.10 *Typical papillary tumour in the wall of a cyst in an elderly woman.*

reason is that cysts are an aberration of involution and less common during the usual child-bearing period. It also has been reported that macroscopic cysts resolve during pregnancy along with the well-recognized improvement in mastalgia and nodularity.

Other cases where cysts contain inspissated pus or infected material are better regarded as a separate group, most of which fall into the categories of duct ectasia, periductal mastitis or chronic cystic disease.

Papillary Tumours associated with Macrocysts

Papillary tumours within the wall of a cyst are rare, yet by no means excessively so. We would see approximately one such tumour a year, yet there is remarkably little written on this subject. Haagensen[4] discusses the concept, regarding them all as duct papillomas within grossly dilated ducts, yet this is not consistent with our experience. Cystic dilation of ducts due to intraductal papilloma (sometimes also called papillary cystadenoma) is commoner than true cysts, but the two conditions are distinct. Cyst puncture and pneumocystography shows no connection with the duct system, nor is there any nipple discharge. Azzopardi[14] mentions that papilloma can be seen within cysts, i.e. of lobular derivation, but gives no details apart from mentioning a single case he had encountered. Devitt[32] discusses the problem of carcinoma *in association with* a cyst.

Papilliferous cysts usually arise in patients a decade or more after the menopause. The patient presents with a soft mass – usually large, often apparently of recent onset. Aspiration yields old blood-stained fluid – cytology will usually show epithelial cells of benign appearance. Pneumocystography will demonstrate the cyst, and a small papilloma within its wall (Figures 9.9 and 9.10). This technique can also give a fair indication as to whether there is invasion outside the cyst wall to indicate malignancy. Fortunately the majority are benign, even in the elderly. In this age group it is best treated by total cyst excision, which amounts to segmental resection. This will provide material for adequate histological assessment in all cases, and definitive treatment in the majority proved benign on histology.

REFERENCES

1. Cooper A. On diseases of the breast. *Cooper Lectures* 1831; 2: 125.
2. Reclus P. La maladie kystique des mammelles. *Revue de Chirurgie* 1883; 3: 761.
3. Bloodgood J. C. The bluedomed cyst in chronic cystic mastitis. *Journal of the American Medical Association* 1929; 93: 1056.
4. Haagensen C. D. *Diseases of the Breast.* Philadelphia, W. B. Saunders, 1986.

5. Bradlow H. L., Rosenfeld R. S., Kream J., Fleisher M., O'Connor J. & Schwartz M. K. Steroid hormone accumulation in human breast cyst fluid. *Cancer Research* 1981; **41**: 105–107.

6. Miller W. R., Humeniuk V. & Kelley R. W. DHAS in breast secretions. *Journal of Steroid Biochemistry* 1980; **13**: 145–151.

7. Bradlow H. L., Schwartz M. K., Fleisher M. *et al.* Accumulation of hormones in breast cyst fluid. *Journal of Clinical Endocrinology and Metabolism* 1979; **49**: 778–782.

8. Narde E., Bigazzi M., Agrimonti F. *et al.* Relaxin and fibrocystic disease of the mammary gland. *First International Conference on Human Relaxin*, Florence, Italy, 1982.

9. Fleisher M., Oettgen H. F., Breed C. N., Robbins G. F., Pinsky L. M. & Schwartz M. K. CEA like material in fluid from benign cysts of the breast. *Clinical Chemistry* 1974; **20**: 41–42.

10. Haagensen Jr D. E., Mazoujian G., Dilley V. G., Pederson C. E., Kister S. J. & Wells J. K. S. A. Breast gross cystic disease fluid analyses. I: Isolation and radioimmunoassay for a major component protein. *Journal of the National Cancer Institute* 1979; **62**: 239–244.

11. Frantz V. K., Pickren J. W., Melcher G. W. & Auchinloss H. Incidence of chronic cystic disease in so-called normal breasts. *Cancer* 1951; **4**: 762–783.

12. Foote F. W. & Stewart F. W. Comparative studies of cancerous versus non-cancerous breasts. *Annals of Surgery* 1945; **121**: 6–53.

13. Hayward J. L. & Parks A. G. Alterations in the microanatomy of the breast as a result of changes in the hormonal environment. In: Currie A. R. (ed.) *Endocrine Aspects of Breast Cancer*. Edinburgh, Livingstone, 1958, pp 133–134.

14. Azzopardi J. G. *Problems in Breast Pathology.* London, W. B. Saunders, 1979.

15. Bradlow H. L., Skidmore F. D., Schwartz M. K., Fleisher M. & Schwartz D. Cations in breast cyst fluid. In: Angeli (ed.) *Endocrinology of Cystic Breast Disease*. New York, Raven Press, 1983, pp 197–202.

16. Dixon J. M., Miller W. R. & Scott W. N. pH of human breast cyst fluid. *Clinical Oncology* 1984; **10**: 221–224.

17. Bradlow H. L., Breed C. N., Nisselbaum J. *et al.* pH as a marker of breast cyst fluid biochemical type. *European Journal of Surgical Oncology* 1987; **13**: 331–334.

18. Miller W. R. & Forrest A. P. M. Androgen conjugates in Human breast Secretions and Cyst Fluids. In: Angeli (ed.) *Endocrinology of Cystic Breast Disease*. New York, Raven Press, 1983, pp 77–84.

19. Dixon J. M., Miller W. R. & Scott W. N. Natural history of cystic disease: the importance of cyst type. *British Journal of Surgery* 1985; **72**: 190–192.

20. Dixon J. M., Scott W. N. & Miller W. R. An analysis of the content and morphology of human breast microcysts. *European Journal of Surgical Oncology* 1985; **11**: 151–154.

21. Fechner R. E. Benign breast disease in women on oestrogen therapy. *Cancer* 1972; **29**: 273–279.

22. Engle E. T., Krakower C. & Haagensen C. D. Oestrogen administered to aged female monkeys with no resultant tumours. *Cancer Research* 1943; **3**: 858.

23. England P. C., Skinner L. G., Cottrell K. M. & Sellwood R. A. Sex hormones in breast disease. *British Journal of Surgery* 1975; **62**: 806–809.

24. Cole E. N., Sellwood R. A., England P. C. & Griffiths K. Serum prolactin concentrations in benign breast disease throughout the menstrual cycle. *European Journal of Cancer* 1977; **13**: 597–603.

25. Devitt J. E. Benign disorders of the breast in older women. *Surgery, Gynecology and Obstetrics* 1986; **162**: 340–342.

26. Jones B. M. & Bradbeer J. W. The presentation and progress of macroscopic breast cysts. *British Journal of Surgery* 1980; **67**: 669–671.

27. Patey D. H. & Nurick A. W. Natural history of cystic disease of the breast treated conservatively. *British Medical Journal* 1953; **1**: 15–17.

28. Tong D. The treatment of solitary cysts in the breast: A new technique. *British Journal of Surgery* 1969; **56**: 885–890.

29. Forrest A. P. M., Kirkpatrick J. R. & Roberts M. M. Needle aspiration of breast cysts. *British Medical Journal* 1975; **3**: 30–31.

30. Cowen P. N. & Benson E. A. Cytological study of fluid from benign breast cysts. *British Journal of Surgery* 1979; **66**: 209–211.

31. Hinton C. P., Williams M. R., Roebuck E. J. & Blamey R. W. A controlled trial of Danazol in the treatment of multiple recurrent breast cysts. *British Journal of Clinical Practice* 1986; **40**: 368–370.

32. Devitt J. E. The clinical recognition of cystic carcinoma of the breast. *Surgery, Gynecology and Obstetrics* 1984; **159**: 130–132.

10   Sclerosing Adenosis

This lesion was first described by Masson in 1923[1] and a number of excellent pathological descriptions have since been published, one such being that by Dawson[2]. It may be regarded as one of the manifestations of ANDI (an aberration of lobular involution; *see* Chapter 3), in which a well-ordered lobular involution is distorted by excessive myoepithelial proliferation. Among surgeons it has received little attention, being known mainly through notoriety as a cause of difficulty for pathologists in the diagnosis of cancer on frozen section. Its surgical implications extend over a wider field for it may simulate cancer clinically, macroscopically and radiologically, as well as histologically. In addition, the condition shows an association with breast pain.

Clinical Presentation

The condition has four separate modes of clinical presentations.

Presentation as a Mass

This may occur at any age from the mid-20s to the postmenopausal age group. The mass tends to be small, 2 cm or less, firm, poorly delineated and attached to surrounding breast tissue. There are no gross signs of cancer – skin retraction or lymphadenopathy – but these would not be expected anyway with a small mass.

Presentation with Pain

This is discussed in more detail in Chapter 7. In brief, it produces the same type of localized persisting pain which is seen in cancer, but sometimes having premenstrual exacerbation. Pressure also often causes exacerbation and, in some patients, it is severe enough to interfere with sleep[3, 4]. The perineural invasion demonstrated histologically in some cases may be an explanation

of the association with pain (Figure 10.1). In a series of 316 consecutive and unselected cases of benign mammary disorders, Davies found that sclerosing adenosis was the condition most frequently found to show actual neural invasion by mammary epithelial cells[5].

Presentation on Mammography

With increasing use of mammography as a screening or semi-screening procedure, the radiological features typical of sclerosing adenosis are being detected more frequently – either in association with a mass or in asymptomatic patients. Where the radiological pattern is indistinguishable from cancer, biopsy is mandatory. Where unequivocal radiological signs of sclerosing adenosis are seen on mammography, 90% will have the condition on histology. Thus in our experience, there is a 10% false negative rate for the mammographic diagnosis.

A Chance Histological Discovery

Small patches of sclerosing adenosis are frequently found on histological section of breast tissue. It

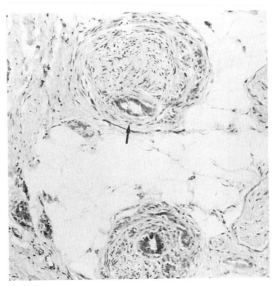

10.1 *Sclerosing adenosis with neural invasion (arrow).*

has been estimated that these occur 20–30 times more commonly than palpable lesions. These small areas found on histology can be ignored.

Frequency of Presentation

In our clinic 43 patients were encountered over a 5-year period. The age range extended from 24 to 71 years. Eleven presented primarily with pain, although 25 of the patients experienced some pain at the site of the lesion. Nine presented with a mass and four were chance histological findings. The rest were detected on mammography. Undoubtedly, there would have been other cases detected on histological examination during this period which the pathologist did not bother to report.

Radiological Criteria

Three patterns of radiographical change are seen[6] (*see also* Chapter 6):

1. Increased density with irregular margins – very similar to cancer but without fine microcalcification.
2. Fine, smooth calcification scattered widely throughout the breast, usually bilateral.
3. Smooth, microcalcifications, up to 10 in number, arranged in a small group. This may or may not be associated with widespread calcification. This pattern cannot be differentiated from that of cancer and biopsy is mandatory.

Pathological Findings

Macroscopic

Careful examination will suggest the diagnosis. The mass is firm, but not as hard or gritty as cancer and it has a nodular, circumscribed appearance rather than the stellate pattern of cancer. Azzopardi points out that examination with a fine hand lens will often demonstrate clearly the nodular and whorled appearance. The nodules have a brownish tinge and the greyish streaks of debris in ductules typical of cancer are not seen.

Microscopic

The pathological criteria outlined by McDivitt et al[7] have been summarized by Davis[5] – nodular epithelial lesions in which fibrosis and myoepithel-

ial proliferation is associated with a stellate or whorled distortion of the normal lobular pattern. This distortion can lead to incorrect diagnosis of malignancy, especially on frozen section. The problem is now well recognized by experienced pathologists, but was the cause of much overdiagnosis of malignancy in the past.

Fisher et al[8] have described 15 cases of a lesion which may be confused with sclerosing adenosis, and they have called them 'non-encapsulated sclerosing lesion of the breast'. They regard it as benign, possibly an incipient form of tubular cancer, but worthy of a separate designation.

The histological similarities between sclerosing adenosis and cancer are illustrated in Figure 10.2, in which the two are shown side by side. Figure 10.3 shows the extensive microcalcification which is the basis of one of the radiological patterns.

Management

When cancer cannot be excluded in a patient with a mass, or mammographic findings, the area must be biopsied. The mass is excised and treated in the usual way for any lump of doubtful pathology. The question of needle biopsy does not usually arise because of the small size of the mass, and even localization for fine needle aspiration may be difficult. It is generally agreed that subclinical lesions are better submitted to paraffin section, and frozen section avoided because of the difficulty of interpretation. With a macroscopic mass frozen section may be used, but it is our view that, if there is any discrepancy between the macroscopic and frozen section assessments, it is

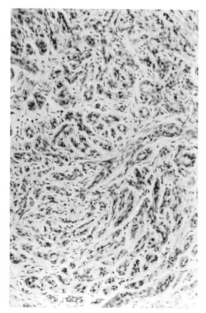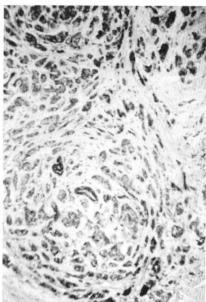

10.2 *Sclerosing adenosis (left) and invasive cancer (right) shown side by side, illustrating difficulties encountered in differentiation on frozen section.*

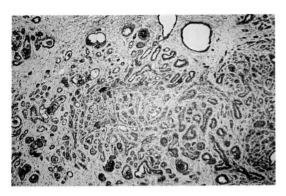

10.3 *Sclerosing adenosis showing numerous areas of microcalcification, providing, the pathological basis for the typical X-ray appearance.*

better to wait for a paraffin section than to proceed to any radical form of surgery on the basis of frozen section. Local excision is adequate management for sclerosing adenosis.

When biopsy is required for a non-palpable, mammographic lesion a standard prearranged procedure involving surgeon, radiologist and pathologist must be followed to ensure that the correct tissue is removed[9]. The steps are described in Chapter 18.

REFERENCES

1. Masson P. *Traite de Pathologie-Medicale.* Paris, A. Malione, 1923.
2. Dawson E. K. Fibrosing adenosis: a little recognised mammary picture. *Edinburgh Medical Journal* 1954; **61**: 391–401.
3. Preece P. E., Fortt R. W., Gravelle I. H., Baum M. & Hughes L. E. Some clinical aspects of sclerosing adenosis. *Clinical Oncology* 1979; **2**: 192.
4. Preece P. E. *A study of the aetiology, clinical patterns and treatment of mastalgia.* MD Thesis, University of Wales, 1982.
5. Davies J. D. Neural invasion in benign mammary dysplasia. *Journal of Pathology* 1973; **109**: 225–231.
6. Evans K. T. & Gravelle I. H. *Mammography, Thermography and Ultrasonography in Breast Disease.* London, Butterworths, 1973.
7. McDivitt R. W., Stewart F. W. & Berg J. W. Tumours of the breast. *Atlas of Tumour Pathology*, Vol 2. Washington DC, 2nd Series Fascicle, 1968, pp 133–137.
8. Fisher E. R. Palekar A. S., Kotwal N. & Lipana S. A non-encapsulated sclerosing lesion of the breast. *American Journal of Clinical Pathology* 1979; **71**: 240–246.
9. Preece P. E., Gravelle I. H., Hughes L. E., Baum M., Fortt R. W. & Leopold J. G. The operative management of subclinical breast cancer. *Clinical Oncology* 1977; **3**: 165–169.

11 The Duct Ectasia/Periductal Mastitis Complex

The terms 'duct ectasia' and 'periductal mastitis' cover the second major group of benign breast disorders – the most important group after those of ANDI. 'Mammary duct ectasia' introduced by Haagensen in 1951[1] is a useful term in that it has a single simple connotation – the presence of dilated mammary ducts – terminology consistent with that of bronchiectasis and sialectasis. To this has been added periductal mastitis to describe the frequent occurrence of periductal inflammation in association with duct ectasia. This term has advantages over others used such as plasma cell mastitis or comedo mastitis because these specific elements are not present in all cases. Hence the condition is best known as the duct ectasia/periductal mastitis complex even though this by no means covers all the pathological or clinical aspects of the disease.

Until recently, there has also been a lack of awareness of the condition and its less common manifestations among both surgeons and pathologists[2]. This is surprising, for a very comprehensive description of the condition was given by Bloodgood, with typical flamboyant style, in 1923[3] and a further description by Haagensen in 1951[1]. We will show later in this chapter that understanding of disease has been held back by the attempts to confine the clinical manifestations within the straight-jacket of a single all embracing disease process or, alternatively, attempts to remove the straight-jacket completely and regard the condition as one aspect of 'fibrocystic disease'. Both approaches are incompatible with the breadth of clinical manifestations or the observed pathology. While the exact aetiology is still uncertain, recent work has demonstrated a number of pathological processes which contribute to the clinical manifestations including duct dilatation, stagnant secretions, epithelial metaplasia, nonbacterial inflammation, bacterial inflammation and periductal sclerosis. These diverse processes, individual but interrelated, explain the protean clinical presentations. Evolution of thought and practice continues and quite recent demonstration of anaerobic bacteria in many cases is having a major impact on understanding and management. This disease complex presents clinically in many ways, at times giving rise to all three common breast symptoms: lump, nipple discharge and pain. The main manifestations are set out in Table 11.1 and any concept of the disease complex must be able to encompass this wide range of clinical presentations. In view of the confusion in nomenclature and understanding, it is useful and salutary to look at it from a historical point of view.

Table 11.1 The clinical spectrum of duct ectasia/periductal mastitis.

Underlying pathology	Clinical manifestations
Duct ectasia	Nipple discharge thick, creamy bloody
Periductal mastitis Single duct	Recurrent subareolar abscess
	Mammary duct fistula
Multiple ducts	Inflammatory and/or abscess formation evanescent recurrent chronic
	Duct fistula
	Mastalgia
Periductal fibrosis Inflammatory	Nipple retraction
Involutional	Nipple retraction
Secondary to nipple discharge	Eczema of the nipple/areola

All the above manifestations may rarely occur in the male.

Historical Survey

This condition has been recognized and well described in the surgical literature over many decades, yet remained unrecognized in clinical practice to a surprising degree. This condition was recorded by many early writers but they were unable, on the whole, to conceive it as a distinct process, confusing it with tuberculosis, galactocele, cystic disease and fat necrosis. Even today, many endocrinological texts confuse the nipple discharge of duct ectasia with galactorrhoea.

John Birkett, surgeon to Guy's hospital and President of the Royal College of Surgeons of England in 1877, gave a description of the condition in his book on breast disease[4]: 'In the breast of a middle-aged woman it is not uncommon to find the ducts dilated and filled with mucous greenish fluid.' Bloodgood described several cases in 1921[5] in a paper dealing primarily with chronic cystic disease. He returned to the subject in 1923 presenting 31 cases. His description could hardly be bettered[3]: 'The characteristic picture when the dilated ducts are situated in the nipple zone is the palpation of a doughy, worm-like mass beneath the nipple. When explored, one can recognize large and small dilated ducts with distinct wall, containing brown, green, milky or cream-like material, of various degrees of viscosity and consistency.' He went on to describe nipple discharge, palpable tumours, some with skin and nipple fixity resembling malignancy, others resembling subareolar abscesses and peripheral breast masses. He even described a case of eczema of the areola apparently due to nipple discharge. Bloodgood made no contribution to aetiology and stated that the condition could be classed as part of chronic cystic mastitis – an area of confusion which persists in some present-day literature. He noted that patients with dilated ducts were often postmenopausal and that the condition seemed to have no relation to parity or breast feeding. He recognized that the condition could present as nipple discharge or a mass which could be evanescent, but that it could also simulate cancer exactly, that it often settled spontaneously and that it had a tendency to be bilateral.

According to Cutler[6], it was James Ewing, of the Memorial Hospital in New York, who drew attention to 'plasma cell mastitis' in the 1920s. It is not surprising that a pathologist should so do, for radical mastectomy was not infrequently carried out mistakenly for a chronic inflammatory mass simulating cancer. He used this term because he was impressed with the number of plasma cells infiltrating these lesions. Cheatle and Cutler[7] recorded it in the literature survey in their book on breast tumours. Adair[8] reported 10 cases from the records of the Memorial Hospital highlighting the clinical problem of inappropriate mastectomy. Further reports added the names comedo mastitis and mastitis obliterans. Each name stressed one

particular aspect of the condition, but the different terminology did little to develop a unifying concept of the condition.

The subject was reviewed from the Mayo Clinic in 1948[9]. This paper gave a good review of the literature and reflected the usual attitude at that time: of 172 cases, the great majority had been identified from a retrospective study of pathology specimens usually found as a chance finding in mastectomy specimens for cancer. Only 19 of this series had undergone treatment for clinical manifestations of the condition.

The increasing recognition of the clinical manifestations was not matched by understanding of pathogenesis, or even of pathology. Rodman and Ingleby[10] tried to produce it experimentally, claiming that a similar condition was produced by injection of pancreatized milk into the mammary duct of rabbits.

Three important papers appeared in 1951 which was a vintage year for this condition. Frantz and her colleagues[11] reported an autopsy study of apparently normal breasts, and found an incidence of substantial duct ectasia of 25% and almost 50% in women over the age of 60. It was clear that the condition of duct ectasia was common, a disease of ageing, and often subclinical.

Zuska et al[12] described the condition now known as recurrent subareolar abscess or mammary duct fistula, recognizing its pathological basis for the first time, and reporting successful management by simple excision or laying open of the fistula. Earlier, Deaver and McFarland[13] had noted that persistent sinuses were sometimes seen after drainage of non-lactational abscesses, but they could only advise wide drainage, antiseptics and simple mastectomy for resistant cases. Even earlier cases of fistula have been reported in France and England in 1835 and 1892[14,15]. Zuska and his co-workers considered the condition to be a complication of duct ectasia ('comedo mastitis') because they saw dilated ducts containing the typical material seen in duct ectasia, which in its thicker form resembles a comedo. They also noted that it occurred in younger women, could be bilateral and was associated with squamous cell lining of the affected duct.

Haagensen[1] also published his first paper on the subject in 1951, and suggested the term 'mammary duct ectasia'. His views are expanded in his textbook[16]. It is surprising that the youngest patient he had seen with the disease was 34 years old, and the mean age of the group was 55. He saw only 67 patients with clinical disease in 30 years' practice, reflecting either the specialized nature of his practice with a bias towards cancer, or suggesting that the disease is becoming more common because we have operated on some 200 cases in 15 years. He supported the classic view that duct dilation was the primary abnormality, leading to stagnation of secretion and nipple discharge, with leakage of material outside the duct leading to a chemical periductal mastitis. He regards it as a rather benign condition and does not discuss severe abscesses, or recurrent inflammation or fistula after surgical excision. He regards recurrent subareolar abscess as a separate condition of trivial importance and criticizes Zuska et al for 'confusing it with duct ectasia'.

Atkins[17] drew the attention of British surgeons to recurrent subareolar abscess with a report of 28 cases. He introduced the unfortunate term 'mammillary fistula' suggesting a fistula into the nipple which soon became corrupted to mammillary duct fistula. The term seems inappropriate because the external opening of the fistula is along the edge of the areola (or more peripheral) and the internal opening is into a duct under the areola rather than within the nipple. It is a term better dropped in favour of the more simple and accurate term 'mammary duct fistula'. He saw the condition in simple mechanistic terms as an obstruction to the exit of the duct, with building up of secretions leading to infection which burst out through the skin. Again he reported it in younger patients, often with inverted nipples, and sometimes beginning during pregnancy and lactation. He recommended a simple laying open technique allowing the wound to heal by granulation. He noted no recurrence but gave no details of follow-up.

Three years later, Patey and Thackray[18] reported a detailed histological study of the ducts excised from seven specimens. They found the terminal portion of the involved duct lined by squamous epithelium instead of the normal columnar epithelium and believed this replacement to be congenital rather than acquired – partly because one case also showed multiple sebaceous glands opening into the track.

Hadfield[19] introduced the operation of major duct excision for a number of benign breast conditions including duct ectasia. He paid tribute to having learned the operation from Adair and Urban at the Memorial Hospital of New York, and 3 years later Urban[20] reported his own technique and results, again giving precedence to Adair. The operation slowly became the standard management for all the syndromes of duct ectasia/-periductal mastitis except localized mammary duct fistula.

Two papers from Sandison and Walker in Glasgow in 1962 and 1964[2,21] did much to increase the knowledge of chronic inflammatory conditions of the breast. They helped to fit periductal mastitis into an overall picture of breast disease and also suggested that recurrent subareolar abscess might have more than one aetiology. It is well worth while studying their papers in detail for their description of the disease complex. However, they do not appear to have used duct excision, preferring wide en bloc excision of diseased tissue. They infer that the results were satisfactory but give no detail of follow-up.

Ewing[22] reviewed the syndrome and the relevant literature to move full circle away from Haagensen, suggesting that mammary duct fistula is not a separate entity, but just a manifestation of duct ectasia. Habif and his colleagues[23] came down strongly in favour of the other view, reporting 146 cases of mammary duct fistula without seeing a single case with dilated ducts. They were all associated with squamous metaplasia of the terminal duct, and these authors fell into the classic error of expecting all manifestations to be based on a single pathological process.

The story is brought up-to-date with the elegant studies of periductal mastitis in the pathogenesis of duct wall disease by Davies[24] and the recognition of the importance of anaerobic bacteria in pathogenesis of abscess formation, both discussed below.

Pathology of Duct Ectasia/Periductal Mastitis

This condition exhibits a paradox. The pathology of the disease at a point in time – surgical biopsy or autopsy – is well established and well described, yet there is almost total ignorance of the sequence of events leading to or from that point in time. It is useful to summarize the position as understood at present and important to recognize that no single pathological process can explain, or should be asked to explain, the whole clinical spectrum. As with other benign breast disorders, it must be considered in relation to interaction of a number of aberrations of normal processes with added complications sometimes pushing it from the area of disorder to disease (see Chapter 3). There are four pathological processes which require consideration, all closely interrelated: duct ectasia with stagnation of secretion and periductal inflammation, which are the two major elements, squamous metaplasia of the epithelium of the terminal duct and periductal fibrosis. A further factor complicating pathogenesis of the clinical syndromes is that the inflammatory process of periductal mastitis may be predominantly chemical, or may have a bacterial element.

Ectatic Ducts

The dilatation may be considerable, varying from just above normal size (about 0.5 mm) up to 5 mm or more. Typically three or four of the ducts are ectatic. It is unusual for more than a few of the ducts to be involved and it is not clear why only some are dilated. Similarly, dilation is often confined to the 2–3 cm closest to the nipple, although it may extend further into the breast; occasionally the dilated ducts extend right to the periphery. Sometimes the wall of the dilated duct is thin and uninflamed; much more commonly the wall is thickened with fibrosis and disruption of the elastic lamina. Although ectatic ducts may look like cysts on section, the ducts are more uniformly dilated than cystic. It is now realized that the two conditions are quite separate, though they frequently coexist. Cystic disease is a condition of lobules, duct ectasia of the ductal system[25]. The secretion in the ducts may be amorphous, representing cellular debris and fatty acid crystals, or cellular, packed with colostrum cells and inflammatory cells. These colostrum cells are thought by many to be macrophages and by others to be myoepithelial cells. Changes in the epithelial cells lining the ducts tend to be non-specific – sometimes hyperplastic in the early stages, later flattened and atrophic or shed completely. Our studies of the duct epithelial cell surface by scanning electron microscopy showed a normal microvillous surface in most cases.

Periductal Inflammation

Histological changes of periductal inflammation with periductal histiocytes and inflammatory cells are usually present with dilated ducts but may be seen whether the ducts are dilated or not. There is sometimes a granulomatous reaction, and often a lipophagic reaction with a picture similar to fat necrosis. Plasma cells may or may not be prominent among the infiltrate. Davies[26] has stressed the relationship of cellular infiltration with focal ulceration, disruption of elastic tissue and subsequent fibrosis. In the presence of clinical periductal mastitis, these changes have spread into the surrounding breast tissue to form an inflammatory mass. Davies[24] has made a detailed study of periductal inflammation in both ectatic and non-ectatic ducts. In the latter group, one sees the paradoxical aspect of this condition – narrow sclerosing ducts – which has led to the old term 'mastitis obliterans' or 'mazoplasia obliterans'. He has demonstrated a striking periductal infiltration by four cell types which can lead to total obliteration of the duct. These cell types seem to derive from macrophages. Their presence is associated with marked damage to the duct wall and epithelial lining. The lumen may be filled with the colostrum cells typical of duct ectasia, but the eventual outcome is fibrosis and obliteration of the ducts. The study shows a predominance of fibrous obliteration occurring in young women although the study was biased towards this group because it derived from biopsy material for benign breast disorders. It was present in a wide variety of benign breast conditions, including those with no clinical evidence of periductal mastitis. It is not clear what relation this intense periductal inflammation and duct wall damage has to the ectatic form of duct disease, but both duct obliteration and duct dilation may be seen to result in different areas of the same breast. This process probably explains the shortening of ducts leading to nipple retraction; it may be part of normal ductal involution or an aberration of that process. Hence, histological periductal mastitis can be seen as a normal process, which may contribute to duct ectasia, to duct obliteration or to duct shortening, and also as a possible precursor of clinical periductal mastitis.

The histological picture of periductal mastitis shows a further spectrum of changes from the 'normal' juxtaductal infiltration of macrophage-derived cells, through a more extensive spread of inflammation characterized by plasma cells or lymphocytes. The final stage is frank abscess formation when more acute inflammatory cells are obvious, often along with lipid-laden foreign body giant cells and granulomas. These latter changes were responsible for confusion with tuberculosis in earlier literature.

Two other aspects of pathology need to be considered in relation to overt inflammatory masses – terminal duct obstruction by squamous metaplasia and the bacteriology of periductal mastitis.

Squamous Metaplasia

The third significant finding which needs to be fitted into the overall pathological picture is the squamous epithelial replacement of the terminal duct described by many workers in patients with mammary duct fistula. Normal squamous epithelium extends into a nipple duct no further than 2 mm from the surface with a sharp linear junction between squamous and columnar epithelium[27]. Patey and Thackray[18] describe this squamous epithelium extending down the duct in surgical specimens for a variable distance into the dilated portion of the duct; they did not find significant squamous down-growth in the fistula itself. They demonstrated fully developed sebaceous glands in the area in two cases and this led them to come down on the side of congenital aetiology. The arguments for a congenital origin of the squamous epithelium put forward by Patey and Thackray are convincing. They found the affected duct lined by squamous epithelium throughout the whole length of the duct from the nipple to the point of junction with the fistula in five of seven cases, and, in the other two cases, the remaining portion of the duct had no epithelium – but was lined by granulation tissue. The squamous epithelium even extended into some secondary branches of the affected duct. It is of interest that only one duct was involved. This might seem to argue against a congenital aetiology, but would explain the usual success of an operation directed towards a single duct. It is also surprising that only one duct should be involved in those cases associated with congenital nipple inversion. Another paper which discusses the problem of squamous metaplasia is that of Habif et al[23] and this paper is worth studying in detail for its pathological material. In contrast to Patey and Thackray, they show cases where more than one duct is lined by squamous epithelium. From their serial section studies, they dismissed the old view – still occasionally resurrected – that mammary duct fistula derives from infection of subareolar sebaceous cysts[28]. Toker[27] argued that it was an acquired condition (although from study of only one case) and likened it to the squamous replacement of columnar epithelium seen in the uterine cervix and other body areas. The duct lined by squamous epithelium is occluded by squamous debris and mechanical obstruction has been regarded as the primary pathological process by some workers. However the 'obstruction' is not sufficient to impede the easy passage of a probe at operation.

Bacteriology

Until recently there has been remarkably little work done on bacteriology of periductal mastitis and it is still a matter of some controversy. For many years it was believed that most cases were sterile early in the disease. In recurrent cases a variety of bacteria had been found. Anaerobes, *Staphylococcus aureus*, *Proteus* sp. and streptococci have been reported. Many are undoubtedly secondary invaders. With the advent of techniques for reliable demonstration of anaerobic organisms, it became obvious that these bacteria were sometimes present in earlier cases. Beigelman and Rantz[29] reported growth of *Bacteroides* sp. and anaerobic streptococci from a breast abscess as early as 1949. A second paper from Los Angeles in 1967[30] reported nine breast abscesses containing anaerobes. More recently, Leach and co-workers[31] studied 15 non-puerperal breast abscesses, although insufficient clinical details are given to determine whether all these abscesses were part of the duct ectasia/periductal mastitis syndrome. It is likely that at least some were because most had inverted nipples and two submitted to duct excision showed down-growth of squamous epithelium. Anaerobes were cultured in eight cases and staphylococci in six. The anaerobes were a mixed group typical of commensals in the oropharynx or vagina, but not those of the colon. *B. melanogenicus* and *B. bivius*, *Peptococcus* and *Peptostreptococcus* spp. were commonly isolated. The same authors have reported anaerobic subareolar abscesses after vaginal manipulation[32] suggesting blood-stream spread of bacteria to settle in the stagnant duct secretions. A more recent paper[33] studied the bacteriology of spontaneous discharge from 51 patients and of pus from 17 patients with abscess or fistula. Bacteria were isolated from 62% of patients with discharge due to duct ectasia and only 5% from those with discharge due to other causes. All the patients with abscesses or fistulae grew bacteria. The bacteria included enterococci, anaerobic streptococci, *Bacteroides* sp. and *Staphylococcus aureus*.

There is clearly room for further investigation into this area since there are still some discrepancies. Some of the more important discrepancies are as follows:

1. The clinical, painful masses of evanescent periductal mastitis resolve without treatment and with surprising rapidity for a bacterial infection. This sequence would be far more compatible with a chemical reaction to leaking duct contents as suggested by Haagensen.

2. Biopsies of masses due to duct ectasia, before overt abscess formation occurs, are rarely followed by wound infection – a situation which contrasts with the high incidence where frank pus is present. This is a surprising finding if there is a high incidence of bacterial colonization of ectatic ducts.

3. Leach et al[31] described typical foul smelling anaerobic pus – something uncommon in our experience.

4. Bundred and co-workers[33] used clinical features and mammography to divide their cases with nipple discharge into those with and those without duct ectasia – criteria which are far from clear-cut. Very careful examination with immediate bacteriological culture for aerobic and anaerobic organisms has failed to

demonstrate bacteria in a significant proportion of our cases on the initial presentation and many such cases fail to respond to appropriate antibiotics. In contrast, it is usual to grow bacteria in recurrent lesions in our experience. It is likely that the truth lies in compromise – in some cases the inflammation is non-bacterial whereas the incidence of bacterial involvement rises with repeated abscesses and drainage. However, there is now no doubt that bacteria play a major role in many of these cases, even from the outset of clinical presentation.

Pathogenesis

The Classic View of the Development of Duct Ectasia/Periductal Mastitis Complex

Each of the 15–20 ducts opening on to the nipple drains a distinct segment of duct and lobular units. The largest ducts normally have a diameter only of the order of 1 mm or less. The lactiferous sinus has a greater potential diameter, but in the resting stage it is collapsed. The subsegmental and terminal ducts become progressively narrower (Figure 11.1a).

In the sequence proposed by Haagensen[1] and developed by Ewing[22] (Table 11.2), the first change to occur is duct ectasia – one or more of the larger ducts dilate, reaching a diameter of 5 mm in gross examples. This is commonly restricted to the portion of the duct deep to the areola (Figure 11.1b). Typically three or four ducts are dilated, the remaining ducts being normal. In a few cases dilation extends peripherally to involve segmental and even subsegmental ducts (Figure 11.1c).

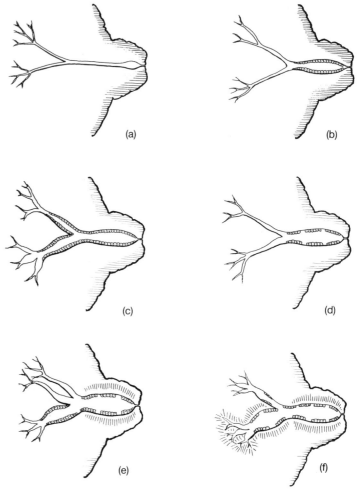

11.1 *The classic view of the pathogenesis of the clinical spectrum of duct ectasia. (See text for alternative theories.) (a) A normal segmental duct, uniformly narrow except for the terminal sinus, and breaking up into subsegmental and finally terminal ducts. (b) The proximal subareolar part of the duct dilates with stagnation of secretion. Intact mucosal epithelium is seen lining the dilated ducts. (c) the dilatation may extend into the subsegmental ducts. (d) The stagnant secretions lead to patchy mucosal ulceration which may give bloody discharge (e) The contents of the duct leak through the ulcerated areas giving a chemical inflammatory response. (f) This may affect subsegmental ducts or even occur peripherally beyond the major duct system. (g) Inflammation leads to fibrosis of the duct wall, as the fibrous tissue contracts nipple retraction is produced.*

Table 11.2 The classic view of the pathology of duct ectasia/periductal mastitis.

Process	Clinical manifestations
Duct ectasia (?A hormonal effect) ↓	
Stagnation of secretions ↓	→ Nipple discharge
Epithelial ulceration ↓	→ Bloody nipple discharge
Leakage of secretion into periductal tissue ↓	→ Evanescent painful mass
Granulomatous reaction + secondary bacterial infection ↓	→ Abscess/fistula
Periductal fibrosis	→ Nipple retraction

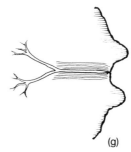

The dilated ducts fill with stagnant secretion which varies from creamy brown or greenish opaque fluid to thick grumous toothpaste-like material which must be squeezed out, leading to nipple discharge, usually of small amounts but sometimes sufficient to cause embarrassment.

Persisting stagnation may lead to loss of the epithelial lining of the ducts and ulceration (Figure 11.1d). This may have two consequences:

1. The ulceration may result in blood-stained nipple discharge and in leakage of stagnant secretions into the periductal tissue.

2. Because these secretions contain fatty acids which are chemically irritant, an inflammatory response, chemical rather than bacterial, may result (Figure 11.1e). This is usually seen beneath the edge of the areola, but in cases where dilatation extends into the subsegmental ducts, periductal mastitis may be seen more peripherally in the breast around large ducts, or even form a granulomatous mass more peripheral to the obviously dilated ducts (Figure 11.1f). This periductal mastitis may be evanescent or recurrent. In severe cases it progresses to abscess formation. When this occurs, simple drainage is unlikely to be curative and a persistent or recurrent sinus is likely to result. Some cases may develop a chronic indurated mass stopping short of abscess formation and the clinical signs in this situation may simulate cancer exactly.

The periductal inflammation leads to fibrosis and, as the fibrous tissue matures and contracts, it leads to nipple retraction (Figure 11.1g).

There are four main theories given to explain the duct dilation. The first sees it as a progressive failure of the muscle wall of the duct, perhaps due to a relaxation effect of progesterone and analogous to the development of varicose veins. The second incriminates failure of absorption of the duct secretion due to inadequate lymphatic flow. The third regards it as an obstructive phenomenon due to blockage of the ducts at their termination by squamous cell debris. In each case, inflammation is seen as a result of stagnation of contents within dilated ducts, with leakage of highly irritant lipid material into the periductal tissue. The fourth theory contrasts sharply with the others – it regards periductal inflammation as the primary process, perhaps a form of autoimmune disease, with muscle damage and duct dilation as secondary phenomena[34].

The Alternative View of the Pathogenesis of the Duct Ectasia/Periductal Mastitis Complex

However, a number of clinical aspects of the condition are incompatible with the classic view of the disease, and it is unlikely that this sequence is correct. There is much evidence to support the last theory of periductal inflammation as the primary condition. For example, inflammatory complications are seen most commonly in early age groups – typically in the 20s or early 30s, while, in contrast, simple nipple discharge due to duct ectasia is more common in the fifth decade. Nipple retraction is commonly seen as a new

development in postmenopausal women, without preceding nipple discharge or inflammatory complication.

For these reasons it seems likely that the duct ectasia/periductal mastitis complex encompasses several different processes, or that individual cases reflect a particular aspect of the disease. Nipple discharge in the premenopausal woman and nipple retraction of the postmenopausal woman may be separate variants, while younger women tend to demonstrate the full picture with the exception of nipple discharge. Perhaps there is a greater obstructive element in young women and this minimizes nipple discharge while aggravating leakage of duct contents into the periductal tissues. The much more complex sequence of events outlined in Table 11.3 fits the clinical spectrum of disease better than the classic view. The full clinical spectrum can only be explained on the basis of several distinct processes, which nevertheless may coexist and interact in some cases. There are distinct processes affecting the young and the old, and perhaps a third process affecting all ages.

Two other aspects of the condition raise clinical problems: the relationship between mammary

Table 11.3 Alternative view of the pathogenesis of duct ectasia/periductal mastitis.

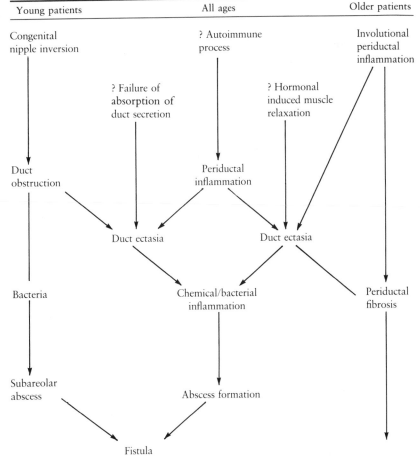

duct fistula and periductal mastitis, and the relation with nipple inversion.

Mammary Duct Fistula

This condition, described by Zuska *et al*[12], is seen in typical form when a young woman develops an abscess under the edge of the areola of one breast. Simple drainage of the abscess results in persisting discharge, or recurrent abscesses presenting at the same point. The condition has been likened to a perianal fistula with a sinus lined by granulation tissue leading down to a dilated sump-like duct (Figure 11.2). Patey and Thackray[18] investigated seven such cases and found the terminal portion of the duct to be blocked by squamous epithelium. They concluded that obstruction of the terminal duct due to desquamation of squamous cells was the cause and that the squamous lining was probably a congenital abnormality.

Other authors have not always confirmed this finding, and one commonly sees cases where secretion can readily be expressed through the terminal duct with no obstruction to the passage of a probe. One study[35] produced experimental evidence which suggested that hormonal effects were more important than obstruction in the pathogenesis. They found that ligation of the mammary ducts in rabbits produced no duct ectasia, whereas administration of hormones (oestrogen, progesterone or gonadotrophin) produced duct ectasia equally alone, or combined with duct ligation. No rabbits developed periductal mastitis. It seems likely that the discrepancies are best explained by at least two separate pathologies underlying mammary duct fistula: a congenital lining of squamous epithelium in the terminal duct and stagnation of duct contents due to duct ectasia. The first is commonest in young women, and is frequently accompanied by congenital nipple inversion. The second is seen in older patients, without nipple inversion. It is important that this dual pathology is recognized – because treatment of multiple duct disease by operation directed towards one duct will lead to recurrence, while failure to recognize the solitary congenital duct abnormality may lead to unnecessarily radical surgery. The consequences of failure to appreciate the overall pathology in the past is vividly illustrated in Sandison and Walker's paper from Glasgow[2]. Of 38 juxta-areolar inflammatory lesions studied, 8 were incorrectly considered to be neoplastic and 7 to be tuberculous, with 9 inappropriate mastectomies. In this series, 12 had shown periductal mastitis without duct ectasia, 12 had shown duct ectasia

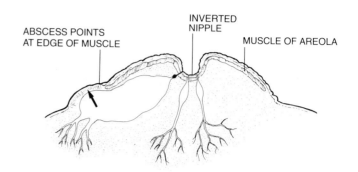

with periductal mastitis, and 14 cases had shown ectopic squamous epithelium. These figures may reflect the relative frequency of the different pathologies underlying periareolar infection.

Nipple Inversion

A number of workers have noted that nipple inversion is commonly associated with both duct ectasia/periductal mastitis and mammary duct fistula. Likewise, periductal mastitis is often associated with, or followed by, the development of retracted nipple. Our experience leaves no doubt that both relationships exist. There is a high incidence of congenital nipple inversion in young girls with recurrent subareolar abscess and we have frequently documented the progressive retraction of a previously normal nipple during the evolution of severe periductal mastitis.

Synthesis of the theories of pathogenesis

Thus the pathogenesis of the duct ectasia/periductal mastitis complex can best be considered from three points of view:

1. An obstructive phenomenon due to squamous metaplasia, either congenital or acquired with duct dilatation and leakage of contents to give secondary inflammation.

2. A primary dilatation of the ducts due to hormone-induced muscle relaxation or to hypersecretion or failure of absorption of duct fluid.

3. A primary inflammatory condition, autoimmune or due to bacterial invasion with secondary duct wall destruction leading to dilatation.

Is it possible to produce a synthesis of these disparate findings and theories which can provide a pragmatic approach to the understanding and management of the disease? A number of facts must be taken into consideration:

11.2 *The basic concept of mammary duct fistula. Squamous debris blocks the duct leading to dilatation of the subareolar portion. Because of the tough muscle of the areola skin, an abscess will tend to burst through the skin at the edge of the areola.*

1. The inflammatory complications are commoner in young women, and nipple discharge and nipple retraction in older women. This has been observed many times and recently given objective confirmation by Forrest's group[36].

2. Acute inflammation occurs frequently in young women with a congenital inverted nipple, but in others of this age group inflammation leads to retraction of a previously normal nipple.

3. Some patients with recurrent subareolar abscess show a definite localized abnormality, squamous metaplasia of the terminal duct, and the condition is cured by excision of that abnormality. A similar clinical picture can develop in women with grossly ectatic ducts and no evidence of squamous epithelial replacement of the terminal ducts.

4. Nipple discharge and retraction often occurs in older women without overt inflammatory episodes.

5. The frequent occurrence of bilateral involvement must be taken into consideration in any discussion of pathogenesis, and the frequency with which the disease starts in the second breast shortly after control of that in the first breast is a striking observation.

It seems to us that the apparently incongruent clinical and pathological features can be reconciled by accepting that we are not dealing with a single stereotyped entity (*see* Table 11.3).

The mammary duct fistula associated with squamous epithelial replacement is one entity, probably congenital in most cases and then usually associated with inverted nipple. In other cases the squamous epithelium may occur as a secondary down-growth – perhaps the result of ulceration due to idiopathic periductal mastitis.

Periductal mastitis can be accepted as a histological abnormality present as a chance finding in one in five cases of benign breast disorder coming to biopsy. It leads to fibrosis and obliteration of ducts. It is probably part of normal involution and may lead to the otherwise asymptomatic nipple retraction of the older woman.

Simple duct dilatation with secretory stagnation can also arise as an asymptomatic development, best regarded as another aberration of involution. The dilatation may result from the same periductal inflammation that may cause duct fibrosis or obliteration, from a hormonal effect or from simple muscle atrophy. There is no gross ductal obstruction and nipple discharge, spontaneous or induced, may be seen.

The aetiology of combined duct ectasia and periductal mastitis is a more difficult problem. Whether it is primarily inflammatory leading to duct damage and dilatation, or primarily duct dilatation giving rise to ulceration and leakage of contents, cannot be determined. The evidence would point at present to both mechanisms being involved – individually, in some cases, and together in others. It is also difficult to be certain at what stage bacterial infection becomes more important than a chemical reaction to leaking duct contents. The evanescent inflammatory masses are probably mainly sterile, but bacteria undoubtedly play a major role in established abscesses. The fact that the bacteria are the same as the flora of the mouth and vagina and that flare-up of abscesses can follow vaginal manipulation suggests that sexual stimulation may be responsible for the organisms reaching the ducts – ectatic ducts provide the soil in which the bacteria can persist or from which they can invade. It is also possible that oral bacteria may be transferred to the nipple, and provides a possible explanation for the frequency of involvement of the contralateral breast.

In each case, symptomatic disease – inflammation, nipple discharge or retraction – must be regarded as the tip of the iceberg of a subclinical histological change. The clinical manifestations of minor degree can be regarded as a benign breast disorder, no more than another minor aberration of the normal processes of cyclical change and involution. It becomes disease only when complicated by the development of severe inflammation.

In the past, pregnancy and breast feeding have frequently been considered as important in the aetiology of duct ectasia. However, the evidence of this is poor and Dixon *et al*[36] found no relation between parity or breast feeding and duct ectasia.

The Clinical Spectrum of Duct Ectasia/Periductal Mastitis (*see* Table 11.1)

Nipple Discharge

Considering the pathology of duct ectasia, it is not surprising that it is sometimes associated with nipple discharge. The commonest complaint is a small amount of purulent discharge, which is confirmed by the patient expressing material from the nipple. Rarely it is so profuse as to cause severe social embarrassment (Figure 11.3). The colour varies over the spectrum seen in the ducts at operation: off-white, creamy, brown, grey or green; sometimes it is as thick as toothpaste (Figure 11.4). Blood-stained discharge is less common than these coloured discharges, although Dixon et al[36] found positive occult blood in about half of their cases with nipple discharge. Certainly, in our experience a blood-stained discharge, even from a single duct, in the older age group (35 and over) is more commonly due to duct ectasia than to duct papilloma. Typically it comes from a number of ducts – it is then even more likely to be due to duct ectasia (Figure 11.5). Patients with nipple discharge and palpable ducts tend to be in the peri- or postmenopausal age group.

Breast Masses associated with Periductal Mastitis (Table 11.4)

Table 11.4. Breast masses associated with duct ectasia/periductal mastitis.

Palpable ducts
Subareolar or periductal mass
   evanescent
   recurrent
   persistent → subareolar abscess
   chronic → simulating cancer
Peripheral mass
   peripheral abscess

Palpable subareolar ducts were described by Bloodgood as very characteristic of this condition. He likened it to a varicocele. This degree of gross duct dilatation is rather uncommon in our experience.

Evanescent Mass

This is a very common presentation of the disease. The patient notices a small, slightly tender mass in the subareolar region. By the time she is seen in a clinic 7–10 days later, the mass has often disappeared. Such rapid development and regression of a breast mass is uncommon in any other breast condition. These masses are typicaly 1–2 cm in diameter, firm, tender and not attached to surrounding tissues. The subareolar situation distinguishes evanescent periductal mastitis from the pain of leakage of fluid from a cyst which is usually a little more peripheral in the breast and is not associated with a small localized mass; in fact a palpable cyst may disappear with the onset of pain. Masses of periductal mastitis may progress to reddening of the overlying skin and still regress in a few days. As Haagensen[16] commented: 'The most remarkable thing about these episodes is the rapidity with which they develop, and, if left alone, the promptitude with which they subside.' This pattern of behaviour makes it very difficult to assess any form of medical treatment. The patients have often been given antibiotics and naturally attribute their improvement to the treatment.

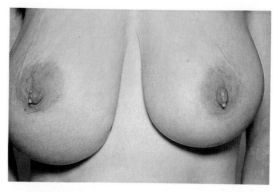

11.3 *The discharge of duct ectasia is often bilateral and sometimes so severe as to be socially embarrassing.*

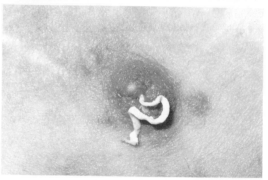

11.4 *Thick grumous nipple discharge of duct ectasia.*

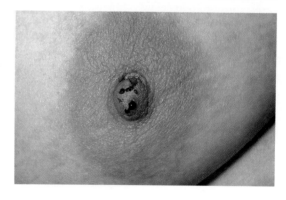

11.5 *Blood-stained nipple discharge from multiple ducts is usually due to duct ectasia.*

Recurrent Mass

While an evanescent mass may not recur, it has a tendency to do so at the same site at intervals of a few months to 10 years or more. The condition also has a tendency to become more severe with each recurrence. There is an appreciable incidence of bilateral involvement and it is not uncommon for the opposite breast to become involved shortly after successful control of one breast, although we have also seen an involvement of the contralateral breast as long as 10 years after the first one.

Persistent Mass

If a mass persists for some weeks, it is usually firm and fairly well defined. Aspiration cytology is characteristic, showing foamy macrophages and inflammatory cells. Cancer cannot be excluded absolutely, but this cytological appearance (i.e. inflammatory cells without epithelial cells) is highly characteristic and justifies a short course of appropriate antibiotics. If the mass does not resolve rapidly, biopsy excision is desirable in women of cancer age group. Provided there is no overt abscess formation, a periareolar biopsy wound will heal satisfactorily and there is no need to perform a formal duct excision. In fact, macroscopically dilated ducts are not particularly common in the presence of a simple periductal mastitis mass.

Some people have split off a condition which has been called granulomatous mastitis[37]. It is far from certain that this is not a variant of periductal mastitis, but it is discussed more fully in Chapter 17.

Chronic Mass

This is the lesion which simulates cancer closely – a hard oedematous mass fixed to skin and with nipple retraction and sometimes with axillary node enlargement. In the past, many such cases were subjected to radical mastectomy because the lesion could show some resemblance to cancer even when cut across. It may also be impossible to distinguish the two on mammography, but aspiration cytology will yield the typical macrophages and inflammatory cells with no epithelial cells, so a presumptive diagnosis can be made and a trial of antibiotics given before biopsy. In these cases, the typical large ducts with their pultaceous contents are more likely to be present. A formal duct excision procedure, together with excision of the mass, is usually indicated. This should be done under appropriate antibiotic cover.

Abscess Formation

Any of these subareolar masses may proceed to abscess formation. The underlying mass becomes attached to the skin which first becomes reddened and then shows bluish discolouration. Nipple retraction will often develop if not already present, and nipple oedema may be marked. These abscesses are associated with discomfort which varies from mild to severe, but not usually as severe as with pyogenic abscess. Aspiration will yield creamy or dirty, watery pus and bacteriological culture may be sterile on the first occasion. If not treated, it will burst spontaneously with considerable relief but a persistent sinus remains, or the abscess recurs sooner or later and usually at the same site. A typical disease sequence is shown in Figure 11.6–11.8. Recurrent abscesses are more likely to grow bacteria – anaerobes or staphylococci as discussed on p. 111. While most sinuses are situated in the juxta-areolar region and are reasonably well localized, more severe abscesses may occur in association with duct

ectasia, sometimes involving most of the breast (Figure 11.9).

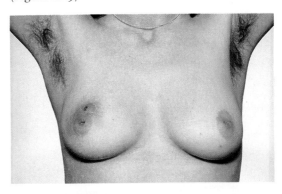

11.6 A 28-year-old woman presenting with a diffuse periareolar abscess which has burst spontaneously while taking antibiotics. Note the bilateral congenital nipple inversion. The patient was successfully treated by major duct excision because of the diffuse nature of the sepsis.

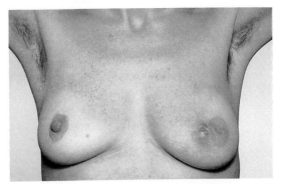

11.7 The patient (as in Figure 11.6) had no further problem with the right breast. Eight years later she presented with a similar condition of the left breast unresponsive to appropriate antibiotics. Treatment was by local drainage, followed by major duct excision 6 weeks later. (This was done in preference to fistulectomy at the patient's request, so that the inverted nipple could be corrected.)

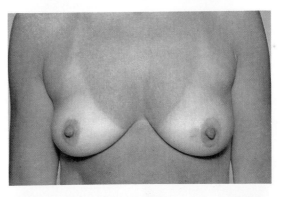

11.8 The result (patient in Figures 11.6 and 11.7) 2 years later. The patient remains asymptomatic. The small scar of conservative drainage is visible medial to the left nipple.

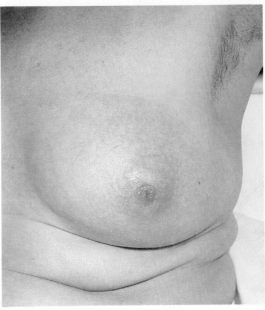

11.9 A diffuse breast abscess associated with duct ectasia. The patient had relatively little pain, despite the gross inflammation.

Peripheral Mass

While most masses arise in relation to major ducts near the areola, similar masses are occasionally seen in the periphery of the breast – two illustrative cases are shown. Figure 11.10 shows a large tender mass in the mid, upper, right breast, which slowly increased in size over 2 months. Mammography and cytology were both consistent with benign diagnosis, but the patient requested excision because of constant aching. Figure 11.11 shows the presence of multiple small abscesses and Figure 11.12 shows the typical histology of intense inflammatory infiltration around duct remnants. The clinical pattern resembles that recorded with 'granulomatous mastitis'.

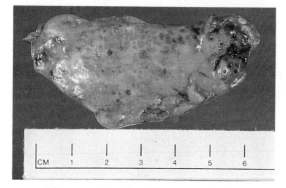

11.10 *A 28-year-old woman with a peripheral mass in the upper aspect of the right breast, due to perilobular mastitis.*

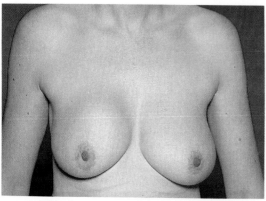

11.11 *The cut specimen from Figure 11.10 showing multiple small abscesses, sterile on culture.*

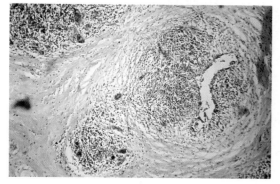

11.12 *The histological picture of Figure 11.11 which shows intense focal inflammation.*

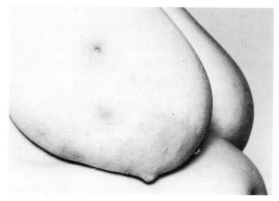

11.13 *Multiple peripheral sinuses following abscesses due to duct ectasia/periductal mastitis. (See text for details.)*

Figure 11.13 shows a 45-year-old woman who presented with recurrent abscesses involving a large area of the upper, outer quadrant of the right breast. Each abscess was painful and discharged to leave a chronic sinus and to be followed by further abscesses. At operation the mammary ducts were grossly distended into the axillary tail and filled with thick, dark-green material. The abscesses were sufficiently incapacitating for the patient to request a large segmental excision. A few further small abscesses later developed adjacent to the excision margin, but were not sufficiently incapacitating to warrant further treatment. This clinical pattern may be confused with hidradenitis suppurativa.

Mammary Duct Fistula

The major papers describing this condition have been outlined in the historical survey. The typical features are classic. A young woman – of average age in the early thirties but sometimes as early as the teenage years – presents with a history of having several abscesses in one breast which had been treated by surgical drainage or have discharged spontaneously. The appearance is so typical that a spot diagnosis can usually be made (Figure 11.14). The features are partial inversion of the nipple and a sinus or scar at the edge of the areola. In cases recurrent on many occasions, the areola is distorted, scarring having reduced the distance between the nipple and the edge of the areola in the radius of the fistula.

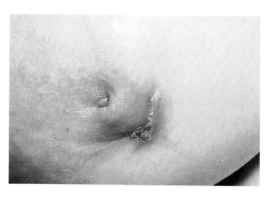

11.14 *The classical picture of late diagnosed mammary duct fistula. (See text).*

A majority of patients developing the condition have nipple inversion, for example 19 of 28 in Atkins' series[17] and 23 of 40 in the series by Bundred *et al*[38]. However, neither states the number of these in which inversion was congenital. In our experience many of the patients have always had inverted nipples, but the history is sometimes vague in patients developing abscesses in their thirties, with inversion of long standing. About one in five of patients first develop an abscess in association with pregnancy or lactation.

Bundred *et al*[38], in a retrospective case note study, reported 13 of 40 patients developing a fistula after breast biopsy – by implication in the absence of an abscess. This is an unusual finding and, in our experience, biopsy of non-suppurative periductal mastitis usually heals uneventfully.

Nipple Retraction

There is a complex relationship between nipple inversion or retraction and the syndrome of duct ectasia/periductal mastitis. It occurs in about one-third of patients requiring surgery for duct ectasia/periductal mastitis but it is difficult to estimate its incidence in patients with asymptomatic duct ectasia. There are at least three aspects of this complex relationship:

1. There can be little doubt that congenital inversion of the nipple predisposes to the development of subareolar abscess and fistula (*see* Figure 11.6 and Table 11.3).
2. There is frequently a close temporal relationship between overt periductal mastitis and the development of nipple retraction. The nipple inversion is characteristically transverse and of minor extent in the early stages (Figure 11.15), but subsequently progresses to more complete retraction over a period of 1 or 2 years. It not infrequently commences following a pregnancy. The initial changes may precede, coincide with, or follow the development of overt periductal mastitis.
3. Nipple retraction is frequently seen as an isolated event, without other evidence of duct ectasia. These cases are usually around or beyond the menopause. The retraction is circular (Figure 11.16) and progresses over 1 or 2 years often followed by the same process in the other breast. It seems likely that this type of retraction is due to the obliterative changes described by Davies[26] where microscopic periductal inflammation leads to disruption and periductal fibrosis without clinical ectasia or inflammation – probably more a normal involutional process than a disease.

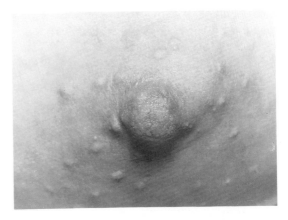

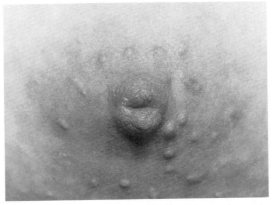

11.15 *The classical transverse central retraction of early nipple involvement in duct ectasia (lower picture). The other nipple developed retraction 2 years later.*

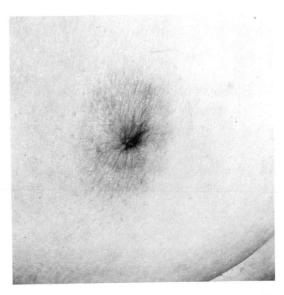

11.16 *Well advanced nipple retraction due to periductal fibrosis in a postmenopausal woman.*

We have previously described the clinical features of nipple retraction in this condition[39]. Thirty patients were seen in a 3.5-year period – an incidence of one case of nipple retraction due to duct ectasia per 100 new patients seen in the breast clinic. The age range of the patients was 25–75 years with a mean of 52 years. The duration of retraction ranged from 3 months to 16 years. The incidence of parity and breast-feeding did not differ from that of other conditions presenting to the breast clinic. Retraction was partial in 12 cases, complete in 18. The left nipple was affected in 14, the right in 11 and was bilateral in 5. Early transverse retraction is easily withdrawn but the eversion becomes more difficult as retraction becomes more complete with the passage of time. However, eversion is still sometimes possible in advanced cases of long duration. The second nipple may show similar changes which may lag months or years behind the first in the development of retraction.

Some clinical features help in the differentiation from carcinoma. Retraction is more likely to be complete in carcinoma and to be accompanied by distortion of the areolar when the breast is examined in different positions, while central and symmetrical retraction favour a diagnosis of duct ectasia. Eversion of the nipple by pressure behind the areola is more likely to be possible in duct ectasia. Pain is of little help in differential diagnosis because two-thirds of patients with nipple retraction due to duct ectasia have no pain. The presence of nipple discharge of the type typical of duct ectasia favours this diagnosis, as does a long history of a year or more – particularly when no mass is palpable. Bilateral retraction favours duct ectasia. However, it must be stressed that no feature is absolutely diagnostic and cancer must always be excluded with care. Mammography will usually exclude cancer in the fatty radiolucent postmenopausal breast, but this may not be so easily achieved in the dense breast of the young patient. Typical radiological features of duct ectasia (*see below*) may be present.

Mastalgia

We believe that a considerable proportion of cases of non-cyclical mastalgia are associated with duct ectasia and periductal mastitis, although it is difficult to prove this except in acute episodes. It would not be surprising if the intense periductal inflammation and subsequent fibrotic process, described by Davies, was a cause of chronic pain.

The evidence associated with the two is derived largely from an association of radiological signs of duct ectasia with pain[40]. Sometimes serial mammograms have shown the subsequent development of typical calcification of this disease at the site of pain.

Eczema

Bloodgood[3] described a case of eczema of the areola which was ascribed to nipple discharge. Azzopardi[25] mentioned similar cases.

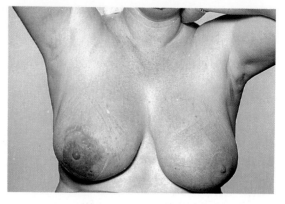

11.17 *Severe, recurrent eczema of the areola and surrounding breast which the patient claimed always followed nipple discharge. Note the scar of a major duct excision on the left breast.*

We have also seen this phenomenon (Figure 11.17 – the 35-year-old woman was adamant that the eczema always followed nipple discharge. After some hestitation, duct excision was performed and the typical changes of duct ectasia were demonstrated. The condition promptly developed on the other side, but again responded to duct excision. Several years later the patient complained of recurrent discharge and recurrent eczema in the right breast. The operation was repeated with a further period of relief. (The question of the reconnection of divided ducts is discussed later.)

While there seems to be good evidence from these cases for an association between eczema and nipple discharge, it is very difficult to exclude a factitial element. However, on balance, we accept the likelihood that some areolar eczema may be due to sensitization of the skin to some element in nipple discharge.

Neonatal Duct Ectasia

The hypertrophy of breast tissue seen in neonates results from the transplacental passage of maternal hormone and both males and females respond in the same way. The degree of secretory change may be sufficient to induce considerable duct ectasia[2]. The changes regress spontaneously in most cases but have been described as a cause of bloody nipple discharge[41].

Duct Ectasia in the Male

The male breast may occasionally show much of the clinical spectrum of duct ectasia/periductal mastitis, including nipple discharge, nipple retraction, recurrent subareolar abscess and bilateral involvement[42]. Tedeschi and McCarthy[43] reported a patient presenting with a tender lump which showed a typical histological picture of periductal mastitis. Habif *et al*[23] also reported two cases. The condition is further discussed in the section on the male breast (*see* Chapter 16).

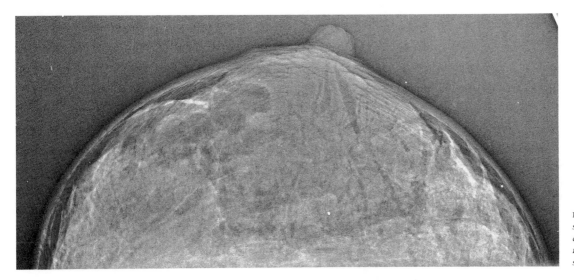

11.18 *Mammogram showing negative shadows due to ducts filled with radiolucent lipoid material – seen just below the nipple.*

Frequency of Duct Ectasia/Periductal Mastitis

Simple duct ectasia is very common, for Sandison[44] found 'gross duct ectasia with much dilated and thickened ducts containing grumous, yellowish green material, ramifying through the fibrofatty parenchyma of the organ' in 11% of women at autopsy with the greatest incidence in the elderly. Clearly the great majority of these had never experienced clinical disease in relation to these ducts. One group[45] encountered 40 cases requiring surgery over a 10-year period, during which time 732 breast operations of all types were performed. The frequency of presenting features in their series and three other series are given in Table 11.5. Dixon *et al*[36] found the mean age of presentation for pain, lump and nipple discharge to be similar at about 40 years, while nipple retraction was seen at a mean age of 53 years. However, in all these series, it is difficult to assess the figures given because it is not possible to differentiate between congenital and acquired nipple retraction, and mammary duct fistula is not considered.

Table 11.5 Presenting features of mammary duct ectasia/periductal mastitis.

	Cromar and Dockerty[53]	Haagensen[16]	Walker and Sandison[21]	Thomas *et al*[45]
No. of patients	24	67	34	78
Mean age	40	50	–	45
Nipple discharge	21	24	47	44
Nipple inversion	42	30	8	32
Mass	100	30	8	32
Sepsis	–	–	9	9

Radiology

The changes on mammography have been described by a number of authors[46]. Nipple retraction will be obvious and prominent ducts will be shown as a conical opacity with the apex of the cone towards the nipple. The individual ducts may be seen leading into this opacity but it is not possible to distinguish radiologically between duct ectasia, intraductal hyperplasia and periductal

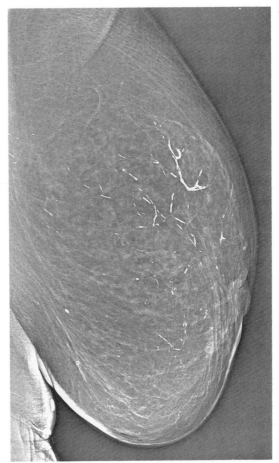

11.19 *Mammogram showing the typical coarse calcification of duct ectasia – some round, some elongated and orientated in the direction of the duct. Note the retracted nipple.*

collagenosis[47]. In a few cases of gross dilatation, the fatty contents may be sufficiently radiolucent to outline the ducts and confirm their ectatic nature (Figure 11.18). Duct ectasia is frequently associated with characteristic coarse calcification. This may be ring-like – the calcification lying on the duct wall – or circular or needle shaped, when the duct contents are calcified (Figure 11.19).

Plasma cell mastitis gives moderately dense opacities, usually in the subareolar region and often flame shaped. Overlying skin and nipple oedema or retraction are sometimes seen (Figure 11.20).

Management of Duct Ectasia/Periductal Mastitis

Medical Management

There can be little hope for efficacious medical management until more is known about the causes of duct ectasia and periductal mastitis, in both its sterile and suppurative form. Because simple duct ectasia with nipple discharge causes trivial symptoms, and other cases are asymptomatic, no active treatment is necessary in many cases. In the more troublesome patients with gross infective lesions, medical management is unlikely to give long-term control, while dilated ducts act as a sump with stagnant secretions forming a nidus for persisting bacterial colonization. It is difficult to assess reports of medical therapy because of the evanescent nature of early periductal mastitis and also because diagnosis is imprecise in the absence of biopsy material. These factors militate against meaningful controlled trials.

Hormone Therapy

Nipple Discharge
Galactorrhea is usually readily distinguished from the nipple discharge in duct ectasia by the volume and consistency of the fluid, but, where any doubts exists, serum prolactin measurement should be performed to exclude a prolactinoma. Bromocriptine is likely to be effective in such a case. We have not seen benefit from bromocriptine therapy in patients with profuse discharge due to duct ectasia and this drug is often poorly tolerated by patients with a normal serum prolactin. J.P. Minton of Columbus, Ohio has reported that nipple discharge may be associated with excess caffeine ingestion. He reports that exclusion of caffeine and other xanthines from the diet may result in resolution of the nipple discharge due to duct ectasia, although it takes 6–9 months for an

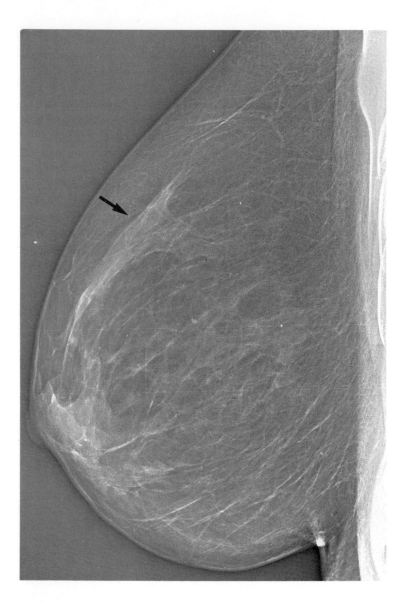

effect to be seen (personal communication). We have no experience of this approach to management.

Painful periductal mastitis
Peters and his co-workers[48] have recently reported rapid resolution of non-puerperal mastitis after prescribing bromocriptine at a dose of 7.5 mg per day for 3 days reducing to 5 mg per day for 11 days. The groups was a mixed one but included some patients with typical periductal mastitis. Symptoms relapsed on stopping treatment but responded again to a 6-months maintenance course of bromocriptine 2.5 mg daily. There is no obvious rationale for this treatment and the results take no account of spontaneous remission, related to the evanescent nature of many early attacks of periductal mastitis. We have not had such satisfactory results but further results of this approach will be watched with interest.

11.20 *Mammogram showing the typical features of subareolar plasma cell mastitis with an associated flame-shaped opacity (arrow).*

Antibiotics

Many patients with painful breast lumps have already been started on antibiotics before attending a breast clinic and will report that symptoms have improved. By the time the patient is seen, it is impossible to determine whether this was spontaneous resolution or the result of antibiotic therapy. However, if the work quoted earlier[33] reflects the bacteriology of mild periductal mastitis, the antibiotics generally used in general practice, such as ampicillin and erythromycin, would not be effective. This suggests that any benefit of such antibiotic therapy may be due to spontaneous resolution. Because anaerobic bacteria and staphylococci are the commonest organisms, metronidazole and flucloxacillin would be the appropriate combination with the addition of a broad-spectrum antibiotic such as erythromycin if these two are not effective. The result of this therapy has been variable in our experience and we are not aware of any reported controlled trial. A controlled trial would be difficult to organize because of the diagnostic uncertainty in pre-suppurative cases. It is likely from general principals that the efficacy of antibiotic therapy is dependent on the underlying pathology. Early bacterial periductal mastitis could be expected to respond while non-bacterial mastitis would not benefit. Advanced cases with grossly dilated ducts might be expected to be resistant because bacteria in the thick duct secretions would not be reached by the antibiotics. This variable response due to diverse pathology would be consistent with our results. In practice, we would recommend the following approach.

Mildly painful and tender masses behind the areola could be observed initially with the likelihood that they would resolve spontaneously. More painful masses should be explored with a 21-gauge needle and any fluid aspirate submitted to cytology and culture with meticulous use of transport medium appropriate to the detection of anaerobic organisms. In the absence of pus, patients are started on a combination of metronidazole and flucloxicillin while awaiting the results of culture. Antibiotics are continued on the basis of sensitivity tests and many of these mild cases respond satisfactorily, especially in the short term. Where there is more than a minimum amount of pus, it is best to proceed to conservative surgical drainage with continuing antibiotic cover. Once a large amount of pus has formed, repeated aspiration is unlikely to lead to resolution but results in destruction of breast tissue and skin with a less satisfactory cosmetic result in the long term. Antibiotic therapy is particularly useful in recurrent inflammation after formal duct excision and a prolonged course – at least 2 weeks and repeated once if necessary – should always be tried before resorting to further surgery.

Surgical Therapy

A striking feature of reports of surgical treatment of the duct ectasia/periductal mastitis complex is the variation in the frequency with which operations are performed and the varying indications given for surgery and for individual operations. Thus Cox et al[49] reviewed 753 consecutive new outpatient referrals to a breast clinic. No operation was performed specifically for this condition, and only one case of mammary duct fistula and one case of duct ectasia was diagnosed, although no fewer than 332 patients in this group had some form of surgical operation. In contrast another recent series[45] reports 78 major duct excisions in a series of 732 breast operations – 40 being for duct ectasia. Urban[20] was able to report 160 major duct excisions in 150 patients, while Hadfield[19] reported 139 similar operations – both authors must now have a very much larger series. We have operated on 200 cases over 15 years, giving an average operation rate of 15 cases per 1000 new referrals to the breast clinic. However, this figure is undoubtedly higher because of the tertiary referrals to our unit, but conversely we find it necessary to operate on only a proportion of clinically significant cases. Indications for surgery in 148 cases of major duct excision in our unit are shown in Table 11.6.

Table 11.6 Indications for operation in the 148 patients undergoing major duct excision.

Indication	Total	Right	Left	Bilateral, same date	Bilateral, different date
Nipple discharge	83	29	41	11	2
Discharge plus subareolar inflammation	9	3	3	0	3
Discharge plus mass	2	1	1	0	0
Subareolar inflammation	32	10	16	4	2
Mass	15	6	9	0	0
Other	7	4	3	0	0
Total	148	53	73	15	7

Recently some workers have reported that surgery can be avoided in most cases by antibiotic therapy. Our own experience does not support this view in the longer term and suggests that the more enthusiastic reports of successful antibiotic therapy reflect cases of mild severity followed for a short time.

Surgeons reporting large series have tended to use the operation very freely, many operations being performed for simple non-bloody discharge or for an otherwise straightforward lump which lies behind the areola. Hadfield[19] and Thomas et al[45] both used total duct excision as the procedure of choice for recurrent subareolar sepsis in preference to the operation of fistulotomy or fistulectomy favoured by other surgeons. With such a diversity of thought and practice, it is not possible to give a consensus from the literature. Hence we give our own views derived from an experience of some 200 operations for duct ectasia and its complications, performed over the last 15 years and from a considerable experience of tertiary referrals of problem cases following earlier surgery.

Indications for Surgery

Surgery may be required in the following clinical situations:

1. Nipple discharge – coloured, opalescent, bloody, serous.
2. Correction of nipple inversion.
3. Diagnosis of a retroareolar mass.
4. Subareolar abscess.
5. Fistula.
6. Eczema.
7. Recurrence after previous surgery.

Non-bloody Nipple Discharge

This condition, typically from several ducts and sometimes bilateral, is a benign condition with no increased cancer risk. It is not normally an indication for surgical treatment. We do not believe that investigation or treatment is necessary except in those rare cases where discharge is so profuse as to require constant wearing of a pad and causes significant social embarrassment. In this situation, we would exclude a prolactinoma, and then offer the patient the operation of total duct excision, bilateral if necessary.

Bloody or Serous Discharge

The management of this symptom is dealt with more fully in Chapter 12. Over the age of 40 years there is a significant risk of cancer or hyperplastic lesions and the operation of total duct excision has some advantages over more conservative procedures. It provides a good histo-logical specimen and relieves the anxiety of the symptom. Where the cause proves to be one which is potentially multifocal, such as duct ectasia or a hyperplastic epithelial lesion, it pre-empts further discharge from other ducts.

Correction of Nipple Inversion

Patients are more likely to request correction of congenital nipple inversion than retraction due to duct ectasia occurring later in life, but some patients request correction of retraction for this condition. Although the results are usually satisfactory, patients seeking correction for cosmetic reasons should be aware of the possibility of nipple necrosis, of interference with sensation, of the inability to breast-feed and the possibility that postoperative fibrosis will lead to late re-inversion.

Because the condition is due to shortening of the ducts, it can only be corrected permanently by a complete division of the subareolar ducts.

We usually do not consider operative correction to be indicated on cosmetic grounds alone, but when patients have had the procedure carried out for complications of periductal mastitis, the resulting correction of nipple inversion has been a much appreciated side-effect. Such patients may then press for operative correction of a contralateral inverted nipple.

Diagnosis of a Retroareolar Mass

The tender acute retroareolar mass of periductal mastitis frequently resolves spontaneously, so surgery should be delayed if aspiration biopsy is suggestive of this diagnosis. Where a mass persists for several weeks, we would treat it by simple excision biopsy, even if dilated ducts filled with pultaceous material are encountered. Primary healing is the rule; only in the presence of an overt abscess is postoperative sepsis likely. If such an abscess is encountered at operation, we would either undertake simple drainage with a view to formal surgery should the problem recur, or proceed immediately to formal total duct excision under appropriate antibiotic cover. We tend to the first course in young women and to the latter in women past the child-bearing period.

Subareolar Abscess

The diagnosis is confirmed by needle aspiration, which also provides a specimen for cytology and bacterial culture. In our experience, aspiration under antibiotic cover rarely leads to resolution of an established abscess and they are best treated by conservative open drainage. Drainage is conservative – unlike puerperal abscess – because the infection is often associated with a single duct system, and it is desirable to confine the process to a single segment. If the abscess leads to a mammary duct fistula it can be treated by fistulotomy. More radical drainage may spread the infection or damage adjacent normal ducts.

Recurrent Abscess with Fistula Formation

This situation provides a difficult problem of surgical judgement, the decision whether a fistula with recurrent sepsis should be treated by fistulotomy or by major duct excision. Some of the factors bearing on this decision are set out in Table 11.17.

Table 11.7. Treatment of recurrent subareolar sepsis.

Suitable for fistulectomy	Suitable for total duct excision
Abscess small and localized to one segment	Abscess large, affecting >50% of areolar circumference
Recurrence always at the same site	Recurrence involving a different segment
Probe passes easily from fistula through nipple at interval operation	Probe may be 'lost' in cavity
Mild congenital nipple inversion or no inversion	Gross nipple inversion
Patient unconcerned about nipple inversion	Patient requests correction of nipple inversion
Younger patient	Older patient
No discharge from other ducts	Purulent discharge from other ducts between episodes
	Recurrence after fistulectomy

When a small localized periareolar abscess recurs at the same point, and a fistula is clearly present, the operation of choice is fistulotomy (or fistulectomy – *see* Chapter 18). It is a simple procedure with minimal complications and a high degree of success. Should it fail (in spite of being carried out correctly), total duct excision can still be used.

Where subareolar sepsis is diffuse rather than localized to one segment or where more than one fistula opening is present, total duct excision is the procedure of choice.

The former situation is likely to be seen in young women with squamous metaplasia or a single duct, the latter in an older woman with multiple ectatic ducts. However, age is not a reliable guide and we would recommend fistula excision as the initial procedure for localized lesions irrespective of age. One exception is where there is marked nipple inversion and the patient wishes to have this corrected. This tips the balance towards total duct excision, particularly if the

patient does not wish to breast-feed in the future. Figures 11.6, 11.7 and 11.8 show a case where duct excision was considered appropriate in a young patient.

Eczema

Where there is good evidence that eczema of the areola follows nipple discharge, total duct excision is the only procedure likely to give relief. However, other forms of eczema and factitial injury should be carefully considered before resorting to surgery, since duct ectasia is a rare cause of areolar eczema.

Recurrence after Previous Surgery

This is considered below.

The Consequences and Results of Operations for Duct Ectasia

Patients should be aware of the consequences of these operations before undergoing surgery, particularly where this is recommended for conditions other than sepsis, because a patient is unlikely to be satisfied if a less than optimal result is obtained. With severe or recurrent sepsis, the morbidity of the disease is such that most patients happily accept the results of surgery which relieves them of their episodes.

Consequences

Cosmesis

In general, the cosmetic effect is excellent when performed for nipple discharge, but less satisfactory when done for sepsis, especially for long-standing sepsis. In the first group the nipple is not distorted and a typical result is shown in Figure 11.21. Satisfactory results may also be

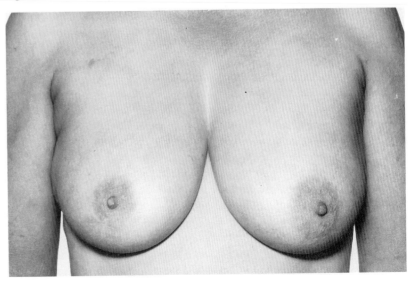

11.21 *A typical long-term postoperative result of (right-sided) major duct excision of nipple discharge. Operation for sepsis often leaves a less satisfactory result.*

obtained when operating for sepsis providing the operation is done before gross scarring has occurred and if the cosmetic result is considered when performing operations (*see* Figure 11.8). Once skin destruction is allowed to occur and multiple abscesses have been drained, severe distortion of the nipple has occurred and cannot be readily corrected. The situation is even worse when recurrent sepsis occurs more peripherally in the breast after duct excision and this is discussed below in relation to operations for recurrent disease.

Although failure to lactate after the operation suggests that glandular atrophy must occur with time, there is no change in size of the breast after the operation.

Sensation

Tactile sensation is usually lost in part over the half of the nipple raised as a flap (Figure 11.22). Multiple incisions around different segments are likely to increase the sensory loss, so should be avoided if possible.

Lactation

Patients cannot breast-feed after this operation and there are few reports of the consequences of pregnancy following duct excision. Urban reported that 4 of his 150 patients became pregnant after the operation. Minimal engorgement occurred following delivery but this rapidly subsided when lactation was suppressed with hormones. Hadfield[50] recommended patients to defer pregnancy for a year after the operation. He reports an unspecified number of pregnancies after the operation. Lactation occurred normally on the unoperated side, but no discharge from the operated breast. When pregnancy occurred within a year of operation, there were varying degrees of enlargement from activity in the operated breast which subsided quickly after delivery.

We also advise our patients to avoid pregnancy for 1 year after operation and have seen no problem under these circumstances. However, one patient became pregnant 4 months after bilateral duct excision for recurrent sepsis. One breast gave no problem but the other became markedly engorged and painful and developed recurrent sepsis which required further surgery after parturition. So our experience would also suggest that there are no untoward effects of pregnancy following duct excision provided the patient waits a year after surgery.

Restoration of Duct Continuity

Duct discharge sometimes recurs after the operation and it must be assumed that occasionally

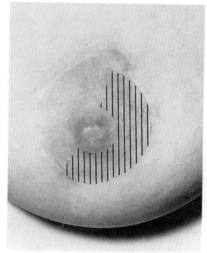
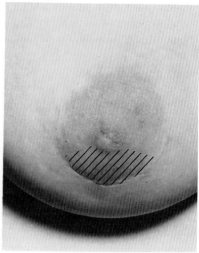

the ducts reconnect to an aperture in the nipple. Indeed one of our patients claimed to successfully breast-feed for 9 months after this operation, but the breast at this time was involutional to palpation compared to the normal breast and we saw no milk from the operated nipple.

Behaviour of Residual Ducts

There is a surprising lack of information about what happens to the remainder of the breast ducts after subareolar duct excision. Haagensen[16] makes no comment nor do the writers of any of the other series. In our experience, the small number of patients coming to further operation have shown that the ducts remain dilated and filled with the same material seen at the primary operation. Since most cases of reoperation have been for recurrent sepsis, this group may behave differently to the majority of patients without further trouble, but the same dilated ducts have also been encountered occasionally where reoperation has been performed for causes other than infection. The fact that dilated ducts can remain in this state for years following major duct excision throws doubt on the suggestion that bacteria can be cultured from most cases of periductal mastitis. In contrast to the persistence of dilated collecting ducts, the minimal response of the breast to pregnancy after long-standing division of the ducts suggests that back pressure may lead to atrophy of the secretory acinar elements of the duct system.

Cancer Risk

The long-standing presence of secretions stagnant in ducts completely obstructed by major duct excision would seem to provide a background for carcinogenesis. However, Haagensen and Urban both state that there have been no excess cases of cancer in their patients having duct excision,

11.22 *Patient following bilateral major duct excision for severe recurrent sepsis multiple on the right side. The stippled area outlines the loss of sensation.*

many of whom were followed for a long time. Our experience would support this although it must be admitted that there are inadequate data based on documented long-term follow-up to provide a definitive answer to the question.

The Results of Operations for Duct Ectasia

Major Duct Excision

Early authors reported excellent results from operations for duct ectasia and periductal mastitis which are somewhat surprising, especially because many such operations were performed before the importance of anaerobic organisms and appropriate antibiotic therapy was realized. Urban[20] concludes his study of 167 major duct excisions by stating that the operation 'results in satisfactory cosmetic appearance. There have been no recurrence of symptoms and no complications in our hands'. Hadfield[50] reported equally satisfactory results. All patients were left with a normal looking breast and nipple, there was no instance of recurrent disease on the operation side, and no case of cancer developing during follow-up of 1–7 years.

More recent series have not been so encouraging. Thomas et al[45] reported good results when the operation was performed for nipple retraction, nipple discharge and subareolar mass, although nine of their patients continued to have nipple discharge for up to 1 year after the operation. One patient required reoperation to correct nipple re-inversion. However, they had 100% recurrent infection following major duct excision for abscess, and two of their patients eventually had a mastectomy.

Browning et al[51] also report a considerable postoperative complication rate, although it is difficult to determine from the paper how many of the patients had trouble following major duct excision and how many had only an excision biopsy.

In our unit 122 patients have had formal examination and follow-up at 1–10 years after major duct excision. Thirty-four patients (28%) had suffered a problem affecting the breast subjected to major duct excision (Table 11.8).

Nineteen of the patients have required further surgery to the breast related to the original operation, eight drainage of an abscess, five required further duct excision, four laying open of the fistula, four biopsies, two mastectomies. Hence it is also our experience that most recurrent problems are related to surgery for subareolar sepsis. This high problem rate falls with increasing

Table 11.8 Breast problems following major duct excision

Mastalgia	9
Infection	9
Discharge	7
Lump	6
Haematoma	3
Recurrent Eczema	1
? Raynaud's disease of the nipple	1

operator experience and is also now lower because of better use of appropriate antibiotic therapy. The interval between operation and development of further problems varies from a few weeks to several years.

Results of Fistulotomy/Fistulectomy

Atkins[17] had no recurrence following his operation of fistulotomy with saucerization, although length of follow-up was not detailed.

Lambert et al[52] reported 48 fistulae: 13 were laid open, 25 excised and allowed to granulate, 8 excised with primary closure. One recurrence occurred 6 weeks after a primary closure. They made no attempt to correct inversion of the nipple. Like many series reporting good results, follow-up is relatively short at a mean of 25 months and the operations were performed in a specialist breast centre. Our experience of tertiary referral cases suggests the results from less specialized centres are far from uniformly satisfactory.

Bundred et al[38] reported 40 patients. Nine patients had fistula excision with wound granulation with one recurrent fistula. Twenty-one had excision and primary closure with only ten satisfactory results. Six patients had fistula excision with primary closure under antibiotic cover (metronidazole and flucloxacillin); all healed primarily. They suggest that primary closure with antibiotic cover may be the procedure of choice, but agree that further experience and longer follow-up will be necessary. Four of their patients had bilateral fistulae. It is clear that laying open of the fistula with curettage or excision of the duct gives good results. If a non-adherent self-dressing technique such as Silastic Foam is used, the wound is painless and the patient can be discharged home and returned to normal activities – 3 or 4 days after operation. Primary closure under antibiotic cover is an alternative, but longer follow-up is necessary to assess its reliability.

Complications of Operations for Duct Ectasia

The complications of fistulectomy are slow healing and recurrent abscess and fistulae. Both are commonly due to inadequate technique.

The complications of major duct excision are haematoma, infection, flap necrosis, nipple inversion, cosmetic deformity, pain and recurrence of the original condition.

Surgery for Recurrence following Operation

The commonest problem calling for further surgery is recurrent infection; less common is persisting nipple discharge or re-inversion of the nipple. The commonest cause of persisting problems following surgery is incorrect or inappropriate surgery. Intractable disease is less common. The first approach to a patient with recurrent problems is careful inspection for evidence of inadequate surgery. If this is found, revisional surgery is usually the best approach. Where surgery appears to have been satisfactory, a trial of prolonged antibiotic therapy for recurrent sepsis is preferable to early operation. The causes of recurrence of symptoms in patients referred to us are shown in Table 11.9.

Persistent Proximal Duct

A common error of inexperienced operators is to leave a residual portion of duct close to the nipple. In the case of fistulectomy, it is essential that the terminal duct be excised or curetted firmly to eradicate the squamous epithelium typically present in this part of the duct. Failure to do so can be detected by careful inspection – when the scar will be seen to fall short of the apex of the nipple (Figure 11.23). This case, recurrent after 'fistulectomy', was cured by reoperation in which the terminal portion of the duct was located by probing and formally excised, together with re-excision of the fistula tract. It is also possible to leave a short section of proximal duct attached to the nipple after a proximal duct excision and this had been the cause of several recurrent cases in our experience (Figure 11.24).

Residual Ducts

It is also common for inexperienced operators to miss some of the breast ducts – those furthest from the incision – when performing major duct excision (Figure 11.25). This must be assumed to be the case when nipple discharge persists immediately following surgery. Details of technique to avoid this are given in Chapter 18.

If the symptoms merit further treatment, operation to remove the residual ducts – usually at the far side of the duct cone from the incision – may be indicated. We have found this necessary occasionally both for eczema of the nipple and for recurrent infection.

Table 11.9 Causes of recurrent disease following fistulectomy and major duct excision for duct ectasia/periductal mastitis.

Persistent proximal ducts
Persistent distal ducts
Persisting or recurrent nipple inversion
Early pregnancy
Contralateral disease
Factitial disease

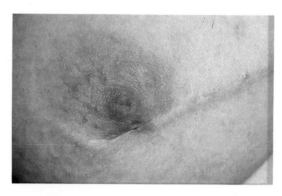

11.23 *A patient with recurrent sepsis following operation for mammary duct fistula. Note that the incision does not reach the centre of the nipple. The causative pathology has not been eliminated.*

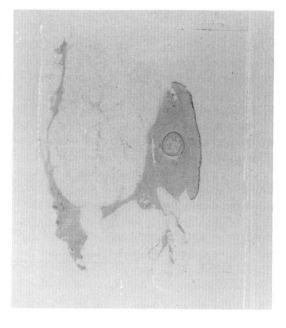

11.24 *Histological section after excision of a persisting fistula. The patient had previously undergone major duct excision but a terminal portion of duct had been left under the nipple.*

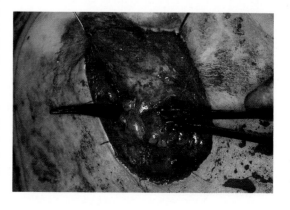

11.25 *At operation for persisting nipple discharge after major duct excision, some ducts have been left at the far end of the dissection.*

Persistent Distal Ducts

The surprising aspect of operations on the major ducts for duct ectasia is that the residual distal ducts give so little trouble. Haagensen noted this as early as 1951 and it has proved to be general experience. Even when dilated ducts are cut across and drain into the wound, late trouble from the residual breast is uncommon. Nevertheless, most authors report recurrent disease in a proportion of cases, some being sufficiently severe to lead to mastectomy. We have seen a number of similar cases – an example, and the way it was managed, is shown in Figures 11.26–11.29. Intensive antibiotic therapy should be the first approach in such cases, but will not control all. It is of interest that some of these inflammatory attacks occurring after duct excision settle without treatment even when quite severe, resolving in 3 or 4 days in exactly the same manner as can be seen in the initial evanescent attacks of periductal mastitis. Once again this seems to be incompatible with heavy bacterial colonization of the residual ducts and suggests a 'chemical' inflammatory response to irritant materials. Where inflammation persists and pus can be aspirated, and antibiotics have not given control, a further wedge excision is the appropriate treatment because inflammatory changes in the residual breast tend to be segmental in outline. At the same time as this wedge excision is carried out under antibiotic cover, the subareolar area should be explored to exclude persisting ducts or a hidden abscess cavity.

We have performed only two mastectomies for duct ectasia. With further experience, we now believe that local incisions under antibiotic cover will control most cases if the proximal duct excision had been correctly performed. However, there are some patients whose disease is sufficiently intractable and peripheral to warrant mastectomy. The complications are not inconsiderable because of scarring of previous operations, and any reconstructive procedure is better delayed to allow all sepsis to settle.

Persisting Nipple Inversion

Correction of nipple inversion requires careful attention to detail during major duct excision. Fistulectomy does not allow correction of inversion. Once nipple inversion is corrected but total duct division, it usually remains everted by a few cases will re-invert after some time – presumably this is due to formation of scar tissue and subsequent fibrous contraction. Persisting nipple inversion leads to collection of grumous material in the inverted cavity which discharges periodically and leads the patient to believe that she has recurrent

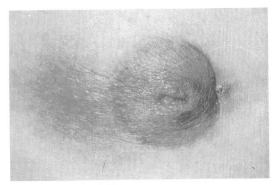

11.26 A patient with recurrent sepsis following major duct excision. Note the nipple inversion has not been corrected.

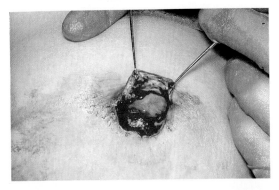

11.27 At reoperation there is a chronic abscess under the nipple with sepsis extending out into the breast. Several ducts had been missed at the original operation.

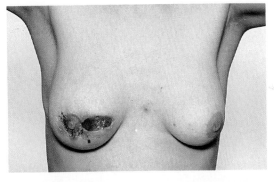

11.28 This was treated by re-excision of the ducts and segmental excision in continuity.

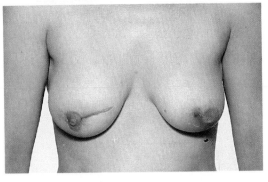

11.29 The patient one year later. The right breast has healed satisfactorily but the patient has developed the same condition in the left breast, reflecting the frequent bilateral incidence of this condition.

duct discharge. The material is sometimes offensive. Collection of material in an inverted nipple undoubtedly predisposes in some cases to further subareolar sepsis, particularly staphylococcal. Presumably organisms ingress through the old duct openings in the nipple.

Hence, for these reasons and for reasons of cosmesis, it is worth taking particular trouble to obtain eversion as detailed in Chapter 18. In some patients, a desire to correct inversion tips the balance from fistulectomy to major duct excision as the primary procedure.

Where persisting nipple inversion is a major problem, reoperation is worth while and should include excision of the central fibrotic portion of the apex of the nipple to allow full eversion and remove the tendency to spontaneous re-inversion.

Early Pregnancy

Pregnancy occurring within a few months of major duct excision will cause engorgement and predispose to recurrent infection. Temporizing treatment with antibiotics and/or drainage is likely to leave a residual fistula which will require further operation after suppression of lactation.

Contralateral Disease

There is a marked tendency for this condition to affect both breasts as illustrated in the cases described earlier. The contralateral disease frequently occurs within a few months of control of the original breast but may be delayed as long as 10 years. It is managed in the same way as unilateral disease, often with a better result because of earlier diagnosis and effective surgery.

Factitial Disease

The problem of self-inflicted disease is discussed in Chapter 17. This question must always be considered when recurrent sepsis becomes a problem after operation for duct ectasia. The presence of bowel organisms, such as *Eschericia coli*, *Streptococcus faecalis* and colonic *Bacteroides* sp. should raise the possibility of a factitial basis. Persistent bleeding from the nipple after major duct excision – particularly if no epithelial lesion was demonstrated – is also suggestive of this condition. Ill-advised mastectomy is likely to be followed shortly by bleeding or other problems with the other nipple so the whole process is repeated.

The patients often seem rather odd, but as is the case with other chronic painful conditions, their psyche may take a turn for the better if the condition is corrected. Most of the cases we have seen where factitial disease has been suspected have been shown to have had inadequate surgery and have healed uneventfully after reoperation.

REFERENCES

1. Haagensen C. D. Mammary duct ectasia – A disease that may simulate cancer. *Cancer* 1951; **4**: 749–761.
2. Sandison A. T. & Walker J. C. Inflammatory mastitis, mammary duct ectasia and mammillary fistula. *British Journal of Surgery* 1962; **50**: 57–64.
3. Bloodgood J. C. The Clinical picture of dilated ducts beneath the nipple frequently to be palpated as a doughy, worm-like mass – the varicocele tumour of the breast. *Surgery, Gynecology and Obstetrics* 1923; **36**: 486–495.
4. Birkett J. *The Diseases of the Breast and their Treatment.* Longman, London, 1850.
5. Bloodgood J. C. The pathology of chronic cystic mastitis of the female breast with special consideration of the blue-domed cyst. *Archives of Surgery* 1921; **3**: 445–452.
6. Cutler M. Benign lesions of the female breast simulating cancer. *Journal of the American Medical Association* 1933; **101**: 1277–1282.
7. Cheatle G. L. & Cutler M. *Tumours of the Breast.* Philadephia, Lippincott, 1931.
8. Adair F. E. Plasma cell mastitis, a lesion simulating mammary carcinoma. *Archives of Surgery* 1933; **26**: 735–749.
9. Tice G. I., Dockerty M. B. & Harrington S. W. Comedomastitis. A clinical and pathological study of Data in 172 cases. *Surgery, Gynecology and Obstetrics* 1948; **87**: 525–540.
10. Rodman J. G. & Ingleby H. Plasma cell mastitis. *Annals of Surgery* 1939; **109**: 921–930.
11. Frantz V. K., Pickren J. W., Melcher G. M. & Auchinloss H. Incidence of chronic cystic disease in so-called normal breasts. *Cancer* 1951; **4**: 762–783.
12. Zuska J. J., Crile G. Jr & Ayres W. W. Fistulas of lactiferous ducts. *American Journal of Surgery* 1951; **81**: 312–317.
13. Deaver J. B. & McFarland J. *The Breast: Its Anomalies, its Diseases and their Treatment.* Philadelphia, Blakiston, 1917.
14. Bonnet. Memoire sur les fistules des conduits du lait. *Archives Générales de Médécine Paris 25* 1835; IX: 451–464.
15. Waters J. J. Mammary sinus subsequent to abscess; treatment by a listerian method; cure. *British Medical Journal* 1892; ii: 209.
16. Haagensen C. D. *Disease of the Breast*, 3rd edn. Philadelphia, W. B. Saunders, 1986.
17. Atkins H. J. B., Mammillary fistula. *British Medical Journal* 1955; 2: 1473–1474.
18. Patey D. H. & Thackray A. C. Pathology and treatment of mammary duct fistula. *Lancet* 1958; ii: 871–873.
19. Hadfield G. J. Excision of the major duct system for benign disease of the breast. *British Journal of Surgery* 1960; **47**: 472–477.
20. Urban J. A. Excision of the major duct system of the breast *Cancer* 1963; **16**: 516–520.
21. Walker J. C. & Sandison A. T. Mammary duct ectasia. *British Journal of Surgery* 1964; **51**: 350–355.
22. Ewing M. Stagnation in the main ducts of the breast. *Journal of the Royal College of Surgeons of Edinburgh* 1963; **8**: 134–142.
23. Habif D. V., Perzin K. H., Lipton R. & Lattes R. Subareolar abscess associated with squamous metaplasia of lactiferous ducts. *American Journal of Surgery* 1970; **119**: 523–526.

24. Davies J. D. *Periductal mastitis.* M.D. Thesis, University of London, 1971.
25. Azzopardi J. C. *Problems in Breast Pathology.* London, W. B. Saunders, 1979.
26. Davies J. D. Inflammatory damage to ducts in mammary dysplasia: a cause of duct obliteration. *Journal of Pathology* 1975; 117: 47–54.
27. Toker C. Lactiferous duct fistula. *Journal of Pathology and Bacteriology* 1962; 84: 143–146.
28. Maier W. P., Berger A. & Derrick B. M. Periareolar Abscess in the non-lactating breast. *American Journal of Surgery* 1982: 144: 359–361.
29. Beigelman P. M. & Rantz L. A. Clinical Significance of Bacteroides. *Archives of Internal Medicine* 1949; 84: 605–631.
30. Pearson H. E. Bacteroides in areolar breast abscesses. *Surgery, Gynecology and Obstetrics* 1967; 125: 800–802.
31. Leach R. D., Eykyn S. J., Phillips I. & Corrin B. Anaerobic subareolar breast abscess. *Lancet* 1979; i: 35–37.
32. Leach R. D., Eykyn S. J. & Phillips I. Vaginal manipulation and anaerobic breast abscesses. *British Medical Journal* 1981; 282: 610–611.
33. Bundred N. J., Dixon J. M., Lumsden A. B., Radford D., Hood J., Miles R. S., Chetty U. & Forrest A. M. P. Are the lesions of mammary duct ectasia sterile? *British Journal of Surgery* 1985; 72: 844–845.
34. Davies J. D. Histological study of mammae in oestrogenized rats after izoimmunization. *British Journal of Experimental Pathology* 1972; 53: 406–414.
35. Tedeschi L. G, Ouzouman G. & Byrne J. J. The role of ductal obstruction and hormonal stimulation in main duct ectasia. *Surgery, Gynecology and Obstetrics* 1962; 114: 741–744.
36. Dixon J. M., Anderson T. J., Lumbsdon A. B. *et al* Mammary duct ectasia. *British Journal of Surgery* 1983; 70: 601–603.
37. Koelmeyer T. D. & MacCormick D. E. M. Granulomatous mastitis. *Australia and New Zealand Journal of Surgery* 1976; 46: 173–175.
38. Bundred N. J., Dixon J. M., Chetty U. & Forrest A. P. M. Mammillary fistula. *British Journal of Surgery* 1987; 74: 466–468.
39. Rees B. I., Gravelle I. H. & Hughes L. E. Nipple retraction in duct ectasia. *British Journal of Surgery* 1977; 64: 577–580.
40. Preece P. E. *A study of the aetiology, clinical patterns and treatment of mastalgia.* MD Thesis, University of Wales, 1982.
41. Stringel G. Infantile mammary duct ectasia – a cause of bloody nipple discharge. *Journal of Pediatric Surgery* 1986; 21: 671–676.
42. Mansel R. E. & Morgan W. P. Duct ectasia in the male. *British Journal of Surgery* 1979; 66: 660–662.
43. Tedeschi L. G. & McCarthy P. E. Involutional mammary duct ectasia and periductal mastitis in the male. *Human Pathology* 1974; 5: 232–236.
44. Sandison A. T. *A postmortem study of the adult breast.* M.D. Thesis, University of St Andrews, 1957.
45. Thomas W. G., Williamson R. C. N., Davies J. D. & Webb A. J. The clinical syndrome of mammary duct ectasia. *British Journal of Surgery* 1982; 69: 423–425.
46. Evans K. T. & Gravelle I. H. *Mammography, Thermography and Ultrasonography in Breast Disease.* London, Butterworths, 1973.
47. Mansel R. E., Gravelle I. H. & Hughes L. E. The interpretation of mammographic ductal enlargement in cancerous breasts. *British Journal of Surgery* 1979; 66: 701–702.
48. Peters F., Hilgarth M. & Brecknoldt M. The use of bromocriptine in the management of non puerperal mastitis. *Archives of Gynecology* 1982; 233: 23–29.
49. Cox P. J., Li M. K. W. & Ellis H. Spectrum of breast disease in outpatient surgical practice. *Journal of the Royal Society of Medicine* 1982; 75: 857–859.
50. Hadfield G. J. Further experience of the operation for excision in the major duct system of the breast. *British Journal of Surgery* 1968; 55: 530–535.
51. Browning J., Bigrigg A. & Taylor I. Symptomatic and incidental mammary duct ectasia. *Journal of the Royal Society of Medicine* 1986; 79: 715–716.
52. Lambert M. E., Betts C. D. & Sellwood R. A. Mammillary fistula. *British Journal of Surgery* 1986; 73: 367–368.
53. Cromar C. D. L. & Dockerty M. B. Plasma cell mastitis. *Proceedings of the Staff Meeting of the Mayo Clinic* 1941; 16: 775–782.

12　Nipple Discharge

Nipple discharge is important when it occurs spontaneously and as the dominant symptom. Spontaneous presentation is important, because a high incidence will be recorded if milky discharge which occurs only following squeezing or expression of the breast, is included in series of patients with nipple discharge. Such a discharge is common in parous women and will often be reported on direct questioning. This is not galactorrhea and can be safely ignored.

Nipple discharge loses its significance when it is accompanied by a dominant lump. The lump then takes precedence in assessment and management. An associated nipple discharge does not increase the likelihood of a mass being malignant, at any age[1].

A patient may complain of discharge because she fears the diagnostic implications, because the amount may be sufficient to cause social embarrassment, or as an incidental accompaniment of other breast symptoms. In general, the patient will delay no longer before presenting with discharge than a lump.

Incidence

Nipple discharge is a relatively uncommon presenting complaint in a breast clinic. Haagensen[2] reported that 3% of patients referred to him complained of nipple discharge. In our clinic there were 259 examples of nipple discharge in 4012 consecutively referred cases – an incidence of 6.4%. Of the 259 14 were found to have cancer, 8 of these had a blood-stained discharge, 15 had a macroscopic duct papilloma (9 blood stained) and 87 were attributed to duct ectasia (15 blood stained). Leis[3] reported that only 8% of 1253 breast operations were performed for the indication of nipple discharge. In a study from Guy's hospital over a 10-year period, 6.6% of referrals were for nipple discharge and of the 6000 oper-

ations performed only 4.5% related to treatment of nipple discharge[4].

Nipple discharge is seen also in males, although only rarely. In a series where 10% of 3787 breast clinic patients complained of a nipple discharge, only 1.5% of the nipple discharge occurred in males and none were associated with cancer[1], although this has not been so in all series (*see* Chapter 16).

Character and Significance of Discharge

Discharges fall into three main groups (Tables 5.1 and 5.2). The character of the discharge should be recorded accurately, because there is a good correlation between macroscopic appearance and underlying pathology. Failure to be specific has lead to confusion in much of the literature.

Blood and Serosanguineous Discharge

Serous discharge is characterized by the yellow colour and sticky quality of serum. Serous, serosanguineous (pink) and heavily blood-stained discharges (*see* Figure 11.5) carry the same significance. They are usually due either to a hyperplastic epithelial lesion or to duct ectasia. The epithelial hyperplasia is usually benign, one or more duct papillomas, less commonly malignant. The risk of malignancy increases with age, being much greater after 55 years than before the menopause. In Selzer's series[1] the overall incidence of cancer in patients presenting only with nipple discharge was 12%. This broke down into 3% in patients under the age of 40, 10% between 40 and 60 and 32% for patients over 60 years.

In those patients with duct ectasia, it is usually assumed that the bleeding arises from areas of ulceration within the stagnant ducts, although we are not aware of any formal study of this question.

In many series, a percentage of cases with

Table 12.1 Relationship of discharge type and pathological diagnosis.

Type of discharge	Main cause	Less common cause
Blood related		
bloody	Hyperplastic lesions[a]	Duct ectasia/pregnancy
serous/serosanguineous	Hyperplastic lesions[a]	Duct ectasia
watery	Hyperplastic lesions[a]	
Coloured opalescent		
creamy, green, brown, black	Duct ectasia	Cyst
Milk	Galactorrhoea of endocrine origin	
	Physiological lactation	

[a] Hyperplastic lesions including hyperplasia, papilloma, carcinoma *in situ* and invasive ductal carcinoma.

Table 12.2 Causes of nipple discharge.

	Blood related			Opalescent	Milk
	Bloody	Serous	Watery		
Physiological					
Neonatal	−	−	−	−	+
Lactation	−	−	−	−	+
Pregnancy	±	−	−	−	+
Postlactational	−	−	−	−	+
Mechanical stimulation	−	−	−	−	+
Hyperprolactinaemia	−	−	−	−	+
Ductal pathology					
Duct ectasia	±	±	−	+	−
Cysts	−	−	−	+	−
Papilloma	+	+	±	−	−
Cancer	+	+	±	−	−

+ = common or likely cause; ± = rare but well defined; − = unusual or unknown.

sanguineous discharge show no clear-cut pathology, even after operations such as major duct excision. Hence, it is not surprising that conditions of low specificity in pathological terms have been invoked to explain the bloody discharge. Older series often specify cystic disease as the cause. Some seem to refer to macroscopic cysts, others to the micropapillomatosis element which we now regard as part of ANDI. With these conditions which are part of the spectrum of normality, specificity as to the cause of bleeding is suspect – and the same must be true of a condition as common as duct ectasia – the diagnosis we believe to be most common. Hence, the cause of some serosanguineous discharges must remain uncertain – even after surgery. At least the satisfactory long-term follow-up of such cases shows that they are not associated with significant pathology which has been missed at surgery.

Haagensen's experience with serous and bloody discharge showed an identical significance for both types[2]. Duct papilloma was the cause in 70% and breast cancer in 10%, with both types of discharge. Likewise, 50% of benign papillomas presented with each type of discharge, and cancer cases with nipple discharge were divided evenly between the two. In the Philadelphia series the incidence of cancer was also the same for serous

or bloody discharge[1]. Our experience is similar, although a higher proportion (29%) of our cases of serous or bloody discharge is associated with duct ectasia. Chaudary *et al*[4] have described the role of routine use of an occult blood test in patients admitted for operation for discharge from a solitary duct. In 292 microdochectomies, 215 were positive for blood – all 16 carcinomas were in this group but, in the benign conditions, the presence of blood did not usefully help to distinguish duct ectasia from benign papillomas.

Blood-stained Nipple Discharge of Pregnancy

A little recognized problem that occurs occasionally in pregnancy is blood-stained nipple discharge due to epithelial proliferation as the breasts respond to pregnancy. This is usually bilateral and occurs in the second or third trimester of the first or second pregnancy. The condition carries no serious significance and requires simple explanation and reassurance that it is self-limiting. It rarely persists more than 2 months postpartum[5]. Further investigation and treatment should be avoided because cytology may be misleading in this situation. It often shows epithelial cell clusters similar to those of intraductal papilloma and the cells may appear cytologically active[6].

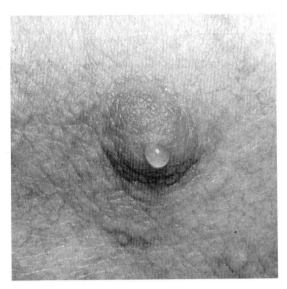

12.1 *Clear watery discharge, distinct from serous and sanguineous.*

Watery Discharge

This is a rare but very distinctive type of discharge (Figure 12.1). It is crystal clear, copious and associated in our experience of two cases with multiple papillomas of the large ducts – macroscopic papillomas in one case and with florid microscopic papillomatosis in the other. Neither has as yet developed cancer (after 5 years of follow-up) although Haagensen believes the large papilloma condition to be premalignant. Lewison and Chambers[7] presented evidence that this type of discharge is associated with breast cancer. Haagensen could only record one such case – associated with papillary intraduct cancer.

Coloured Opalescent Discharges

It is generally agreed that all coloured opalescent discharges, after sanguineous discharges and milk

have been excluded, may be put into a single group in relation to significance – in particular, they are associated with no increased cancer risk. Such discharges are common in late reproductive life, often intermittent, sometimes persisting and occasionally very profuse. Multiple ducts of one or both breasts are often involved and with discharge of differing appearance from individual ducts. They show a wide range of colours and consistency from a creamy purulent appearance through yellow, brown, green and black. In general, the brown, green and black discharges tend to be of fluid consistency, the creamy discharge is more grumous – sometimes as thick as toothpaste (*see* Figure 11.4). The coloured discharges resemble the range of appearances seen in cyst fluid (*see* Figure 9.3). They are most commonly due to duct ectasia. At operation for duct ectasia, it is noticeable that some ducts are of normal calibre and others dilated, while the dilated ducts of the same breast will show material of widely differing appearance – creamy brown or green are commonly present in adjacent ducts. Nipple discharge associated with duct ectasia is dealt with further in Chapter 11.

In some cases, nipple discharge is clearly due to cysts, since occasionally a ductogram for nipple discharge will show the dye entering a cyst from the duct (Figure 12.2).

Coloured discharges are usually readily distinguished from sanguineous ones – but where a brownish discharge causes difficulty a chemical test for blood is helpful.

Galactorrhoea

The thin, off-white, modestly opalescent quality of human milk is characteristic. There is a 'grey'

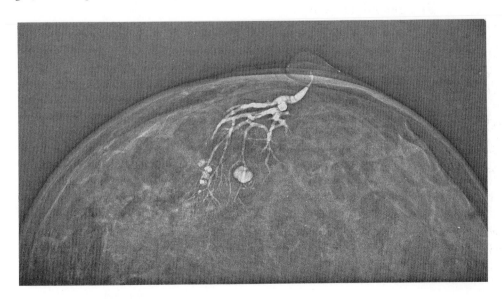

12.2 *Duct injection for nipple discharge showing communication with small cysts.*

area between milk and the thicker creamy discharge of duct ectasia, but it is not commonly difficult to distinguish the two.

Physiological Galactorrhoea

Galactorrhoea is defined as milk secretion unrelated to breast feeding. Many patients complaining of milky discharge are suffering from physiological rather than pathological conditions. Drugs also commonly lie behind milk discharge. Pathology within the breast is so rare within this group that the cause should be sought elsewhere.

Milk production may continue long after lactation has ceased and a regular menstrual cycle has been re-established. This discharge is usually bilateral and may occasionally be copious. It is of no pathological significance and is usually due to stimulation of the breast by continued maternal attempts at expression. This is sometimes carried out in the belief that it will prevent further milk production, or that milk should not be allowed to lie in the breast. Milky discharge associated with other mechanical forms of stimulation is occasionally encountered, explaining the anecdotal reports of successful breast-feeding in the absence of prior pregnancy, and even reports of successful suckling by men!

Treatment is by reassurance and explanation of the sequence of events, that the condition is self-limiting and that cessation of expression or other mechanical stimulation will allow resolution. Occasionally, physiological milk discharge is seen at the extremes of reproductive life. At the menarche, during the period of rapid breast development, and at the menopause, squeezing of the breasts may produce small quantities of fluid. Again, explanation and reassurance is all that is required.

The appearance of 'witch's milk' in the neonate has been dealt with in Chapter 2 and is due to the transplacental transport of maternal lactogenic hormones.

Secondary Galactorrhoea

The appearance of a milky discharge is occasionally seen apart from the conditions mentioned above. A careful history and examination will usually reveal the cause (Table 12.3). These causes are mostly related to those situations in which there is an increase in the levels of circulating prolactin. The important causes are prolactinoma, a tumour which is being recognized with increasing frequency, and medications. Vorherr[8] reviewed the literature and gives a list of 17 causes of galactorrhoea. It is likely that some of these are in reality pituitary microadenomas secreting prolactin, a condition which was unrecognized at

Table 12.3 Causes of galactorrhoea.

Physiological
Mechanical stimulation
Extremes of reproductive life (puberty, menopause)
Postlactational
Stress

Drugs
Associated with hyperprolactinaemia
   dopamine receptor-blocking agents
     phenothiazines, e.g. chlorpromazine
     haloperidol
     metoclopramide, domperidone
   dopamine-depleting agents
     reserpine
     methyldopa
Others
   oestrogen
   opiates

Pathological
Hypothalamic and pituitary stalk lesions
Pituitary tumours
   adenoma
   microadenoma
Miscellaneous
   ectopic prolactin secretion (e.g. bronchogenic
     carcinoma)
   hypothyroidism
   chronic renal failure

the time of the original descriptions. The diagnosis of prolactinoma is suggested by the history of galactorrhoea, amenorrhoea and relative infertility. If the tumour is large, expansion of the pituitary fossa, and possible erosion of the floor of the sella may be seen on radiography and help to confirm the diagnosis. More often the lesions are microadenomas and skull radiology is normal; diagnosis is then dependent on dynamic hormonal studies of prolactin, and on computerized tomographic (CT) scanning of the pituitary fossa. The galactorrhoea disappears following appropriate treatment with bromocriptine or surgical removal of the adenoma[9].

Drug-induced galactorrhoea is not uncommon and occurs with a number of tranquillizing agents, particularly of the phenothiazine group, oral contraceptives and antihypertensives as well as drugs which have a direct action on the hypothalamic pituitary axis such as domperidone and metoclopramide[10]. The mechanism of action of some of these changes is obscure. Drugs which have been implicated in the production of galactorrhoea are listed in Table 12.3.

Pathology Underlying Nipple Discharge
Duct Papilloma

Solitary Duct Papilloma

The commonest hyperplastic lesion causing a serous or sanguineous discharge is duct papilloma:

single or multiple. In about half the cases, the discharge is bloody – in the other half it is serous. A subareolar lump is palpable in less than half of the cases. The history is sometimes a long one; the discharge may have been present for several years.

The typical ductal papilloma is just 2–3 mm in diameter (Figure 12.3), but as it grows it elongates and extends along the duct system so that it may be 1 cm or more long. Larger papillomas tend to cause, and lie within, a local pocketing of the duct, a diverticulum which alters the normal line of the duct. Fine probes passed into the duct tend to get side-tracked into these diverticula. The papilloma has a narrow fragile stalk and delicate fronds. The narrow stalk predisposes to torsion, which may result in infarction and this is not uncommonly seen on histology. It is presumably the reason why bloody discharge frequently remits spontaneously, particularly in young women. The sequence of events is summarized in Figure 12.4. The delicate fronds account for the marked tendency to haemorrhage. As the papilloma elongates and grows along the ducts, torsion becomes less likely but partial ischaemia may lead to fibrosis and adhesion to the duct wall, making differentiation from papillary carcinoma more difficult. Typical small lesions have many fronds with a fibrovascular core and a covering of regular epithelium, although mitoses may be quite frequent.

Although a well known lesion, solitary papilloma is relatively uncommon. There were only 15 solitary duct papilloma cases in the 259 nipple discharge patients in our Cardiff study and the figure of 29% of operations for nipple discharge is similar to the 37% operations for nipple discharge described by Leis[3]. Most papillomas appear in the fourth and sixth decades with a peak age incidence in the fifth decade. However, it has a wide range of age incidence and we have seen it at the age of 16 and in an octogenarian. Sandison[11], in his postmortem study of 800 women, found an

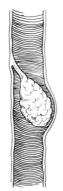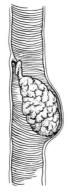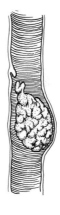

12.4 *Schematic representation of torsion and infarction of a duct papilloma.*

incidence of duct papilloma of 1.6%. This suggests that many papillomas go undetected through life.

The usual location of a duct papilloma is in the subareolar major ducts, within 5 cm of the nipple. Occasionally, it develops in the terminal subareolar duct, when it may distend the nipple or prolapse through the duct orifice on to the nipple (*see* Chapter 14).

When this occurs, it requires separation from a distinct entity – erosive papillomatosis (Chapter 14). The characteristic feature of a prolapsed ductal papilloma is that the surface of the nipple is unaffected. With erosive papillomatosis, the nipple itself is eroded. Haagensen[2] gives clear guidelines for distinguishing the two.

Macroscopic papillomas are usually solitary, but it is not uncommon to find two or three distinct papillomas in the one segment of duct (*see* Figure 12.3). These are better included in the 'solitary' group than the 'multiple papilloma' group, which tend to involve a number of ducts and to be more peripheral. Duct papillomas are sometimes bilateral – 7 of 173 in Haagensen's series; bilateral involvement was simultaneous in one case. In the remainder, the average time to presentation in the opposite breast was 8 years.

Solitary intraduct papilloma is not usually considered to be premalignant. Many recent studies have shown no increased incidence of cancer, but it must be admitted that there is a paucity of sound long-term follow-up data. The recent ACP consensus statement puts papilloma with a fibrovascular core in the group with a slightly increased risk of cancer (*see* Chapter 4).

Multiple Duct Papillomas

In about 10% of duct papillomas the lesions are found to be multiple, usually two or three, often in the same duct. However, the term 'multiple duct papilloma' is better reserved for the very rare and more distinctive group where more than one duct system is involved, the papillomas are

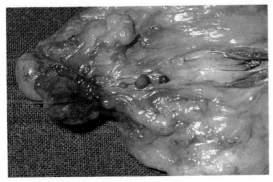

12.3 *Microdochectomy specimen opened to show three small duct papillomas.*

large and palpable and distributed more peripherally in the breast. Nipple discharge is less common in this group than in the solitary papilloma of the central ducts. Haagensen[2] described 53 examples of this condition and found the mean age to be younger than those with solitary papilloma; a tumour was usually palpable and only a minority of patients described nipple discharge. Haagensen considered such lesions premalignant, as 15 of his 39 patients developed carcinoma; also there was a high rate of recurrence unless an adequate excision is done. In our experience this syndrome was associated with a watery discharge.

Papillary Carcinoma

Papillary carcinoma is the usual type of malignancy associated with nipple discharge. However, most papillary carcinomas do not present in this way – only 26% of Haagensen's cases presented with a nipple discharge. In 80% it was sanguineous or serosanguineous, in the remaining 20% the discharge was serous. This diagnosis becomes much more likely over the age of 50 than in younger patients. This condition is outside the scope of this book, and an excellent description can be found in Haagensen's textbook[2].

Duct Ectasia

It is uncommon for more than a few of the 15–20 ducts to be affected. The ducts are usually about 2–5 mm in diameter, often very thin walled but sometimes become thick walled. The fluid may vary from thin to thick to grumous – toothpast-like which has to be squeezed out. The colour of the discharge varies – usually creamy coloured but it is often brown or greenish. Analysis of the discharge shows fatty crystals and large foamy macrophages and much amorphous cell debris. Pigmented cells termed 'ochrocytes' by Davies[12] are also presumed to be macrophages which have ingested the ceroids produced by degeneration of the fatty material in the ducts which gives this type of discharge its wide variety of colour. The pathology is dealt with in detail in Chapter 11.

Cysts

It is uncertain how commonly cysts are the cause of nipple discharge. They are undoubtedly responsible in some cases, because injection for nipple discharge may show the duct communicating with the cyst (see Figure 12.2). Sometimes aspiration of the cyst will be followed immediately by discharge of similar material through the

nipple – presumably release of intracystic tension allows the draining duct to open. The frequency of multiple duct involvement with coloured opalescent discharge suggests that duct ectasia is the commonest cause, as does the frequency of ectatic ducts at operation where this type of discharge has been seen.

The situation is confused by the fact that cysts have often been regarded in the past as an extreme form of duct ectasia – especially in the American literature. It is now well demonstrated that cysts arise from lobules, and have a different pathogenesis to duct ectasia.

Physical Examination and Investigation of Nipple Discharge

The history will cover duration, frequency, associated symptoms and precipitating causes. In women with a milky discharge, particular attention needs to be paid to a history of mechanical stimulation of the breast and of medication.

Physical Examination

A useful sequence is as follows:

1. Inspection – this should reveal whether discharge is from a solitary duct (and, if so, which duct) or from multiple ducts, and the colour and nature of the fluid. It is usually most convenient for the patient to express a little fluid herself while the physician watches. Where discharge is scant, a magnifying glass may be useful. Where no discharge is produced, inspection of the brassière may reveal enough fluid to determine whether or not it is sanguineous.
2. Palpate slowly and systematically around the areola to determine where pressure will produce discharge and which duct is involved. If this is successful, a smear may be taken for cytology. When the segment has been localized, feel carefully for a palpable mass or dilated duct, especially under the areola.
3. Careful standard examination of both breasts.

Mammography (see Chapter 6)

Mammography is advisable in all patients over 30 years with nipple discharge, and particularly so where the discharge is serous, bloody or watery. The most important finding is microcalcification along the line of ducts as it may draw attention to an otherwise unsuspected intraduct carcinoma.

This may occur even in young women. Prominent ducts may be noted together with the coarse large calcifications which are typical of duct ectasia (*see* Figure 11.19).

Duct Injection

Small papillomata may be demonstrated by cannulation of the duct and injection with contrast material, but false positives and false negatives are not uncommon. Debris or blood clot may masquerade as papillomas, while others may be missed in dilated ducts. Duct injection is distinctly uncomfortable for the patient and, for this combination of reasons, we do not use the procedure as a routine investigation, but reserve it for unusual or difficult cases. It rarely, if ever, alters management. Those who advocate its routine use[13] recommend it for all spontaneous discharges and, if no pathology is demonstrated, will use it repeatedly until something is found or the patient refuses further examination.

Exfoliative Cytology

This investigation will sometimes indicate intraduct carcinoma as the cause of the discharge. However, there are too many false negatives for this to be regarded as a completely reliable investigation. For example, Kjellogren[14] found a 16% false negative and a 4% false positive rate. Aspiration cytology of any associated mass is obviously appropriate (*see* Chapter 5) and is considered more reliable[15].

More recently investigation has been directed to cytology of nipple aspirates obtained by suction rather than of discharge. As King *et al*[16] have shown, it is possible to identify atypical cells as well as those which are unequivocally malignant. However, satisfactory specimens were obtained in less than half of the patients they studied so the value of this technique in routine practice is limited. Because of the very glandular epithelium in pregnancy, false positives are particularly likely at that time.

Cytology may be helpful in confirming duct ectasia. Large foamy macrophages with few, if any, epithelial cells are typically seen.

We regard cytology of the discharge as useful in those over 35 years old, but as with other tests for malignancy, negative results should be ignored. Indeed Leis[3] has shown that sanguineous discharge may be found to be due to cancer, in spite of negative physical examination, mammography and cytology.

Management

The philosophy of management of serous or serosanguineous nipple discharge has changed radically in the last 50 years. Opinion regarding the likelihood of it being due to cancer was sharply divided early in this century. Judd[17], in 1917, reported a 57% incidence of cancer in 100 cases at the Mayo Clinic. At about the same time, Bloodgood[18] regarded it as an innocuous symptom due to duct papilloma and not duct carcinoma. Two papers in the 1930s played an important role in influencing the vogue for mastectomy which dominated the mid-decades of this century. In 1930, Adair reported 108 cases from the Memorial Hospital, with 47% malignant. In 1931, Cheatle and Cutler[19] argued strongly from pathological evidence that benign papillomas could progress to papillary carcinoma. This led to simple mastectomy being the standard treatment for blood-related discharge in many clinics.

However, in the last 30 years, a more conservative approach has become accepted, resulting particularly from the studies of Haagensen in the USA and Hedley Atkins[20] in the UK, who both recognized that those patients whose discharge was due to duct papilloma were cured by removing the papilloma. Both recommended conservative operations, Atkins developed the operation of microdochectomy and Haagensen[2] used a procedure intermediate between the microdochectomy of Atkins and the major duct excision operation of Urban[21].

More recent series have given a better indication of the likely pathology of these blood-related discharges. Leis' study of 560 patients undergoing breast surgery for discharge showed that only 20% of those with blood-related discharge had cancer or a premalignant condition[3]. Funderburk and Syphax[13] give a clear breakdown of the causes of 167 cases of nipple discharge. Of 46 which were opalescent or green, none had cancer or hyperplasia; but of 121 patients with a clear, serous or bloody discharge, 11 had cancer, 11 had 'papillomatosis' (hyperplasia) and 59 had a duct papilloma. All series show a marked relationship between the incidence of cancer and increase in age, as discussed earlier in this chapter.

More recently, non-sanguineous discharges have also become better recognized and management of nipple discharge is now related to a number of factors, particularly the type of discharge, the age of the patient, and whether a blood-related discharge can be localized to a single duct.

General Principles of Management

Nature of the discharge
Milk. Look for a cause outside the breast.
Coloured, opalescent discharges. These have no serious significance. Treat only if causing social embarrassment. In doubtful cases, exclude blood by a chemical test.
Blood-related discharges. These cause much more concern to the patient and are associated with cancer risk – minimal in young patients but more significant with increasing age.

Age of the patient
This is important only in blood-related discharges, because of cancer risk. No active treatment is necessary in young patients if the discharge ceases spontaneously, but surgical biopsy is usually indicated over the age of 40 years – irrespective of investigations and even if the discharge has ceased. In Leis' series of patients with blood-related discharge found to have cancer, 11% had no mass, 11% had a negative mammogram and 16% had negative cytology.

Localization
If the discharge can be localized to a single duct, microdochectomy gives satisfactory results in younger patients with minimal interference to the breast. In older patients, major duct excision may

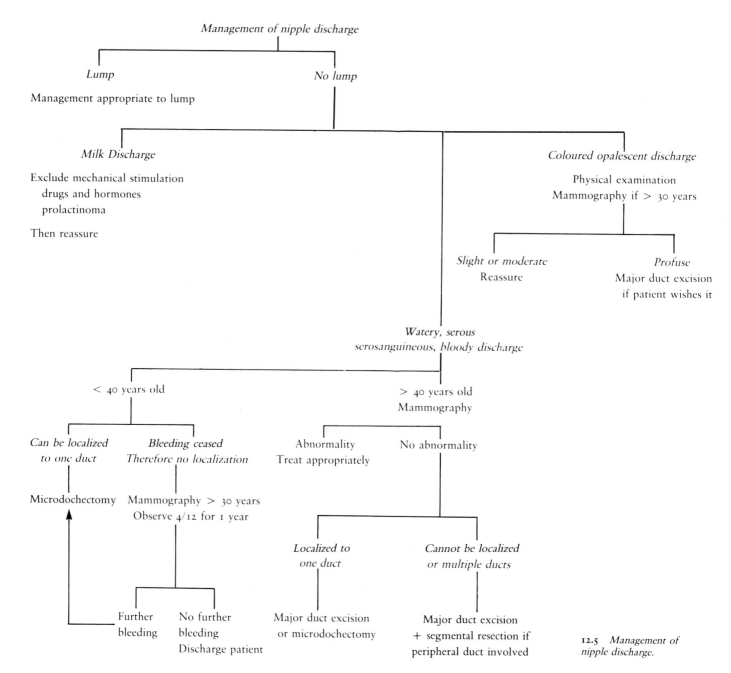

12.5 *Management of nipple discharge.*

be preferable irrespective of whether the discharge is localized to one duct.

Specific Details of Management

The management of nipple discharge is summarized in Table 12.4 and Figure 12.5.

Table 12.4 Management of milky and opalescent discharge.

Milk discharge (galactorrhoea)
eliminate mechanical stimulation
stop or change medication
measure serum prolactin
reassure
Coloured opalescent discharge
exclude blood
mammogram to exclude other pathology
(over age 30 only)
reassure
major duct excision if socially embarrassing.

Blood-related Discharge – Serous, Serosanguineous, Sanguineous, Watery

Under the age of 30, risk of malignancy is low so the patient may be safely observed after full assessment as above. If discharge persists, and a solitary duct can be identified, the procedure of choice is microdochectomy (*see* Chapter 18). If the discharge ceases and does not recur within a year, no further follow-up is indicated.

For patients over 45, the risk of malignancy dictates the need for operation and our preferred operation is a formal excision of the major duct system on the affected side (*see* Chapter 18), with urgent paraffin section. It is important to remember to mark the terminal part of the ducts immediately behind the nipple so that the pathologist can orientate the specimen. The advantages of this approach are that it is not essential to isolate a solitary offending duct, it deals with multiple papillomas if these are present

and gives maximum histological information, and it deals with duct ectasia if this proves to be the cause. If dilated blood-filled ducts are found extending into the periphery of the breast, the excision should be extended to a segmental resection (*see* Chapter 18).

Patients between 30 and 45 are suitable for either approach. In general, they may be treated as for the under-30 age group, but may be moved towards major duct excision by additional factors, e.g. strong family history of breast cancer, a particularly worried patient, or coexisting nipple inversion which the patient wants corrected.

Coloured Opalescent Discharge

This only requires treatment if the amount of discharge is personally embarrassing with the need to constantly wear pads. The only effective procedure is a total duct excision.

Galactorrhoea

The management is that of the underlying cause. Prolactinomas are treated by bromocriptine or surgical excision. For drug-induced problems, an alternative medication is usually available if the galactorrhoea remains unacceptable. For physiological discharge, reassurance and cessation of mechanical stimulation should prove sufficient.

Follow-up

Patients who prove to have solitary duct papilloma have insufficient increase in the risk of subsequent malignancy to justify routine follow-up (*see* Chapter 4). Patients with multiple papillomas do have an increased risk[22] and should be kept under annual review with biennial mammography. Because the risk is small, long term and affecting both breasts, long-term follow-up is more appropriate than mastectomy.

REFERENCES

1. Selzer M. H., Perloff L. J., Kelley R. I. & Fitts W. T. The significance of age in patients with nipple discharge *Surgery, Gynecology and Obstetrics* 1970; **131**: 519–522.
2. Haagensen C. D. *Diseases of the Breast*, 3rd edn. Philadephia, W. B. Saunders, 1986.
3. Leis H. P. *Diagnosis and Treatment of Breast Lesions*. London, H. K. Lewis & Co., 1970.
4. Chaudray M. A., Millis R. R., Davies G. C. & Hayward J. L. Nipple discharge. The diagnostic value of testing for occult blood. *Annals of Surgery* 1982; **196**: 651–655.
5. O'Callaghan M. A. Atypical discharge from the breast during pregnancy and/or lactation. *Australia and New Zealand Journal of Obstetrics and Gynaecology* 1981; **21**: 214–216.
6. Kline T. S. & Lash S. R. The bleeding nipple of pregnancy and the post partum period. *Acta cytologica (Philadelphia)* 1964; **8**: 336.
7. Lewison E. F. & Chambers R. G. Clinical significance of nipple discharge. *Journal of the American Medical Association* 1951; **147**: 295–299.
8. Vorherr H. *The Breast, Morphology, Physiology and Lactation*. New York, Academic Press, 1974.
9. Scanlon M. F., Peters J. R., Picton-Thomas J. *et al*. The management of selected patients with hyper-prolactinaemia by partial hypophysectomy. *British Medical Journal* 1986; **291**: 1547–1550.
10. Hall R., Anderson J., Smart G. A. & Besser M. *Fundamentals of Clinical Endocrinology*, 3rd edn. Tunbridge Wells, Pitman Medical, 1980.
11. Sandison A. T. An autopsy study of the human breast. *National Cancer Institute Monograph* No.

8, US Department of Health, Education and Welfare. 1962.

12. Davies J. D. Pigmented periductal cells (ochrocytes) in mammary dysplasias: their nature and significance. *Journal of Pathology* 1974; **114**: 205–216.

13. Funderbunk W. W. & Syphax B. Evaluation of nipple discharge in benign and malignant disease. *Cancer* 1969; **24**: 1290–1296.

14. Kjellogren O. The cytologic diagnosis of cancer of the breast. *Acta Cytologica* 1964; **8**: 216–223.

15. Rimsten A., Skoog V. & Stenkvist B. On the significance of nipple discharge in the diagnosis of breast disease. *Acta Chirurgica Scandinavica* 1976; **142**: 513–518.

16. King E. B., Chew K. C., Petrakis N. L. & Ernster V. L. Nipple aspirate cytology for the study of breast cancer precursors. *Journal of the National Cancer Institute* 1983; **71**: 1115–1121.

17. Judd E. S. Intracanalicular papilloma of the breast. *Journal Lancet* 1917; **37**: 141.

18. Bloodgood J. C. Benign lesions of female breast for which operation is not indicated. *Journal of the American Medical Association* 1922; **78**: 859–863.

19. Cheatle G. L. & Cutler M. *Tumours of the Breast.* Philadelphia, J. B. Lippincott Co., 1931.

20. Atkins H. & Wolff B. Discharges from the nipple. *British Journal of Surgery* 1964; **51**: 602–606.

21. Urban J. A. Excision of the major duct system of the breast. *Cancer* 1963; **16** 516–520.

22. Carter D. Intraductal papillary tumours of the breast – A study of 78 cases. *Cancer* 1977; **39**: 1689–1692.

13   Infection of the Breast

Infection of the breast may occur as a localized phenomenon or as part of a systemic illness. The common acute infective conditions are usually easy to diagnose; the importance of the rarer infections of the breast lies in the similarity of their presentation to a carcinoma – a painless indurated mass. There are a number of specific infective conditions which are now uncommon in the UK and are of historical interest. Tuberculosis remains important in British practice with respect to immigrant populations, particularly from the Indian subcontinent. The other infections are interesting curiosities.

Studies based on hospital experience are likely to give a distorted picture of the true incidence of breast infection. In hospital practice, non-puerperal abscess is more common than lactational abscess[1], but in general practice a survey showed 80% of infective episodes were puerperal[2].

Lactational Breast Infection

Epidemiology

Lactational mastitis is a common condition which has been described as occurring in up to 9% of puerperal women[3] but seems far less common today, an opinion shared by Benson[4]. Our experience (Figure 13.1) gives an indication that puerperal breast infection remains a significant, and possibly increasing, problem. Newton and Newton[5] halved the incidence of breast abscess during postnatal hospitalization from 0.82% to 0.47% by routine administration of penicillin. Although puerperal breast infection is sometimes described in sporadic and epidemic forms, the pathological processes within the breast are identical. The epidemic form is seen in institutional outbreaks in which the organism is transmitted from infant to infant by cross-infection and thence to its mother.

Prophylaxis

Attention to detail in the care of the breast during pregnancy and lactation can do much to reduce the chances of developing infection. Good hygiene and avoidance of breast engorgement or cracked nipple are important. During pregnancy daily washing will remove the dried secretions which will otherwise collect on the nipple. After feeding the infant, the nipples should be dried and a bland moisturizing cream applied after expression of any segments of the breast that have not been adequately emptied during feeding.

Pathology

The organism most commonly implicated is *Staphylococcus aureus* which presumably gains entry via a cracked nipple (p. 152). Occasionally, the infection is haematogenous. Milk provides an ideal culture medium, so bacterial dispersion in the vascular and distended segment is easy. In the early

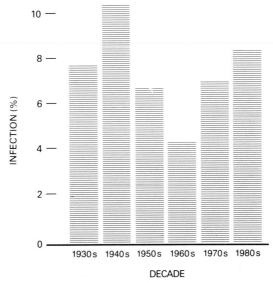

13.1   *Incidence of puerperal infection, reported retrospectively by 425 patients undergoing 1000 pregnancies between 1930 and 1988.*

stages, the infection tends to be confined to a single segment of the breast and it is relatively late that extension to other segments may occur. The pathological process is identical to acute inflammation occurring elsewhere in the body, although the loose parenchyma of the lactating breast and the stagnant milk of an engorged segment allows the infection to spread rapidly if unchecked. Because this is an infection of breast parenchyma, the bacteria are excreted in the milk.

Bacteriology of Lactational Abscess

The vast majority of lactational breast abscesses are caused by *Staphylococcus aureus*. In the early, commonest type of abscess, this is most likely to be hospital acquired. The antibiotic resistance of the organisms will reflect this. Many hospital staphylococci are now penicillinase producing. In the study of Goodman and Benson[6], all the hospital acquired infections were *Staphylococcus aureus* and, of the 98 hospital acquired infections, only 50% had penicillin-sensitive organisms. A wide variety of organisms may occasionally be encountered. Typhoid is a well recognized cause of breast abscess in countries where this disease is common. This is a particularly important diagnosis to make because the organism is secreted in the milk.

Clinical Features

Nursing mothers are most vulnerable to breast abscess at two stages:

1. During the first month of lactation following the first pregnancy when, due to inexperience, the nipples are more likely to be damaged and hygiene inadequate. Eighty-five per cent of lactational breast abscess occur during the first month after delivery[5].
2. At weaning when the breasts are more likely to become engorged. An additional factor after about 6 months is that the baby's teeth increase the likelihood of nipple trauma.

The patient complains of a painful red swollen breast associated with constitutional upset and fever. The local signs of infection vary greatly with the stage of infection. In early cases, a little cellulitis or nothing at all is found; in neglected cases a fluctuant abscess with overlying skin necrosis may be observed (Figure 13.2). In patients who have already had treatment, the signs may have been masked by antibiotics leading to a mass without the classic signs of infection, and which may or may not be tender.

Figure 13.3 shows the sites of breast abscesses.

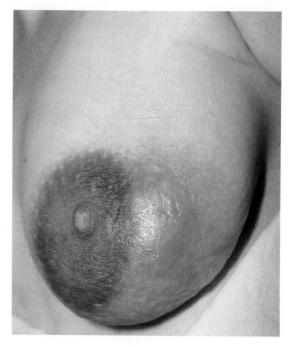

13.2 *Late lactational abscess with skin necrosis.*

Most lie in the parenchyma. Abscesses in the less common sites, such as the retromammary space, periareolar region or subcutaneous tissue, should alert the clinician to the possibility of an underlying pathology.

Management

The clinical problem may be resolved into three categories: cellulitis without pus formation; uncertain; abscess.

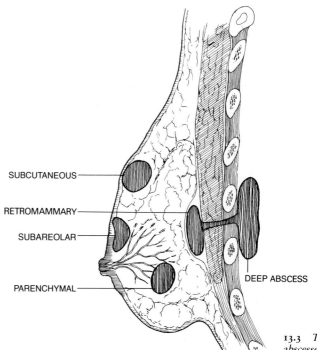

13.3 *The sites of breast abscesses.*

The importance of an accurate assessment of the situation cannot be over-emphasized. Surgery in the early cellulitic phase is meddlesome and unnecessarily destructive; continued antibiotic therapy in the presence of an abscess may lead to unnecessary tissue destruction by the disease process. Test needle aspiration of the cellulitic area should be performed. It is wrong to wait for the development of fluctuation and pointing before proceeding to drainage, because further destruction of breast will occur. The aspiration of pus will indicate that an abscess has formed; the absence of pus indicates that the condition is still in the cellulitic phase. In either event the opportunity should be used to carry out bacteriological examination of the aspirated material.

A useful bonus of this approach is that the rare case of inflammatory carcinoma may be diagnosed on the smear, thus avoiding operation in this difficult condition (Figure 13.4).

Treatment

Taylor and Way[7] clearly enunciated the principles of treatment: curtail infection and empty the breast. The methods of achieving this differ in the cellulitic and abscess stages.

Curtailing infection

Cellulitic phase. During the cellulitic phase, treatment with antibiotics may be expected to give rapid resolution. The predominance of *Staphylococcus aureus* allows a rational choice of anti-

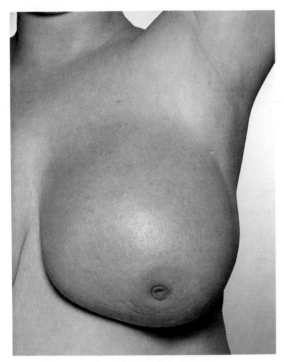

13.4 *Inflammatory carcinoma of the breast.*

biotic without having to wait for the results of bacteriological culture. A penicillinase-resistant antibacterial should be given; flucloxacillin 500 mg four times daily will prove satisfactory but, if the patient has a penicillin sensitivity, erythromycin is a satisfactory alternative. If rapid improvement does not occur, repeated aspiration will usually reveal the presence of pus. After 24 hours, the results of culture should give guidance to a possible change in antibiotic therapy if the lesion is not improving and no pus is found on repeat aspiration. If resolution is proceeding satisfactorily, no further action is required.

Antibiotics are secreted in milk so tetracyclines, aminoglycosides, sulphonamides and metronidazole should be avoided because of their possible ill-effects on the child. Penicillin, cephalosporins and erythromycin, however, are considered safe. Such a regimen will prove adequate in most cases but in 5–10% an abscess will develop[8,9], although Bates *et al*[2] found that 24% failed to respond to antibiotics and progressed to abscess formation.

Abscess phase. Once abscess formation has occurred, which is likely after 48 hours, use of antibiotics may cause a temporary regression of the symptoms without sterilizing the abscess and lead to a protracted illness. Newton and Newton[5] observed that the introduction of antibiotics led to delayed resolution of the abscess. In cases where the development of an abscess is uncertain, aspiration should resolve the point. Where an abscess has formed, surgical intervention is required, with antibiotic cover to reduce systemic infection and local cellulitis. Our preference is for open drainage and packing (*see* Chapter 18), but Benson and Goodman[6] have argued for a policy of immediate closure under antibiotic cover. The results they describe suggest that this approach is as good as the convention approach. Unfortunately, the study of Benson and Goodman[6] was uncontrolled and gave no indication as to how patients were allocated to the different treatment groups. Overall, the patients require a longer course of antibiotics than if open drainage is instituted, when antibiotics may be avoided altogether in some patients. We still prefer conventional open drainage, but accept the case that primary closure may have a role. The selection of antibiotics should follow the guidelines given in the cellulitic phase. In the absence of systemic symptoms, a well-localized abscess should be drained and antibiotics withheld. Aspiration of the abscess alone is unlikely to be adequate: breast abscesses are frequently multilocular and the aspirating needle may be obstructed by necrotic tissue.

Emptying the Breast

This important aspect of the management of puerperal breast infection is sometimes ignored. The breast may be emptied either by suckling or by expression. Rowley[11] in 1771 described and illustrated the use of a breast pump which is similar to some still in use today. Although bacteria are present in the milk, no harm appears to be done to the infant if breast-feeding is continued[9].

After draining an abscess, suckling may be difficult for a few days for mechanical reasons on the affected side, but the mother should be encouraged to feed on the unaffected side. The infected breast, however, should be emptied either by manual expression or by a pump.

Suppression of Lactation

Following development of a breast abscess, patients are often advised to abandon breast-feeding[12]. This advice is given on the grounds that:

1. The bacteria are excreted in the milk and may then infect the infant.
2. Continued pain makes it difficult to empty the affected breast satisfactorily, thus causing further engorgement and stasis leading to rapid spread of the infecting organisms.

There is no real basis for these views – with skilled nursing assistance the infant may be safely fed on the contralateral breast and the affected breast may be expressed by pump until such time as feeding can be recommenced[13]. Indeed, except when the presence of the cavity makes suckling impossible, there is no indication to remove the child from the affected breast. The bacteria in the milk do not appear to harm the child. A leading article in the *British medical Journal*[14] reviewed the evidence and concluded that mothers with breast abscesses should be encouraged to continue breast-feeding. Our own approach is in-line with this policy.

If it is decided to abandon breast-feeding, lactation should be suppressed as quickly as possible. The most effective suppressant currently available is bromocriptine 2.5 mg twice daily for 14 days[15]. The engorged breast should be emptied as far as possible mechanically. Fluid restriction and firm binding are not necessary.

Non-lactational Breast Abscess

Non-lactational breast abscess is normally a manifestation of periductal mastitis. This is discussed fully in Chapter 11. A number of rarer causes need to be considered. The average age of these patients tends to be older than the average for patients with lactational infection (Figure 13.5). Many of these patients are nulliparous suggesting a different source of infection, a view confirmed by the quite different bacteriological findings.

Neonatal

Neonatal breast abscesses (Figure 13.6) may be regarded as a variant of lactational abscess in the sense that maternal hormonal influences cause the presence of sufficient milk to predispose to this condition. If this condition is encountered, care needs to be taken to ensure that as little tissue damage as possible is caused either by disease or surgery. It is easy to remove the whole breast disc at this stage – leading to secondary amastia. The incision should avoid the breast bud behind the nipple and no tissue should be excised. Neonatal abscess is as common in boys as in girls.

In adolescence and adult life

Acute abscesses occurring outside the puerperium may occur as part of a haematogenous spread or more often as an abscess of an overlying skin structure such as a sebaceous cyst. More often such episodes are examples of periductal mastitis

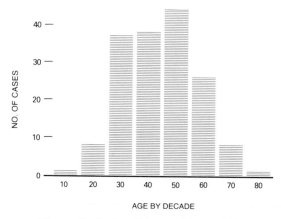

13.5 *The age distribution of 160 non-lactational abscesses – Cardiff series.*

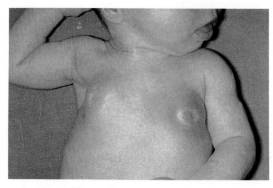

13.6 *Neonatal breast abscess.*

which may become secondarily infected. Trauma is another factor that needs to be considered. Closed trauma may cause a haematoma which may become secondarily infected, but penetrating injuries are a more common source of trouble. Foreign bodies occasionally lodge in the breast, often accidentally, but sometimes they are self-inflicted. In any case of recurrent atypical abscess, the possibility that it is self-inflicted needs to be considered, although confirmation may be exceedingly difficult[16]. Infected retained foreign bodies may lead to persistent sinuses until they are removed.

Bacteriology

A non-lactational pyogenic abscess may occur in the course of any septicaemic episode and the involved organism will reflect the underlying cause. The bacteriology is much more variable with this type of abscess so that selection of a broad-spectrum antibiotic is advisable unless information regarding other septic foci is available. Recently, attention has been drawn to the importance of anaerobic infections in non-puerperal breast abscess. Leach et al[17] described 15 cases of non-puerperal breast abscess and found anaerobic organisms in 8. Hale et al[18] described 3 cases of anaerobic infection in nulliparous women and identified the cause as Bacteroides sp. Leach[19] has since described anaerobic abscesses occurring in women with inverted nipples following surgical manipulation and postulated that the anaerobic bacteraemia leads to subsequent breast abscess. In view of the likelihood of finding anaerobic bacteria[16] in this situation[19], it would seem advisable to add an agent such as metronidazole to the antibiotic regimen used in the treatment of non-puerperal breast infection.

Non-puerperal staphylococcal abscess is sometimes encountered without predisposing cause – even after the menopause.

Recurrent Subareolar Abscess

Haagensen[20] has drawn attention to this condition, which is described more fully in Chapter 11.

Treatment is as conservative as possible with drainage (or aspiration) of the initially sterile abscess (which may become secondarily infected). If a fistula becomes established, careful excision of the fibrous track and the affected milk sinus proves adequate in most cases.

Specific Infections of the Breast

Tuberculosis

Tuberculosis is an uncommon condition in the UK today, but was more frequent in the earlier part of this century. Scott in 1904[21] reported that 1.5% of the breast cases seen at St Bartholomew's Hospital were due to tuberculosis. This represented one case for every 40 new cancers seen. In India it is still a relatively common condition: Rangabashyam et al[22] reviewed 215 cases of breast disease over a 5-year period in Madras and had 7 cases of tuberculous disease (3%) while Banerjee et al[23] found 1.06% of all breast lesions were due to tuberculous mastitis. Alagaratnam and Ong[24] reported that they still found one case per year in Hong Kong. Although tuberculosis is now seen mainly in the less developed countries, it is still not uncommon in recent immigrants to the UK[25]. However, not all granulomatous lesions of the breast prove to be tuberculosis. In the past, the foreign body granulomas of periductal mastitis were frequently confused with tuberculosis.

In most patients, the diagnosis is relatively straighforward as they have evidence of tuberculosis elsewhere. However, in a few patients breast disease is the first manifestation. Tuberculosis may appear as sinuses, ulcers, contracted breast or as a cold abscess. The condition appears to occur more frequently during pregnancy[26,27]. Pathological examination of the tissue shows granulomatous reactions which are indistinguishable from those seen in other granulomatous diseases. Diagnosis is dependent on identifying the organism either in the sections or on culture. It follows that the clinician needs to be aware of this rare disease and plan the appropriate bacteriological investigations in suspected cases.

Treatment is difficult; a prolonged course of antituberculosis chemotherapy may effect a cure, but may lead to a scarred and deformed breast. Wilson and MacGregor[27] claim that even with chemotherapy lesions tend to persist and recur if pregnancy ensues; they advise simple mastectomy, a view echoed by Rangabashyam et al[22]. However, Alagaratnam and Ong[24] were able to treat all but 4 of their 16 cases without resorting to this procedure. Banerjee et al[23] obtained good results from chemotherapy in their 18 patients, only 2 of whom required mastectomy. Certainly the long-term results of surgery are good, even in the days before effective chemotherapy[28], but it would seem reasonable to pursue a course of modern antituberculosis therapy before resorting to surgery. If mastectomy is required, it would seem appropriate to consider a reconstructive procedure at a later date.

Other Mycobacteria

Mycobacterial species, apart from tuberculosis, also occasionally cause problems in the breast. Leprosy has been described and is usually accompanied by other manifestations of the disease[29]. Clegg et al[30] have described atypical mycobacterial infection occurring around prostheses used in augmentation mammoplasty.

Syphilis

This disease is now very rare but deserves a mention if only for historical reasons. The breast used to be regarded as a common site of extragenital chancres. Fitzwilliams[28] quoted the findings of Buckley who described 1148 examples of nipple chancre.

Tertiary syphilis may effect the breast either as a diffuse fibrotic reaction or as a gumma. The gumma usually appears as a discrete lump which disappears when appropriate antisyphilitic treatment is instituted.

Today, these conditions are a medical curiosity, but awareness of the possibility of a primary chancre needs to be considered because early treatment is curative.

Actinomycosis

Actinomycosis occasionally occurs in the breast. It is not different to actinomycosis elsewhere in the body and is characterized by induration, sinus formation and excretion of sulphur granules. There is usually actinomycosis elsewhere, but sometimes the breast is the first or only part afflicted[31].

Mycotic Infections

Mycotic infections occasionally occur and have been reviewed by Symmers[31]. Salfelder and Schwartz[32] speculated on the rarity of mycotic infection of the breast and considered that many cases were overlooked. Subsequently a further report of a case of blastomycosis[33] has been made. Pityrosporum infection of the breast has also been recorded[34]. Three cases of fungal infection complicating augmentation mammoplasty have been reported[35].

Protozoan Infections

These are extremely rare in developed countries. However, in the less developed countries where the appropriate conditions are common, they are met from time to time when they presumably represent metastatic septic foci. Marsden et al[36] have however described two cases of Leishmaniasis of the nipple which they considered to have been directly infected – one from the mouth of her suckling child.

Helminthic Infection

Filaria

This is relatively common in the Orient and is clinically easily confused with carcinoma. In Madras, there were 5 cases in the 215 cases of benign disease described by Rangabashyam et al[22]. The pathological process appears to be confined to the superficial dermal layers and lymphatics, the glandular tissue being spared. In the early stages, appropriate antifilarial therapy is effective although, when secondary damage has occurred, simple mastectomy may be indicated in occasional patients. Filaria is the most frequently reported infestation of the breast and may take a variety of forms. The adult worm may appear at the nipple[37], or a granulomatous reaction may present as a mass[38,39]. Most of the reports emanate from south-east Asia but Periar[39] records examples occurring in France.

Other Infestations

Hydatid disease may rarely occur in the breast in parts of the world where this is common, although it was known as an entity to Sir Astley Cooper[40] who clearly described a case in his work. Such an event occurs in less than 0.5% of patients with hydatid cysts[41]. The lesion is usually cystic and the diagnosis made on aspiration. If the possibility is considered prior to this, replacement with hypertonic saline seems appropriate and a local excision of the cyst should prove curative for the local disease, although it should always be assumed that it is secondary to internal hydatid disease – usually of the liver.

Cysts due to cysticerous have also been reported[26,42]. Guinea-worm infection has also been reported. The adult worms may be seen on mammography[43].

Viral Infections

Mastitis is frequently described as a complication of mumps. The incidence is uncertain because the only symptom, swelling and tenderness of the breast, is such a common one that recognition that this is a separate condition may be difficult. Phillip et al[44], in their study of a mumps epidemic in an isolated Eskimo population, reported that 15% of 158 women had mastitis. The ages of the affected patients ranged from 12 to 61; the incidence of mastitis was 31% of women over 15 years old. As the majority of women in this age group would be menstrually active, it is difficult to be certain that the symptoms were not related to cyclical discomfort rather than mumps-specific mastitis. We have never seen a case which could be attributed to mumps.

Infections of Associated Structures

Skin Lesions

The breast is covered by normal skin and any cutaneous infection may occur on the breast. Perhaps the commonest of these is an infected sebaceous cyst. Furuncles and carbuncles may also occur occasionally. There is not usually any problem with diagnosis because they are clearly dermal in origin.

Hidradenitis suppurativa may occur. When it occurs in association with axillary disease,

diagnosis is not a problem. Isolated hidradenitis, particularly in the intermammary cleft but also sometimes of the inframammary fold, may cause difficulty. When this condition occurs in the skin overlying the breast, differentiation from an underlying peripheral duct ectasia with periductal mastitis may be difficult. It is dealt with more fully in Chapter 17.

Pilonidal Abscess

In the series of mammary duct fistula described by Patey and Thackray[45], it is recorded that loose hairs were found in a lactiferous sinus of one of their patients. They also record that they found loose hairs in a normal lactiferous sinus. Because there are no hair follicles in the nipple, it seems that this event is analogous to the classic pilonidal sinus. A case which appears to be pilonidal abscess occurring in the breast has been reported in the UK[46]. Bowers[47] has described three cases of periareolar pilonidal abscess acquired as work-related disease in sheep shearers and barbers.

REFERENCES

1. Scholefield J. M., Duncan J. L. & Rogers K. Review of hospital experience of breast abscess. *British Journal of Surgery* 1987; 74: 469–470.
2. Bates T., Down R. H. L., Tant D. R. & Fiddian R. V. The current treatment of breast abscess in hospital and in general practice. *Practitioner* 1973; 211: 541–547.
3. Fulton A. A. Incidence of puerperal and lactational mastitis in an industrial town of some 43,000 inhabitants. *British Medical Journal* 1945; 1: 693–696.
4. Benson E. A. Breast abscesses and breast cysts. *Practitioner* 1982; 226: 1397–1401.
5. Newton M. & Newton N. R. Breast abscess. A result of lactation failure. *Surgery, Gynecology and Obstetrics* 1950; 91: 651–655.
6. Goodman M. A. & Benson E. A. An evaluation of current trends in the management of breast abscesses. *Medical Journal of Australia* 1970; 1: 1034–1039.
7. Taylor M. D. & Way S. Penicillin in treatment of acute puerperal mastitis. *British Medical Journal* 1946; 2: 731–732.
8. Devereux W. P. Acute puerperal mastitis. Evaluation of its management. *American Journal of Obstetrics and Gynecology* 1970; 108: 78–81.
9. Marshall B. R., Hepper J. K. & Zirbell C. C. Sporadic puerperal mastitis: an infection that need not interrupt lactation. *Journal of the American Medical Association* 1975; 233: 1377–1379.
10. Benson E. A. & Goodman M. A. Incision with primary suture in the treatment of acute puerperal breast abscess. *British Journal of Surgery* 1970; 57: 55–58.
11. Rowley W. *A Practical Treatise on Diseases of the Breast of Women*. London, Newberry & Ridley, 1772.
12. Vorherr H. Contraindications to breast feeding. *Journal of the American Medical Association* 1974; 227: 676.
13. Applebaum R. M. The modern management of successful breast feeding. *Pediatric Clinics of North America* 1970; 17: 203–225.
14. Editorial. Puerperal mastitis. *British Medical Journal* 1976; 1: 920–921.
15. Walker S. Inhibition of puerperal lactation. *Scottish Medical Journal* 1980; 25: 595–598.
16. Rosenberg M. W. & Hughes L. E. Artefactual breast disease: a report of three cases. *British Journal of Surgery* 1985; 72: 539–540.
17. Leach R. D., Eykyn S. J., Phillips I. & Corrin B. Anaerobic subareolar breast abscess. *Lancet* 1979; i: 35–37.
18. Hale J. E., Perinpanayagam R. M. & Smith G. Bacteroides: An unusual cause of breast abscess. *Lancet* 1976; ii: 70–71.
19. Leach R. D. Vaginal manipulation and breast abscesses. *British Medical Journal* 1981; 282: 610–611.
20. Haagensen C. D. *Disease of the Breast*, 3rd edn. Philadelphia, W. B. Saunders, 1986.
21. Scott S. R. Tuberculosis of the female breast. *St Bartholomew's Hospital Reports* 1904; 40: 97–122.
22. Rangabashyam N., Gnanaprakasam D., Krishnaraj B., Manohar V. & Vijayalakshmi S. R. Spectrum of benign breast lesions in Madras. *Journal of the Royal College of Surgeons of Edinburgh* 1983; 28: 369–373.
23. Banerjee S. N., Ananthakrishnan N., Mehth R. B. & Parkash S. Tuberculous mastitis: A continuing problem. *World Journal of Surgery* 1986; 11: 105–109.
24. Alagaratnam T. J. & Ong G. B. Tuberculosis of the breast. *British Journal of Surgery* 1980; 67: 125–126.
25. Apps M. C. P., Harrison N. K. & Blauth C. I. A.

Tuberculosis of the breast. *British Medical Journal* 1984; **288**: 1874–1875.

26. McKeown K. C. & Wilkinson K. W. Tuberculous disease of the breast. *British Journal of Surgery* 1952; **39**: 420–429.

27. Wilson T. S. & MacGregor J. W. Tuberculosis of the breast. *Canadian Medical Association Journal* 1963; **89**: 1118.

28. Fitzwilliams D. S. L. *On the Breast.* London, William Heinman, 1924.

29. Furniss A. L. Leproma occurring in a female breast presenting as a carcinoma. *Indian Medical Gazette* 1952; **87**: 304.

30. Clegg H. W., Foster M. T., Sanders W. E. & Baine W. B. Infections due to organisms of the mycobacterium fortuitum complex after augmentation mammaplasty: clinical and epidemiological features. *Journal of Infectious Diseases* 1983; **147**: 427–433.

31. Symmers W. S. The breasts. In: Payling Wright G. (ed.) *Systemic Pathology*, Vol. 1. London, Longman Green, 1966, pp. 953–955.

32. Salfelder K. & Schwartz J. Mycotic 'pseudotumours' of the breast. *Archives of Surgery* 1975; **110**: 751–754.

33. Seymour E. Q. Blastomycosis of the breast. *American Journal of Roentgenology* 1982; **139**: 822–823.

34. Bertini B. Cytopathology of nipple discharge due to pityrosporum orbiculare and cocci in an elderly woman. *Acta Cytologica* 1975; **19**: 38–42.

35. Williams K., Walton R. L. & Bunkis J. Aspergillus colonisation associated with bilateral silicone mammary implants. *Plastic Reconstructive Surgery* 1983; **71**: 260–261.

36. Marsden P. D., Almeida E. A., Llanos Cuentas E. A. *et al.* Leishmania braziliensis infection of the nipple. *British Medical Journal* 1985; **290**: 433–434.

37. Lahiri V. L. Microfilariae in nipple secretion. *Acta Cytologica* 1975; **19**: 154.

38. Chen Y. Filarial granuloma of the female breast. A histopathologic study of 131 cases. *American Journal of Tropical Medicine and Hygiene* 1981; **30**: 1206–1210.

39. Periar J. M. Dirofilariasis of the breast in France. *American Journal of Tropical Medicine and Hygiene* 1980; **29**: 1018–1019.

40. Cooper A. *Illustrations of the Diseases of the Breast.* London, Longman & Co., 1829.

41. Dew H. R. *Hydatid Disease.* Sydney, Australia Medical Publishing Co., 1928.

42. Leggat C. A. C. Cysticercosis of the breast. *Australia and New Zealand Journal of Surgery* 1983; **53**: 281.

43. Stelling C. B. Dracunculiasis presenting as a sterile abscess. *American Journal of Roentgenology* 1982; **138**: 1159–1161.

44. Philip R. N., Reinhard K. R. & Lackman D. B. Observations on a mumps epidemic in a 'virgin' population. *American Journal of Hygiene* 1959; **69**: 91–111.

45. Patey D. H. & Thackray A. C. Pathology and treatment of mammary duct fistula. *Lancet* 1958; ii: 871–874.

46. Goepel J. P. Trichogranulomatous mastopathy: an unusual cause of nipple bleeding. *Postgraduate Medical Journal* 1980; **56**: 850–851.

47. Bowers P. W. Roustabouts' and Barber's breasts. *Clinical and Experimental Dermatology* 1982; **7**: 445–448.

14 Disorders of the Nipple and Areola

The nipple and the areola constitute an area of skin modified by the underlying breast tissue and ducts. In addition, the nipple has an extensive network of smooth muscle whose fibres are mainly arranged in circular fashion. The areola surrounds the nipple, both having more pigment than the surrounding skin, and contains the glands of Montgomery which provide a protective lubrication during lactation. The areola also has circular smooth muscle fibres and may contain auxiliary breast tissue which secretes milk during lactation.

Nipple Inversion and Retraction

The failure of full nipple eversion during breast development is common, is termed 'inversion' and is dealt with under congenital conditions (Chapter 15) together with absent and supernumerary nipples.

Nipple retraction is an acquired condition and occurs after previous normal nipple development. The patients will give a clear history that a previously normal nipple has changed shape, and become retracted.

Bryant[1] made an appeal for careful assessment of nipple retraction over a hundred years ago pointing out that many cases were not due to malignancy – the erroneous view that most cases of recent nipple retraction are due to malignancy is still widely held. However, recent changes in the appearance of the nipple portend an underlying pathological process which requires evaluation. The principal diagnoses to be considered are malignancy and duct ectasia. The presence of a clinical lump associated with nipple changes increases the likelihood of an underlying carcinoma, but is also seen with periductal mastitis. In the absence of either clinical or mammographic malignancy, recent nipple retraction is likely to be due to the periductal fibrosis part of the duct ectasia syndrome (see Chapter 11) and as such may be considered to be within the range of normal involution.

Few women are sufficiently concerned to wish to undergo surgery for retraction alone. For those cases due to duct ectasia, a formal excision of the major ducts is necessary; the details are given in Chapter 18.

Assessment of Nipple Retraction

Although the early retraction of duct ectasia typically produces a transverse crease (see Figure 11.15), in established cases the appearance is not sufficiently clear-cut to allow reliable distinction from cancer. If the changes are bilateral the diagnosis is more likely to be duct ectasia. Carcinoma is uncommon when the retraction has been present for more than one year, but even in duct ectasia the signs may be of recent onset. Associated masses may be difficult to assess clinically, but aspiration cytology is usually diagnostic. Cancer will give atypical epithelial cells while typical inflammatory cells (macrophages and foam cells) occur in patients with duct ectasia and periductal mastitis. Similarly, cytology of any associated discharge may provide helpful information. Mammography is helpful because it will usually show the typical features of cancer, or a notable absence of these features in patients with duct ectasia. In patients where doubt as to the underlying diagnosis remains, a rare event, biopsy of the associated mass or the duct system will provide the definitive diagnosis. Excision of the major duct system has the added advantage that the inverted nipple can be corrected by duct excision. The pathology, differential diagnosis and management of nipple retraction due to the duct ectasia complex are considered more fully in Chapter 11.

Cracked Nipples

Cracked nipples are the bane of nursing mothers, for these are the source of entry of bacteria in lactational breast infection.

Pain in the nipple on suckling is a common event in the first few days of breast-feeding and may occur in up to 17% of nursing mothers[2]. In most of these, careful examination, using a magnifying lens if necessary, will reveal a small erosive lesion[3]. The mechanism suggested is that during vigorous suckling the skin of the nipple exposed between tongue and hard palate is subjected to a high negative pressure – if the milk does not flow easily the infant will suck harder – which produces a small blood blister. This lesion usually regresses spontaneously but, if the trauma is repeated, especially if the nipple skin becomes macerated due to the moist environment that often occurs, the lesion may progress to the typical fissure often referred to as a cracked nipple, seen about one week postpartum. This is often infected with either bacteria or with *Candida* sp.

As in many conditions, prevention is better than cure so recognition of predisposing factors is important. Good hygiene and a pattern of cleaning in the pre-confinement period is helpful. The nipples should be washed gently in water and dried secretions removed. The breasts are then dried by dabbing rather than rubbing. Care needs to be taken in establishing suckling – the infant will find an over-engorged breast difficult to empty and short or inverted nipples may also lead to over-vigorous suckling. If one breast is painful, feeding should commence on the unaffected side, so that by the time the infant is applied to the affected breast, the draught reflex will allow easy flow of milk. After feeding the breasts should be cleaned and dried carefully – and kept as dry as possible until the next feed.

In the established case, correct feeding habits need reinforcing and in addition an antibiotic-based cream should be applied to the nipple – if candidal infection is suspected a nystatin-containing cream should be used. With care the fissure will heal and breast-feeding can be maintained although manual expression for a few days may be necessary. Neglect at this stage may lead to the development of an abscess as described in Chapter 13. If nipple inversion is the problem leading to difficulty with suckling the use of nipple shields may be helpful[4].

Nipple Crusting

This symptom usually represents dried up secretions. Sometimes it hides an underlying nipple lesion such as Paget's disease, eczema or erosive adenomatosis.

Erosive Adenomatosis

This is a rare condition which is also described as papillary adenoma, florid papillomatosis of the nipple, subareolar papillomatosis and erosive adenomatosis of the nipple[5]. This condition is termed 'adenoma' by Haagensen[6] who points out the difficulties of diagnosis and records that many of the early cases were treated by radical mastectomy in the belief that the lesion was a carcinoma. It usually presents as a papilliferous lesion of the nipple, often with ulceration which may be concealed under a crust[7] (Figure 14.1). This condition is sometimes painful, the commonest descriptions being burning or itching[8], although Perzin and Lattes[7] only recorded pain in 1 of their 51 cases. Our own experience with this condition would favour the latter view that it is relatively painless. On examination, the whole nipple may be indurated, has an expanded appearance and may be ulcerated. The main differential diagnosis are prolapsing intraductal papilloma, Paget's disease of the nipple, artefactual disease and eczema. The differential diagnosis from Paget's disease can only be made with certainty by biopsy, although the characteristic clinical features are different. Erosive adenomatosis does not extend on to the areolar as does Paget's disease, and it has the appearance of a deeper lesion eroding through the nipple – early Paget's disease is superficial in appearance. When a papilliferous lesion erodes through the nipple duct, it is more likely to represent this condition than an intraductal papilloma (Figure 14.2). An intraductal papilloma tends to expand the nipple rather than erode it, but if a papilloma prolapses through the opening of a duct, the nipple remains normal – it is not ulcerated.

Azzopardi[5] describes this lesion as being an extensive ramifying proliferation of two-layered tubules: an outer layer of myoepithelial cells

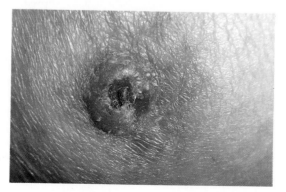

14.1 *Erosive adenomatosis of the nipple.*

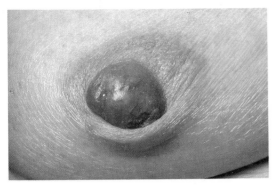

14.2 *A large benign papilloma of the terminal duct, distending the nipple of an elderly woman.*

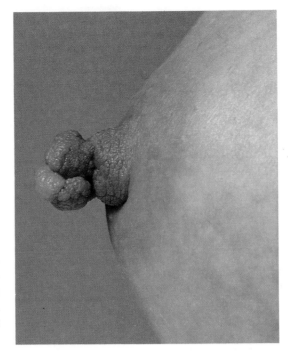

14.3 *Benign pedunculated fibroepithelial polyp.*

and an inner layer of cuboidal cells. Although associated malignant breast disease has been described, this lesion is not usually regarded as premalignant[7]. Erosive adenomatosis is adequately treated by local excision of the affected part of the nipple; there is no need to remove the whole nipple as advocated by some[9].

Syringomatous Adenoma

Rosen[10] has described a benign infiltrating lesion of adnexal skin origin which he differentiates from erosive adenomatosis, in four women and one man. It is more likely to recur than erosive adenomatosis so adequate treatment may require nipple resection. We have no experience of this condition.

Simple Fibroepithelial Polyp

This not uncommon condition was first described by Hutchinson[11] who thought they arose from Montgomery's tubercle, although they are found more frequently on the nipple than the areola. They are pedunculated dry lesions resembling the skin tags seen elsewhere in the body (Figure 14.3). Neurofibromas occurring at this site may also be pedunculated. They are readily treated by local excision and do not recur.

Eczema

This may occur in a form localized mainly or completely to the nipple and areola (Figures 14.4 and 14.5) and requires to be distinguished from Paget's disease and erosive adenomatosis which also have an eczematous appearance. Paget's disease and eczema can usually be differentiated on clinical grounds (Table 14.1). In spite of this, Paget's disease is still often neglected because of an erroneous diagnosis of eczema. It is important

to think of Paget's disease in every inflammatory condition of the nipple and areola and to be aware of the range of appearances of Paget's disease (Figures 14.6 and 14.7). Even so, biopsy in all cases is the safest course to follow. The typical Paget cells usually allow the pathologist to make the diagnosis without difficulty.

In patients with eczema of the nipple and areola, the condition is bilateral and in many patients there is evidence of eczema elsewhere. When this is not the case, eczema is usually symmetrical and does not extend beyond the areola (Figure 14.5). The possibility of an artefactual syndrome (*see* Chapter 17) should not be overlooked.

Treatment in cases of eczema follows the same guidelines as eczema elsewhere in the body.

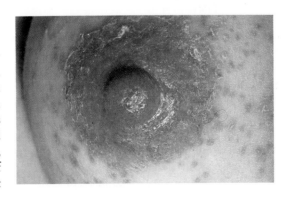

14.4 *Eczema of the nipple and areola – note the uniform involvement*

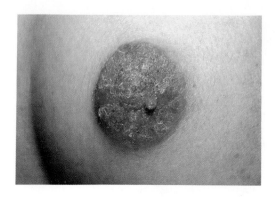

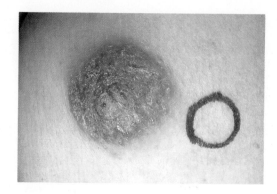

14.5 *Eczema of both areolae, with an unrelated benign cyst in the right breast.*

Table 14.1 Clinical features of eczema of the nipple and Paget's disease.

Eczema	*Paget's disease*
Usually bilateral	Unilateral
Intermittent history, with rapid evolution	Continuous history with slow steady progression
Moist	Moist or dry
Indefinite edge	Irregular but definite edge
Nipple may be spared	Nipple always involved and disappears in advanced cases
Itching common	Itching common

Leiomyoma

Leiomyoma of the nipple is surprisingly uncommon in view of the large quantities of smooth muscle that are present. When it occurs it appears as a smooth round lump, obviously within the skin of the areola or nipple. It can occur at any age, is usually about 6–7 mm in diameter and may have been present for some years. Haagensen[6] distinguishes between this superficial leiomyoma, arising in the smooth muscle of the nipple and areola, and deep leiomyoma which arises from smooth muscle associated with blood vessels. Both are adequately treated by local excision.

Traumatic Lesions

The nipple is occasionally the site of trauma and the condition of jogger's nipple is well recognized[12]. This lesion is presumably the result of constant friction of an unprotected warm and moist nipple on ill-fitting clothing. It is sometimes severe enough to produce bleeding. A related condition is cyclist's nipple[13] which appears to be a cold injury with the subsequent pain lasting for several days. An entertaining traumatic lesion is the recently described tassle dancer's nipple[14]; the rings placed in the nipple may produce unusual radiological artefacts[15]. Artefactual trauma of the nipple is also seen occasionally (*see* Chapter 17).

Raynaud's Phenomenon

Raynaud's phenomenon has also been described in the breast. It is probably more common than is usually recognized. In one series from New Zealand, it was thought that up to 1 in 20 pregnant women had symptoms suggestive of Raynaud's phenomenon during cold weather[16]. The nipple necrosis described after vasopressin is also presumably due to vascular spasm[17].

Professor O'Higgins (personal communication) has provided details of a 53-year-old patient who had Raynaud-like changes that were subsequently shown to be due to pagetoid infiltration by intraduct cancer. The patient described sudden episodic pain in the nipple associated with sequential white and bluish-purple colour changes. The areolar glands usually became prominent and the nipple partially inverted. The symptoms recurred randomly day or night, and were not related to ambient temperature.

We have seen a similar case after major duct excision, which was related to cold. Even though the patient was warmly clothed, the nipples were subjectively intensely cold and objectively so to examination. The attacks gradually abated over a period of 4 to 5 years.

Various sensations of irritation, pricking, burning and cold are sometimes described around the perimenopausal period and may result from the normal periductal fibrotic process of involution. Paget's disease must always be considered in the differential diagnosis.

Montgomery's Glands

Montgomery, an Irish obstetrician, in 1837 gave a classic description of the changes in the areolar tubercles occurring during pregnancy. These structures, which now bear his name, had in fact been described by Morgagni in 1719. There are three types of gland in the areola: (1) Apocrine sweat glands; (2) Modified sebaceous glands; (3) Rudimentary mammary glands.

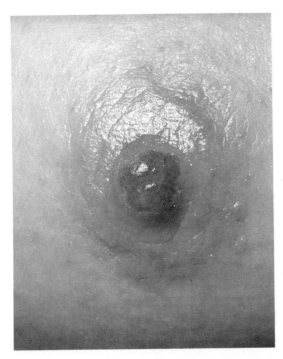

14.6 *The moist, erosive form of early Paget's disease. It is correctly managed by early biopsy.*

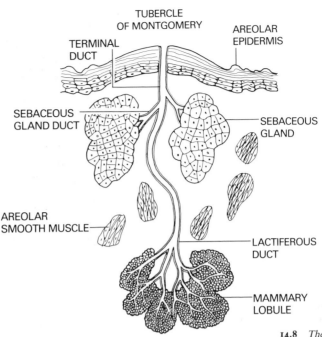

14.8 *The anatomy of the subareolar glands. (After Smith et al[19].)*

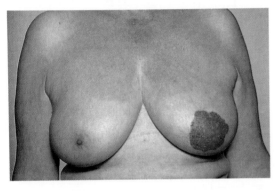

14.7 *More advanced, 'dry' form of Paget's disease. The nipple is disappearing.*

There is clear evidence that aprocrine sweat glands are a normal finding in the areolar skin[18]. The modified sebaceous glands which lie under the tubercles of Montgomery are similar to sebaceous glands elsewhere, except that they are associated with a lactiferous duct extending from a more deeply placed mammary gland[19]. The rudimentary mammary glands and the sebaceous glands both undergo changes during pregnancy which lead to typical changes in the tubercle described by Montgomery. The position and relative sizes of these glands are depicted in Figure 14.8.

In addition to the areolar glands, there are dermal sebaceous glands of the nipple and occasional deep ectopic sebaceous glands which open into the main breast ducts. These are discussed below and in Chapter 11 in relation to the aetiology of mammary duct fistula.

When the detailed anatomy of the glandular components of Montgomery's tubercles are considered, the clinical problems of retention cysts and milk-like discharge are not surprising. It is perhaps more surprising that discharge from the tubercles is as rare as it seems to be in the literature[20]. Infection of the tubercles may mimic subareolar abscess associated with duct ectasia and the persisting lesion suggests a mammary duct fistula, although it will present on the areola rather than at the periphery of the areola as occurs with mammary duct fistula.

We have encountered one case of repeated bleeding from a Montgomery gland in a 16-year-old girl. No obvious cause was found and micro-injection of the affected duct origin showed a blind ending duct (Figure 14.9; case of Mr P. Braithwaite).

Sebaceous Cyst of the Nipple

This rare condition presents as a painless lump palpable immediately below and attached to the nipple (Figure 14.10). Because this lies deeper than the dermal sebaceous glands of the nipple, its origin can be explained by the findings of Patey and Thackray[21] that ectopic sebaceous glands may occasionally be found deep in the nipple, opening into the terminal portion of the duct. It is satisfactorily treated by excision. However, this is obviously a more extensive operation than that necessary for a retention cyst of the dermal

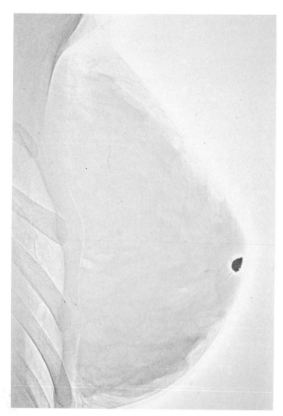

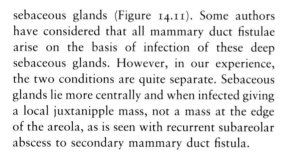

14.9 *Microinjection of a subareolar gland which presented with bleeding from the areola.*

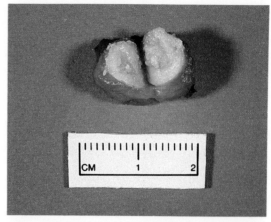

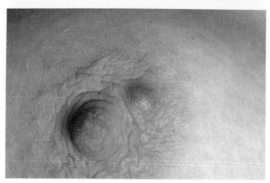

14.10 *A sebaceous cyst presenting as a lump within the nipple – treated by conservative enucleation.*

14.11 *A retention cyst of Montgomery's gland.*

sebaceous glands (Figure 14.11). Some authors have considered that all mammary duct fistulae arise on the basis of infection of these deep sebaceous glands. However, in our experience, the two conditions are quite separate. Sebaceous glands lie more centrally and when infected giving a local juxtanipple mass, not a mass at the edge of the areola, as is seen with recurrent subareolar abscess to secondary mammary duct fistula.

Viral Infections

Molluscum contagiosum occasionally occurs in the skin of the nipple when it produces a discrete lump which may ulcerate[6]. It is readily recognized on histopathology. It is uncommon[22] which is perhaps surprising as this pox virus is usually transmitted sexually. Herpes virus lesions[23] and genital warts of the nipple (condyloma accuminatum)[24] are also seen occasionally.

REFERENCES

1. Bryant T. On the diagnostic value of the retracted nipple as a symptom of breast disease. *British Medical Journal* 1866; **2**: 635–637.
2. Gans B. Breast and nipple pain in early stages of lactation. *British Medical Journal* 1958; **2**: 830–832.
3. Gunther M. Sore nipples. Causes and prevention. *Lancet* 1945; **ii**: 590–593.
4. Waller H. The early failure of breast feeding. A clinical study of its causes and their prevention. *Archives of Diseases in Childhood* 1946; **21**: 1–12.
5. Azzopardi J. G. *Problems in Breast Pathology*. London, W. B. Saunders, 1979.
6. Haagensen C. D. *Disease of the Breast*, 3rd edn. Philedelphia, W. B. Saunders, 1986.
7. Perzin K. H. & Lattes R. Papillary adenoma of the nipple (florid papillomatosis, adenoma, adenomatosis). *Cancer* 1972; **29**: 996–1009.
8. Taylor H. B. & Robertson A. G. Adenomas of the nipple. *Cancer* 1965; **18**: 995–1002.
9. Blamey R. W. (Ed.) *Complications of Breast Surgery*. London, Baillière Tindall, 1986.
10. Rosen P. P. Syringomatous adenoma of the nipple. *American Journal of Surgical Pathology* 1983; **7**: 739–745.
11. Hutchinson J. Polypoid outgrowths of the nipple areola. *Archives of Surgery, London* 1897; 37–39.
12. Levit F. Jogger's nipples. *New England Journal of Medicine* 1977; **297**: 1197.
13. Powell B. Bicyclist's nipples. *Journal of the American medical Association* 1982; **249**: 2457.
14. Collins R. E. C. Breast disease associated with tassle dancing. *British Medical Journal* 1981; **283**: 1660.
15. Healey T. Nipple piercings – unusual artefacts. *Radiography* 1979; **45**: 164–165.
16. Hood L. Raynaud's phenomenon of the nipple. *New Zealand Medical Journal* 1983; **84**: 294–295.

17. Reddy K. R., Iskandarani M., Jeffers L. & Schiff F. R. Bilateral nipple necrorsis after vasopressin therapy. *Archives of internal Medicine* 1984; **144**: 835–836.
18. Craigmyle M. B. L. *The Aprocrine Glands and the Breast.* Chichester, John Wiley & Sons, 1984.
19. Smith D. M., Peters T. G., & Donegan W. L. Montgomery's areolar tubercle. A light microscopic study. *Archives of Pathology and Laboratory Medicine* 1982; **106**: 60–63.
20. Heyman R. B. & Rauch J. L. Areolar gland discharge in adolescent females. *Journal of Adolescent Health Care* 1983; **4**: 285–286.
21. Patey D. H. & Thackray A. C. Pathology and the treatment of mammary duct fistula. *Lancet* 1958; **ii**: 871–873.
22. Carrahlo G. Molluscum contagiosum in a lesion adjacent to the nipple. Report of a case. *Acta cytologica (Baltimore)* 1974; **18**: 532–534.
23. Quinn P. T. and Lofberg J. V. Maternal herpetic breast infection: Another hazard of neonatal Herpes Simplex. *Medical Journal of Australia* 1978; **2**: 411–412.
24. Wood C. Condyloma accuminatum of the nipple. *Journal of Cutaneous Pathology* 1978; **5**: 88–89.

15 Congenital and Cosmetic Aspects

The breast, like other physical features, exhibits a wide range of appearances. There is variation in size, shape and, to some extent, position. The borderline of what is socially and cosmetically acceptable is one of perception because the variants retain normal function. The descriptive terms used by plastic surgeons to describe some of these appearances and the techniques used for their correction are beyond the scope of this book and are adequately dealt with in plastic surgical literature.

Developmental Anomalies

The development of the breast has been described in Chapter 2. The foetal mammalian milk line runs from the base of the upper limb bud to the base of the lower limb bud (*see* Chapter 2). In most adult mammals, breast tissue is confined to this line but, in some, breast tissue is found in other sites: either the milk line is more extensive or breast tissue migrates. Examples of these ectopic sites are the labia in whales and dolphins, the scapular region in nutria, abdominal midline in the possum, dorsal thigh in the viscaccia, and the acromium in a species of lemur.

Supernumerary Breasts

The incidence of supernumerary breasts, defined as structures which produce milk under appropriate hormonal influences, remains uncertain although the condition has been recorded since antiquity. Statues of both Artemesia and Diana of Ephesus represent these ancients as having supernumerary breasts. The great majority of accessory breasts develop along the milk line, but ectopic milk-producing structures have been described at all the ectopic sites that occur in the mammals described above. Fitzwilliams[1] gave a

good account of many of the earlier descriptions. Darwin was clearly aware of the existence of polymastia and used the condition as an illustration of an atavistic phenomenon[2].

The commonest site of accessory breasts is in the axilla. It is remarkable how often these remain unnoticed until the second or third pregnancy (Figure 15.1). These accessory glands do not always have nipples and may be quite troublesome during pregnancy and lactation.

It is presumably because of hormonal stimulation that accessory breasts are more frequently recorded in women than in men (there being no embryological reason to suppose a difference).

Treatment is only indicated if the accessory breast proves troublesome to the patient, the treatment then being surgical excision. It needs to be borne in mind that any condition, including cancer, may occur in an accessory breast. Many examples of accessory breast remain undiagnosed until removed with a clinical diagnosis of lipoma which is found to contain mammary tissue.

Accessory breast tissue may be isolated or may be connected to an accessory nipple. In the former case, the breast will involute soon after

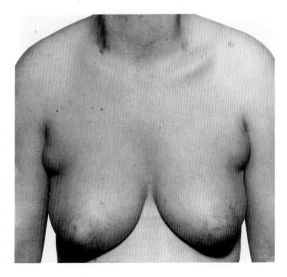

15.1 *Accessory (axillary) breasts. First noticed at time of lactation following first pregnancy.*

parturition, in the latter an active secreting gland may produce sufficient milk to sustain the infant.

Supernumerary nipples may occur in association with accessory glandular breast tissue or more commonly occur alone.

Polythelia and Supernumerary Nipples

Some authors use these terms synonymously; others reserve polythelia for those examples of more than one nipple appearing on the same breast mound[1]. We seen no benefit in the distinction and regard the terms as interchangeable. This condition is as common in men as in women, the extra nipples usually appearing along the milk line.

The reported incidence of supernumerary nipples varies greatly in the literature. The condition is usually considered to be more common in Oriental populations[2]. Mehes[3] screened 4000 neonates in Hungary and found an incidence of polythelia of only 0.2% and described an association with renal abnormalities. This association is supported by the findings of another study which found an incidence of supernumerary nipples in 16% of patients with end-stage renal failure, but only 2% of control patients[4]. Two other studies have failed to confirm the findings. In one study of 1691 births, an incidence of 2.5% supernumerary nipples was found[5]. Robertson et al[6] found an incidence of 1.2% in 2875 black children with no evidence of associated renal anomalies. The balance of evidence suggests that supernumerary nipples are common and parents may be reassured that they are of no significance. Extra nipples are most commonly found on the lower part of the breast, chest wall and upper abdomen and are often mistaken for naevi (Figure 15.2). No treatment is required for this condition, except when it is accompanied by active breast tissue or if the patient finds it cosmetically unacceptable

Nipple Inversion

Nipple inversion is a common finding. The causes may be congenital, periductal inflammation or tumour infiltration. The last of these is beyond the scope of this book but in our series represents only a small percentage of observed nipple retraction.

The distinction between inversion and retraction is rather arbitrary: we use inversion to describe the nipple that did not protrude at the time of adolescent development and retraction for those cases in which a previously everted

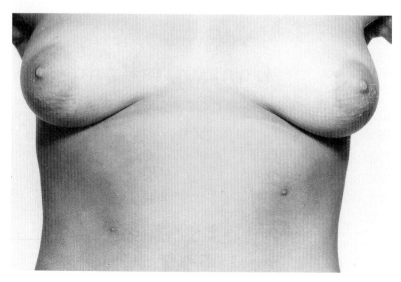

15.2 *Supernumerary nipples.*

nipple is affected by an underlying pathological process.

Congenital

During foetal life, the nipple is represented by a central depression which persists after birth until development of the underlying breast produces elevation of the areola. Subsequent retraction of the surrounding smooth muscle leads to flattening of the mound and protrusion of the nipple[7].

Schwayer et al[8] in his study of 339 breasts found 6 with inversion of the nipple (a prevalence of 1.8%). There was no difference in the constituents of the areola, mammary ducts, smooth muscle or collagen, but there was a deficiency in the supporting stroma immediately behind the nipple. An alternative view is to regard the inversion as due to the failure of the smooth muscle bundles of Sappy (circular) and Myerholtz (radial) to relax[9]. In any event it appears that inversion is best regarded as failure of normal eversion to occur.

The true incidence of congenital nipple inversion is hard to determine because it seems likely that such women are more disposed to periductal inflammation – the second most common cause of nipple inversion. The findings are usually bilateral, but often to different degrees, and it is not rare to find one side completely inverted and the other normal.

Problems related to inverted nipples are functional, in association with breast feeding and cosmetic.

Inverted nipples and breast-feeding
The problems associated with breast-feeding have been reviewed by Inch[10]. Waller[11] found that nearly 40% of young women in their first pregnancy had at least a minor degree of failure of normal protrusion of the nipple, but maintained

that this should not be considered a contraindication to breast-feeding, as so many maintain. He recommended a 'pinch test' to assess protrusion, and patients failing this test were given a glass (Woolwich) shield to wear during pregnancy, the purpose of which was to gradually stretch and loosen the non-protractile nipple. Of patients with poorly protractile nipples treated in this way, only 44% were deemed to have breast-fed successfully.

In contrast, Hytten[12] found that only 14% of 2461 primiparae had unsatisfactory nipples, and only 16% of these had breast-feeding problems as a direct result. Of those with normal nipples, 3.5% had similar problems. Thus, although antenatal examination of the nipples might have some predictive value, most patients with poor nipples will have no related problems with breast-feeding.

These findings may be explained by cineradiographic[14] and ultrasound studies[15] of breast-feeding. These show that the nipple itself plays a relatively small part in the anatomical aspects of suckling. The infant makes a 'teat' from the surrounding breast tissue as well as the nipple, in a ratio of about 3:1. Thus mothers with inverted nipples should be encouraged to ensure that the baby has an adequate mouthful of breast to form the teat, and be reassured that the contribution of the nipple is relatively small. Correct positioning during feeding is perhaps the most important factor and the patient should be given skilled help from a midwife before starting to breast-feed.

Inverted nipples and cosmesis

Treatment consists of reassurance that there is no serious underlying disease and, when the cosmetic defect is severe, consideration of surgical correction. Sometimes the situation may be improved by repeated massage, although there are few data from controlled studies to support this. In severe cases surgical correction may be requested. Pitangay[9] has described a procedure of dividing the muscle bundles without damaging the lactiferous tissues – an important consideration in young women who may still wish to feed their children. However, the large number of procedures described for congenital inverted nipple suggest that none of them is ideal, and there is considerable doubt about the efficacy of procedures which do not divide the ducts. Our own views on surgical management are given in Chapter 18.

Following Periductal Inflammation

Periductal inflammation is discussed more fully in Chapter 11. Inversion due to periductal inflammation is often accompanied by thickening of the ducts in and behind the nipple, a feature which can be readily appreciated by rolling them between finger and thumb. There may be a history of acute attacks of periductal mastitis, but more frequently this is a smouldering process which goes unrecognized until the inverted nipple, often unilateral, is remarked upon and the patient fears the onset of a malignant process.

The histological features in these cases are associated with periductal inflammation, often a plasma cell infiltrate, ductal dilatation and shortening.

Assessment is made by history, examination, mammography in patients over 30 years and cytology of any associated discharge or mass. If the cosmetic defect is significant and the patient requests correction, the operation of major duct excision (Chapter 18) is satisfactory – the more conservative procedures that can be effective in congenital inversion are unsatisfactory in this group of patients.

Amastia and Hypoplasia

Amastia is a rare condition and is presumably due to failure of the milk line to develop or to its complete involution. It is not surprising that such an obvious abnormality was recorded in biblical times (Song of Solomon, viii 8). The condition, however, is quite uncommon and is usually unilateral. Some of the cases have absence of the pectoral muscles and associated syndactyly (a condition known as Poland's syndrome following his description in 1841). In spite of its popular eponym, this condition was apparently first described in 1839 by Floriep. The terminology has been challenged and, although Ravitch[11] has argued that the term should be abandoned, descriptions of Poland's syndrome persist. The familial nature of this condition was first remarked upon in 1894 by Whyte and, more recently, it has been established that it is transmitted as an autosomal dominant feature[17].

Congenital absence of the breast is as common in boys as in girls but its exact incidence is unknown.

Treatment is surgical and a moderately satisfactory breast reconstruction can be obtained using a latissimus dorsi mycutaneous flap to provide added bulk and to replace the missing pectoralis major muscle[18]. If the nipple/areola complex is also missing a nipple sharing operation may be performed as a secondary procedure.

Hypoplastic breasts of a lesser degree are not uncommon and there is some evidence of an association with mitral valve prolapse. Patients attending for breast augmentation have a higher incidence of mitral valve prolapse; patients with a diagnosis of mitral valve prolapse have been found to have smaller breasts than controls, the putative defect occurring during a time of mesenchymal development in the sixth week[19].

Athelia

Absence of the nipple is an extremely rare event and usually is associated with absence of the breast. Occasional examples of imperforate nipple have been reported as a cause of failure to lactate with an engorged breast. It is difficult to be certain that these obstructed nipples were not secondary to trauma (such as burns) or a disease process such as squamous metaplasia of the lactiferous sinus.

Asymmetry

Minor degrees of asymmetry are very common and the patient may be reassured. When the discrepancy is great (Figure 15.3), surgical correction may be indicated to equalize the breasts. Augmentation of the smaller breast, reduction of the larger breast, or both procedures may be required to obtain a satisfactory result.

More severe cases may be partially expressed examples of Poland's syndrome or follow trauma (usually burns or surgery) in childhood when the breast bud is damaged.

Fusion of the Breasts

There is a wide variation of normality in the placing of the breasts on the chest wall. With one extreme, the breasts are fused in the midline (Figure 15.4). This can cause difficulty and discomfort with clothing, and it is worth while separating the breasts by a simple plastic procedure (Figure 15.5).

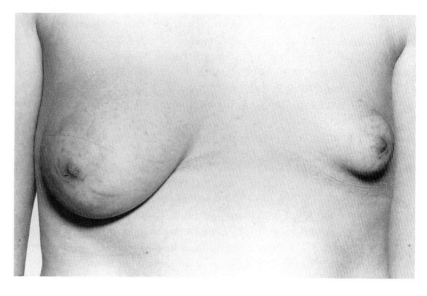

Hypertrophic Abnormalities of the Breast

An otherwise normal breast may enlarge for no discernible reason at several stages in childhood and adolescence. This excludes those cases due to excessive hormone production in childhood and in none of the conditions described below has any abnormality of circulating hormones been demonstrated.

Neonatal Enlargement

Reference has already been made to neonatal hypertrophy in Chapter 1. It is normal to have some palpable breast tissue at birth and for this to disappear by the age of 6 months, although it tends to remain longer in girls than boys[20]. Cases have been described in which the genitalia as well as the breasts are fully developed very early in childhood and, in these cases, a search for an underlying abnormality should be made.

15.3 *Marked asymmetry of breasts for which plastic surgery is indicated.*

15.4 *Fused breasts.*

15.5 *Postoperative result of patient in Figure 15.4.*

15.4

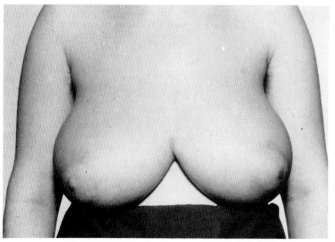

15.5

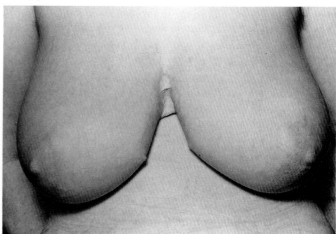

Prepubertal (Premature) Thelache

It is not uncommon to see precocious enlargement of the breast at about the age of eight. This is often unilateral. It is of no significance in the absence of other signs of precocious puberty and in 50% of cases it is the first sign of early puberty[20].

The clinical appearances are of a firm discoid lesion behind the nipple, not unlike that found in the pubertal boy with gynaecomastia. The importance of the lesion is in recognizing it for what it is – normal breast tissue! Surgical removal of the mass is a disaster because it represents the whole of the developing breast. Removal will result in secondary amastia on the affected side. In a review of the natural history of this condition in 46 cases, 32% regressed completely over a 2-year period, 57% remained unchanged and 11% underwent progressive enlargement[22].

Pubertal Asymmetry

The breasts do not always develop synchronously and parents sometimes seek advice about a unilateral lump. The same considerations apply to this condition as to the prepubertal variety – biopsy and excision must be avoided.

Postpubertal Hypertrophy

Adolescent (Virginal) Hypertrophy

The normal development of the breast occasionally continues unchecked so that huge breasts result (Figure 15.6). This condition was reported in 1669[23]. This condition is usually bilateral but occurs as a unilateral disease sufficiently often to imply that it is due to local factors rather than a hormonal imbalance. No hormonal problem has been identified in these patients except possibly a rather high rate of infertility[2]. However, episodes of epidemic breast enlargement which seem to be caused by exogenous steroids rather militate against the view that hypertrophy is not a hormonal event. Epidemics of breast enlargement attributed to steroids present in chicken meat have been reported from Italy[24] and Puerto Rico[25]. Gigantomastia may also occasionally be induced by drugs such as D-penicillamine[26]. As the breasts enlarge and become pendulous, the nipple and areola may stretch to an extent where they are recognized with difficulty. The superficial veins enlarge and palpation reveals general firmness with a varying degree of nodularity, sometimes minimal, sometimes very marked. The weight results in back pain, the characteristic grooving of the shoulders by the brassière straps, and even orthopnoea. Once a significant degree of hypertrophy has become established, regression does not seem to occur[2].

Hypertrophy in Pregnancy

Very occasionally, bilateral or unilateral gross hypertrophy occurs in relation to pregnancy – usually the former. The aetiology is uncertain. Treatment of this condition should follow the same guidelines as adolescent hypertrophy,. It may progress to the stage where infarction may occur.

Treatment of Hypertrophy

When the enlargement of the breast occurs rapidly, medical treatment with danazol[26] and bromocriptine[27,28] may be tried but insufficient data exist to give clear guidelines as to their use. Dihydrogesterone has also been recommended, both before and for 6 months after surgery[29]. On general principles, danazol is probably the drug whose pharmacology is best documented, and is the first choice on the basis of safety and lack of side-effects.

If the bulk of the enlarged breasts causes enough trouble a reduction mammoplasty is indicated. It is usually advised that the operation is deferred to the age of 17, but this is purely arbitrary. When selecting an operative technique, it is desirable to use one in which the nipple/areolar complex is transferred with underlying breast tissue, so that the patient may keep her options with regard to subsequent breast-feeding. Occasionally the breasts continue to enlarge and further resections

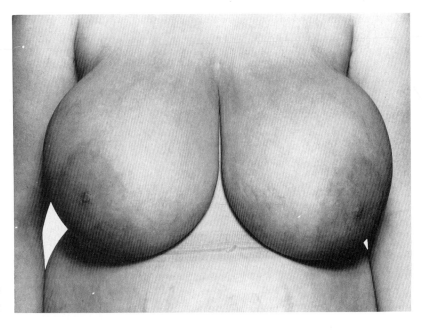

15.6 *Adolescent hypertrophy. This degree of enlargement causes great psychological and physical embarrassment.*

may become necessary. In some of the more extreme cases occuring in pregnancy, more than one resection may be needed if further progression occurs[2]. Usually a combination of anti-hormone therapy and surgery is required to curtail the problem and the patient should be warned that a similar event may occur in subsequent pregnancies. Some authors suggest that the appropriate treatment is bilateral total mastectomy with reconstruction[30].

Histology

The microscopic findings of the resected breast tissue are remarkably normal, the great size seeming to be due to an increase in stromal rather than glandular tissue[2].

Excessive Postlactational Involution

Women not uncommonly complain that after pregnancy and lactation, their breasts involute excessively and are much smaller than before. This is to be regarded as physiological. If the involution is marked and the psychological distress is great, augmentation mammoplasty is well justified. It is usually performed by submammary or subpectoral silicone implants.

Cosmetic Aspects

The normal breast has a variety of shape, size and firmness which is not constant even in the same woman. In a cosmetically orientated society it is not surprising that some women express dissatisfaction with the state of their breasts. When the changes are gross, associated with the conditions outlined above, then the need for corrective surgery is self-evident.

A patient may express her dissatisfaction by stating her breasts are: too small, too large, drooping, asymmetrical or the wrong shape. The need for change may be initiated by a desire to alter her body image, to save a failing marriage or for employment in the entertainment industry. It is impossible to give general guidance and each patient must be treated on her own merits. In general, patients who want cosmetic surgery for themselves do better than those who want it for other reasons. A policy of gentle dissuasion will usually result in the right decision which should not be made at the first interview.

Selection of patients for treatment with less clear-cut abnormalities is in the realm of the plastic and cosmetic surgeon and beyond the scope of this book. The interested reader may refer to the appropriate texts for further details but a brief account is given here.

Augmentation

In the past, a variety of substances have been injected into the breast. The best known of these are paraffin and silicone-based agents. Although these occasionally gave good short-term results, the long-term effects were disastrous. The patients developed hard lumpy breasts and not infrequently developed sinuses. It is not unknown for a mastectomy to have to be performed for the complications of this approach. This method has now been abandoned but occasional patients still present with ongoing problems (see Chapter 17).

The development of a silicone envelope which could be filled with a silicone gel, or saline was subsequently developed for placement in the retromammary area. The earlier thin-walled prostheses were liable to rupture – particularly when decompressed during aeroplane flights. The phenomenon of bleeding, i.e. the extrusion of the gel through the membrane, was also described. Some of these problems have been averted by the use of thicker-skinned envelopes.

The prosthesis is placed in either a retromammary or retropectoral pocket prepared by blunt dissection. This has the effect of projecting the breast tissue forward. There is clearly a limit to the size of the pocket, and thus the prosthesis that can be inserted, but the development of tissue expansion has made it possible to extend the role of this type of surgery.

Complications

A number of potential problems remain for the patient and her attendants after this type of surgery.

Deflation

Even the thicker-walled prostheses deflate occasionally. This usually occurs spontaneously and is more commonly seen in the older prostheses filled with saline, e.g. the Varifil prosthesis. The mechanism of this event is not clear but seems likely to be due to the folding of the envelope (the so-called fold flaw defect), if it is not completely filled. In the prostheses that have been removed, a small hole has been found so that the fault does not seem to be with the valvular mechanism used for filling the prosthesis.

If the prosthesis that ruptures is filled with saline, the fluid is resorbed and the only real problem is the embarrassment of the patient. The old prosthesis may be removed and a new one re-inserted at any time. If the ruptured prosthesis contained silicone, then this may cause a marked granulomatous foreign body reaction and, if re-exploration is delayed, removal may be difficult.

Capsular contraction

This complication is the real scourge of augmentation mammoplasty. A tight fibrous capsule forms around the prosthesis and, as it contracts, the prosthesis is squeezed into a spherical shape. The mechanism of its occurrence is unknown. Postulated theories include infection, haemorrhage, ischaemia due to a tight pocket, and leaking of silicone through the envelope with production of a foreign body reaction. None of these theories entirely fits the observed facts. We have removed a number of prostheses associated with capsular contraction. Portions of the capsule have been sent for bacteriological examination and been negative on each occasion. Histological examination has failed to show any evidence of a foreign body reaction. As regards the ischaemic theory and the tight pocket, it needs to be pointed out that capsular contraction is most common after submammary insertion and that placement in a subpectoral pocket (which may be quite tense) is associated with a reduced incidence of early capsular contraction.

The problem of capsular contraction is a continuing one and, until it is solved, the long-term results of augmentation mammoplasty will remain unpredictable.

Treatment of capsular contraction consists of reassurance and explanation, or capsulotomy. The capsule can be ruptured by external pressure if it is in the submammary plane. It is not possible to do this if the prosthesis is placed subpectorally. If the capsule cannot be ruptured by the closed technique, an open capsulotomy may be needed. In very severe cases the prosthesis will require removal.

Less Common Complications

Occasionally the prosthesis migrates, usually into the axilla. If the pocket is tight, pressure necrosis may occur leading to skin ulceration and extrusion of the prosthesis.

Infection of a foreign body is as disastrous at this site as elsewhere. The only action is to remove the prosthesis to allow the infection to settle.

After an interval of 6 months it may be possible to re-insert the prosthesis.

Assessment of subsequent disease

The majority of women requesting augmentation mammoplasty are young. They will not differ from other women in their subsequent development of breast symptoms. The presence of a prosthesis, particularly if capsular contraction is present, may make assessment more difficult, may compromise adequate mammography although with attention to detail this may be circumvented, and adds a new danger to any form of biopsy (aspiration, needle or open) – rupture of the prosthesis. However, concealment of breast disease is not a major problem because the breast tissue lies in front of the prosthesis.

Reduction Mammoplasty and Correction of Ptosis

The physical, cosmetic and psychological consequences of very large and heavy breasts are great, and patients should be made aware of the benefits of reduction mammoplasty. Unlike other forms of cosmetic surgery, patients rarely regret competently performed reduction mammoplasty. A wide variety of techniques has been described and these aim to reduce the size of the breast and to correct ptosis. Skin, subcutaneous fat and breast tissue are excised to a preplanned pattern and the nipple transposed upwards on a de-epithelialized pedicle to its new position. The pedicle may be superiorly, centrally or inferiorly based depending on the reconstruction employed. Alternatively the nipple areola complex may be replaced as a free graft. The very wide variety of techniques available attest to the fact that none of them produces entirely successful results. Provided a satisfactory cosmetic result is achieved, the long-term results are good and in most cases postoperative assessment straightforward.

The immediate postoperative complications of haematoma, fat necrosis and infection may lead to later difficulty in assessing the breast for subsequent disease if they lead to excessive scarring – features which may also cause mammographic difficulties. With such patients a case can be made for routine mammograms 6 months after operation to provide base-line films for later comparison.

REFERENCES

1. Fitzwilliams D. C. L. *On the Breast.* London, William Heinemann, 1924.
2. Haagensen C. D. *Disease of the Breast,* 3rd edn.
Philadelphia, W. B. Saunders, 1986.
3. Méhes K. Association of supernumerary nipples with other anomalies. *Journal of Pediatrics* 1979; 95: 274–275.
4. Matesanz R., Teniel J. L., Garcia-Martin F. *et al.*

High incidence of supernumerary nipples in end stage renal failure. *Nephron* 1986; **44**: 385–386.

5. Mimoumi F., Merlob P. & Reisner S. H. Occurrence of supernumerary nipples in newborns. *American Journal of Diseases of Children* 1983; **137**: 952–953.

6. Robertson A. , Sale P. & Sathyanarayan. Lack of association of supernumerary nipples with renal anomalies in black infants. *Journal of Pediatrics* 1986; **109** 502–503.

7. McFarland J. Residual lactation acini in the female breast. Their relation to chronic cystic mastitis and malignant disease. *Archives of Surgery* 1922; **5**: 1–12.

8. Schwager R. G., Smith J. W., Gray G. F. & Goulan D. Inversion of the human female nipple, with a simple method of treatment. *Plastic and Reconstructive Surgery* 1974; **54**: 564–569.

9. Pitangay I. Reconstruction of congenital nipple deformities. In: Chang W. H. J. & Petry J. J. (eds) *The Breast, an Atlas of Reconstruction.* 1984, pp 355–361.

10. Inch S. Inverted nipples and breast feeding. In: Chalmers, Enkin & Kierse (eds) *Effective Care in Pregnancy and Childbirth.* Oxford, Oxford University Press, 1988, in press.

11. Waller H. The early failure of breast feeding. A clinical study of its causes and their prevention. *Archives of Disease in Childhood* 1946; **21**: 1–12.

12. Hytten F. Clinical and chemical studies in human lactation: IX Breast feeding in hospital. *British Medical Journal* 1954; **2**: 1447–1452.

13. L'esperance C. M. Pain or pleasure. The dilemma of early breast feeding. *Birth and the Family Journal* 1980; **7**: 21–26.

14. Ardran G. M., Kemp F. H. & Lind J. A cineradiographic study of breast feeding. *British Journal of Radiology* 1958; **31**: 156–162.

15. Weber F., Woolridge M. W. & Baum J. D. An ultrasonographic analysis of suckling and swallowing in new born infants. *Pediatric Research* 1984; **18**: 806.

16. Ravitch M. M. Poland's syndrome – A study of an eponym. *Plastic and Reconstructive Surgery* 1977; **59**: 508–512.

17. Nelson N. M. & Cooper G. K. N. Congenital defects of the breast – an autosomal dominant?

South African Medical Journal 1982; **61**: 434–436.

18. Bostwick J. *Aesthetic and Reconstructive Breast Surgery.* St Louis, CV Mosby, 1983.

19. Rosenberg C. A., Derman G. H., Grubb W. C. & Buder A. J. Hypomastia and mitral valve prolapse. Evidence of a linked embryologic and mesenchymal dysplasia. *New England Journal of Medicine* 1983; **309**: 1230–1232.

20. McKiernan J. K. & Hull D. Breast development in the newborn. *Archives of Disease in Childhood* 1981; **56**: 525–529.

21. Marshall W. A. & Tanner J. M. Variations in pubertal changes in girls. *Archives of Disease in Childhood* 1969; **44**: 291–303.

22. Mills J. L., Stolley P. D., Davies J. & Moshang T. Premature thelarche. Natural history and etiologic investigation. *American Journal of Diseases of Children* 1981; **135**: 743–745.

23. Durston W. Concerning a very sudden excessive swelling of a woman's breasts. *Philosoph Transact for Anno 1669.* London Royal Society, 1670.

24. Fara G. M., Del Corvo G., Bernuzzi S. *et al.* Epidemic of breast enlargement in an Italian school. *Lancet* 1979; **ii**: 295–297.

25. Bongiovanni A. M. An epidemic of premature thelache in Puerto Rico. *Journal of Pediatrics* 1983; **103**: 245–246.

26. Taylor P. J. Successful treatment of D-penicillamine induced breast gigantism with danazol. *British Medical Journal* 1981; **282**: 362–363.

27. Kullander S. Effect of 2Br alpha ergocryptin (CB134) on serum prolactin and clinical picture in a case of gigantomastia in pregnancy. *Annales Chirugiae et Gynaecologie Fenniae* 1976; **65**: 227–233.

28. Hedberg K., Karlsson K. & Lindstedt A. Gigantomastia during pregnancy: effect of a dopamine agonist. *American Journal of Obstetrics and Gynecology* 1979; **133**: 928–931.

29. Mayl N., Vasconez L. O. & Jurkiewicz M. J. Treatment of macromastia in the actively enlarging breast. *Plastic and Reconstructive Surgery* 1974; **54**: 6–12.

30. Stavides S., Hacking A., Tiltman A. & Dent D. M. Gigantomastia in pregnancy. *British Journal of Surgery* 1987; **74**: 585–586.

16   The Male Breast

The development of the male breast is identical to that in the female before puberty. It develops ductal structures but, in the absence of oestrogenic stimulation, lobular structures are not formed. The incidence of absent breast or nipple or supernumerary nipples is similar to that found in the female.

Gynaecomastia

Gynaecomastia is defined as an enlargement of the ductal and stromal tissue of the male breast which is palpably and histologically different from the surrounding subcutaneous fat. It may range in size from a small retroareolar button of tissue to enlargement indistinguishable from the normal female breast[1].

Gynaecomastia is the commonest condition affecting the male breast. The term was used by Galen to describe the changes that would now be described as pseudo-gynaecomastia. The term appears to have been reintroduced in the 1860s[2,3]. The alternative form of gynaecomazia is now regarded as obsolete. It may be either primary (physiological) or secondary (to a defined extramammary stimulus). It requires careful distinction from pseudo-gynaecomastia in which the external appearance suggests the presence of breast tissue, but palpation (and histology) reveals that the swelling is all fat with no increase in breast tissue.

Clinical Presentation

The patient usually presents with a swelling of the breast, often unilateral (Figure 16.1) which is frequently tender. He may be concerned about the tenderness itself, cosmetic appearance or the possibility of underlying malignancy. In many cases, especially in secondary gynaecomastia, changes are asymptomatic and are noted by the attending physician. Examination reveals a firm disc of retroareolar tissue which is mobile and often tender. There is usually a clear, but not sharp, demarcation of the firm, often slightly tender, breast tissue from softer surrounding fat. It needs to be distinguished from carcinoma of the male breast and pseudo-gynaecomastia, retroareolar fat deposition in obesity. The hallmark of gynaecomastia is its concentricity, if an eccentric mass is found an alternative diagnosis should be considered. At the initial assessment careful examination is needed to decide whether the enlarged breast is due to breast tissue or to fat. In cases where clinical examination leaves doubt, mammography will allow quantification of the amount of fat and breast parenchyma.

Histology

The enlargement of the breast in gynaecomastia is due to a proliferation of loose periductal connective tissue, together with a variable degree of multiplication, elongation, or branching of ducts. There is also periductal, or more widespread, infiltration by plasma cells, lymphocytes, and large mononuclear cells[4]. The changes seen

16.1   *Unilateral, pubertal gynaecomastia in a male.*

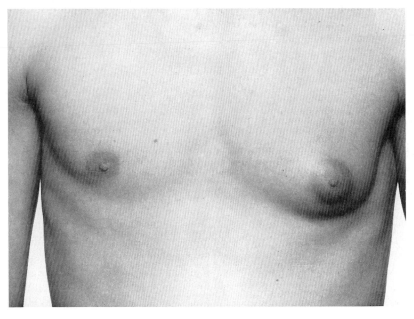

in the stroma are quantitative rather than qualitative. Acinar formation seems to occur only after long-term oestrogen treatment or in Klinefelter's syndrome[5]. Anderson and Gram[6] described 6 cases of focal lobular formation in a series of 76 surgical resections in whom they failed to identify a source of oestrogens and so concluded that oestrogenic stimulation was unnecessary for acinar formation. In view of the obscure source of some exogenous oestrogens[7], this view must remain unproven. Azzopardi[8] has commented on the lack of periductal elastic tissue in these patients in comparison to the female.

The histological incidence of gynaecomastia at autopsy has been estimated by Sandison[5] as 4% and by Anderson and Gram[9] as 55%. However, Anderson and Gram[9] described three phases of gynaecomastia: active, inactive and intermediate. Only a few (7%) of the cases were active or intermediate so that there is less discrepancy than is immediately apparent.

Incidence

A review of the literature will reveal conflicting information on the incidence and significance of gynaecomastia. Specialist endocrinologists who see a selected group of patients may consider the development of gynaecomastia to be of sinister significance[10]. In one series it was considered that 27 out of 46 cases had endocrine causes susceptible to, or curable by, endocrine therapy[11].

Two studies, however, have established that mild forms of gynaecomastia are very common although presentation as a clinical complaint is far less frequent. Nydick et al[12] showed in their study of 1855 boy scouts, that the overall incidence between the ages of 10 and 16 was 38%; this reached a maximum of 65% in the 14-year-old boys which had dropped to 14% in those of 16 years. Nuttall[13] in his study of 306 men showed that an incidence of 17% in youths in their late teens gradually increased in the following decades so that the incidence was 57% in those over 50 years. The overall incidence was 36% and in the vast majority bilateral disease existed. Figure 16.2 combines the findings of Nydick et al[12] and Nuttall[13].

The literature, however, provides conflicting information on the laterality of gynaecomastia; for example, in his study of the radiology of this condition Dershaw[14] found 28 had unilateral disease, 4 had symmetrical involvement and 8 had bilateral but asymmetrical involvement. In another radiological study, 63% of 94 patients had bilateral but usually asymmetrical involvement[15]. The variations in these reports probably reflect

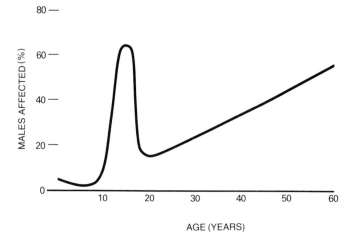

referral patterns as diagnostic doubt is likely to be increased when the condition is unilateral.

Primary gynaecomastia is usually considered under the headings neonatal, pubertal and senescent, although, as can be seen from the foregoing, it would be better to regard it as a continuum with a peak at puberty, which falls in the late teens to be followed by steadily increasing incidence with age, as illustrated in Figure 16.2.

Aetiology

Because of the clear relationship between the incidence of gynaecomastia and hormonal events, the role of an endocrine abnormality in gynaecomastia needs to be seriously considered.

Androgen Physiology

The major androgen in the adult human male is testosterone produced by the testes; the adrenal gland produces an insignificant amount of this hormone. The active hormones are dihydrotestosterone, produced peripherally from testosterone at its site of action, and androstenedione which is derived from the adrenal cortex. Both testosterone and androstenedione may be converted to oestrogens by peripheral aromatization.

Hormonal Defect in Gynaecomastia

The putative hormonal defects in gynaecomastia have been well studied. Prolactin appears to have no influence on the development of gynaecomastia[16,17], although Lee[18] recorded a transient rise in prolactin levels just prior to the development of gynaecomastia. Most patients with gynaecomastia have normal prolactin levels; few men with hyperprolactinaemia and/or galactorrhoea develop gynaecomastia. A number of studies have shown a relative alteration in circulating sex steroids in patients with gynaecomastia. Lee[18] prospectively studied 29 boys, 20 of whom subsequently developed gynaecomastia. Those who did

16.2 *The age incidence of gynaecomastia found on routine examination (Derived from Nydick et al[12] and Nuttall[13].)*

so had a transient increase in oestrogen levels before the gynaecomastia became clinically apparent. Moore et al[17] studied 30 pubertal boys with gynaecomastia and 20 without and demonstrated a lower Δ^4-androstenedione/oestrone and oestradiol ratio (the testosterone/oestrone ratio remaining normal) in the affected boys and postulated that the cause was peripheral conversion of adrenal androgens to oestrone and oestradiol.

Pirke and Doerr[19] have shown that the androgen/oestrogen ratio falls with increasing age: an observation which fits well with the observation of increasing incidence of gynaecomastia with age[13]. Despite these somewhat inconsistent results, it seems likely that the development of gynaecomastia is the result of a relative increase in the levels of circulating oestrogens with respect to androgens and that, in most cases of primary gynaecomastia, this is the operative mechanism. It seems likely that examples of secondary gynaecomastia are due to a similar perturbation of hormonal equilibrium. The mechanisms by which these changes may occur have been reviewed by Wilson et al[20]. Unilateral gynaecomastia presumes a local factor – presumably related to hormone receptors or local hormone conversion but remains an endocrinological enigma.

Physiological Gynaecomastia

Infantile

A small percentage of male neonates have noticeable breast enlargement due to circulating maternal hormones. This resolves by the age of 4 months. It is usually bilateral but may be unilateral. No treatment beyond reassurance of the mother is required.

Adolescence

This is a common age to develop gynaecomastia. Nydick et al[12] in their study of 1855 boy scouts aged between 10 and 16, found a 38% incidence of gynaecomastia. They have shown that the majority resolved within 6 months, although 27% of cases persisted for 2 years and 8% for 3 years. In 25% of cases, the disease was unilateral but, when bilateral, the sides were usually affected to different degrees and the onset was usually asynchronous.

Adult

Asymptomatic gynaecomastia in the adult usually persists unless a reversible underlying cause is found. When symptomatic it runs a variable course and often undergoes spontaneous remission – although examination will reveal persisting enlargement of the breast disc.

Secondary Gynaecomastia

A number of disparate conditions are associated with gynaecomastia as summarized in Table 16.1. When the clinical sign of gynaecomastia is so common in healthy men, care needs to be taken in ascribing such findings to underlying pathology or medication. A number of well-described associations do, however, merit some discussion.

Table 16.1 Causes of secondary gynaecomastia.

Decreased androgens
  Reduced production
    congenital anorchia
    chromosomal abnormalities,
      e.g. Klinefelter's syndrome
    bilateral cryptorchidism
    viral orchitis
    bilateral torsion
    granulomatous disease
    renal failure
  Androgen resistance
    testicular feminization

Increased oestrogens
  Increased secretion
    testicular tumours
    carcinoma lung
  Increased peripheral aromatization
    adrenal disease
    liver disease
    starvation re-feeding
    thyrotoxicosis

Drug induced
  see Table 16.2

Tumours

A number of tumours which secrete hormones may be associated with gynaecomastia. Both teratomas and seminomas of the testis may secrete sufficient oestrogens to produce gynaecomastia. Bronchogenic carcinoma is a well-recognized source of ectopic hormone production and may also produce hormones with oestrogenic activity. Tumours of the pituitary and hypothalamus may also produce gynaecomastia – presumably mediated via the testis by gonadotropic hormones. Oestrogenic precursors produced by adrenal tumours are considered an excessively rare cause of gynaecomastia[1].

Klinefelter's Syndrome

This chromosomal anomaly, when an apparent male has an XXY karyotype, is due to nondisjunction of the parental sex chromosomes. The clinical features of the syndrome are testicular atrophy, eunuchoid habitus with female hair distribution and gynaecomastia. Confirmation of the diagnosis depends on chromosomal examination. The gynaecomastia in this condition is unusual in that the patient may develop lobular structures[5], and is associated with an increased incidence of carcinoma[21].

Secondary Testicular Failure

Testicular damage from any cause may result in decreased testosterone production and a change in the androgen/oestrogen ratio. The absolute levels of oestrogen do not need to be raised for gynaecomastia to occur. Viral orchitis, most commonly due to mumps, is the most frequent cause of testicular atrophy but a variety of causes should be considered.

Liver Failure

With the exception of drug-induced changes, this is probably the commonest cause of secondary gynaecomastia. The failing liver fails to eliminate androstenedione which is then available for peripheral conversion to oestrogens[22].

Starvation Re-feeding

The mechanism by which this occurs is probably related to the fatty liver change that occurs in such patients. Originally described in liberated prisoners of war[23], it may also be seen in patients who have been severely ill on intensive care units.

Drugs

A large number of drugs have been implicated in the development of gynaecomastia (Table 16.2). When the finding of gynaecomastia is as common as it appears to be, isolated case reports need to be treated with scepticism. However, a number of clear associations can be accepted, the effect produced either by a relative increase in oestrogenic activity or inhibition of androgenic activity. Administration of female sex hormones, for example stilboestrol in treatment of prostatic cancer, will

not surprisingly lead to increased breast development. Perhaps more surprising is that enough oestrogen may be absorbed from topical preparations to cause gynaecomastia[24, 25]. Some other drugs may have oestrogenic effects; well-known examples of this group are digitalis and marijuana.

Some drugs have antiandrogenic effects either as part of their intended therapeutic action, e.g. cyproterone used for prostatic cancer, or as an unwanted and unexpected effect as seen with cimetidine or spironolactone (Figure 16.3). Although it is usual to ascribe the cause to the drug administered, it is sometimes due to metabolites, e.g. it is tetrahydrocannibol rather than its parent that is responsible for marijuana-induced gynaecomastia. Conversely, the gynaecomastia of spironolactone, almost universal when used for treating hepatic ascites, may be avoided by administration of its active metabolite sodium canrenoate[26].

Assessment of Gynaecomastia

Clinical

In the majority of patients, history and examination will reveal the likely cause of the gynaecomastia. The age of onset, relation to drug ingestion and underlying ill health are the main pointers from the history. Examination of the liver, testes and chest as well as the gynaecomastia itself are clearly important.

Investigation

Investigation should be confined to liver function tests and a chest radiograph in the older patient, unless there is reason to think that there is an underlying endocrine abnormality, when more sophisticated investigations may be indicated.

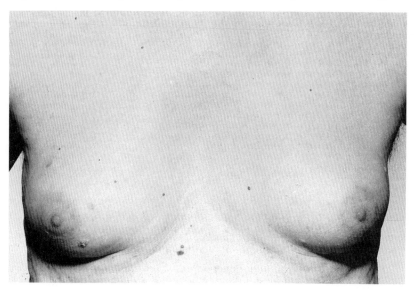

16.3 Bilateral gynaecomastia due to spironolactone therapy.

Table 16.2 Drugs associated with gynaecomastia.

Drug	Mechanism
Androgens	? Peripheral aromatization
Cyproterone Spironolactone	Antiandrogens
Digitalis Cannibis Griseofulvin	Bind to oestrogen receptors and oestrogenic activity
Phenothiazines Reserpine Tricyclics Cimetidine Methyldopa Isoniazid Metoclopramide	Disturbance of gonadotrophin control

After Hall et al[1].

Exclusion of Malignancy

In addition to clinical and endocrinological studies of male patients with breast disease, aspiration, cytology and radiology should be used to exclude malignant disease in the older patient. This is particularly important in the absence of a well-defined cause, in unilateral disease and when the palpable mass is eccentric instead of having the usual concentricity.

The role of mammography in the male breast has been reviewed by Dershaw[14]. Gynaecomastia appears as a flame-shaped opacity extending into the surrounding fat. It is possible to distinguish those patients on oestrogens when the breast takes on the appearance of the female. Cases of pseudo-gynaecomastia can be readily identified by the absence of breast tissue. Malignancy can usually be diagnosed by mammography.

Treatment

The management of gynaecomastia is governed by two premises. First, the majority are due to minor hormonal imbalances or to drugs and carry no serious significance. Secondly, a serious cause should be considered in each case and, in the older patient, breast cancer excluded. In the majority of cases reassurance that this is a benign self-limiting condition which is not premalignant will suffice. A minority of patients will require treatment either for tenderness or for cosmesis.

Treatment of Primary Gynaecomastia

For the minority of patients in whom firm reassurance proves inadequate a number of options are open.

Drug Therapy

A hormonal basis for gynaecomastia is widely accepted[20] so it is not surprising that attempts have been made to correct the putative abnormality. What is surprising is that no agent has been studied in a systematic manner. Testosterone has been reported to be of variable value but occasionally produces a dramatic effect[27]. Eberle et al[28] treated four pubertal patients with dihydrotestosterone heptanoate, which does not undergo peripheral aromatization, and claimed good results. The clinical improvement was associated with falls in circulating oestradiol, LH, FSH and free testosterone. There had been no return of symptoms during a follow-up period ranging between 5 and 15 months. Other drugs whose use has been reported are clomiphene[29,30] and tamoxifen[31,32] which act as anti-oestrogens, and danazol, an antigonadotrophin which has a weak androgenic effect. These reports are of a few patients only with a number of hetergeneous causes and the results are variable from one report to another. For example, Stephanas et al[29] reported that 18/19 patients responded to clomiphene 50 mg daily whereas Plourde et al[30] found a similar dose unsatisfactory in a group of 12 patients.

Tamoxifen 10 mg twice daily has been reported to be beneficial in both secondary[31,32] and primary gynaecomastia[33] but, as with clomiphene, small uncontrolled studies are reported. Parker et al[34] reported a cross-over study of 10 men between the ages of 54 and 80. Seven regressed, one of whom recurred after cessation of treatment. No patient responded to the placebo. Buckle[35] reported the results of danazol treatment in 42 patients: 25 had marked regression of the gynaecomastia and 10 moderate regression. The dosage used in adults was 100 mg three times daily increased to 200 mg three times daily if no response was seen, continued for between 4 and 6 months followed by maintenance at the lower dose for 4 months. In adolescents the dosage used was 100 mg twice daily. Side-effects were acceptable and no patient stopped treatment on account of these. The levels of testosterone fell during treatment as did the levels of gonadotrophins – oestrogen levels were not measured. Our own experience in 18 cases is that half of them obtain useful relief of symptoms. Tenderness disappears rapidly in those who are going to respond but there has been slower change in the patients whose main complaint is cosmetic. We have used varying doses between 100 mg and 200 mg three times daily with no definable side-effects. A typical course is 100 mg three times daily for 4 weeks then 100 mg twice daily for 8 weeks. Age of onset and duration of symptoms were not predictive of those who were going to respond. We have recently reviewed our own experience of danazol in 18 patients with a median age of onset of 21 years (range 12–54). It was unilateral in 11, painful in 14, focal in 5 and diffuse in 13. Seven patients had a complete response and three a partial response. Treatment failed in six patients and two failed to take the tablets. There were no side-effects. The time to response was 6–12 weeks, and there was no recurrence at a median follow-up of 8 months, extending to 18 months.

Surgery

When reassurance is inadequate, and drug treatment either inappropriate or unsatisfactory, surgical removal of the breast tissue is indicated. Although the operation is usually described as a subcutaneous mastectomy, it is important to leave a small area of subareolar breast tissue as overzealous resection will replace the cosmetic deformity of a swelling with one of a hollow. In obese patients particularly the cosmetic benefit may be marginal, and the patient should appreciate the difficulty in judging the right amount of tissue. Too much or too little removed from the obese is likely to leave a dissatisfied patient. In other cases, the gynaecomastia may merge with firm subcutaneous fat rather than form a localized protrusion (Figure 16.4) and these cases are also unlikely to get a satisfactory cosmetic result from surgery.

Details of the surgical procedure will be found in Chapter 18.

Radiotherapy
Prophylactic irradiation therapy of breast tissue to prevent the gynaecomastia which regularly accompanies the use of oestrogens in the management of prostatic cancer is now only of historical interest but does appear to have been effective[36].

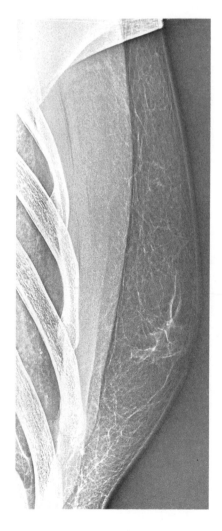

16.4 *Xerograph of juvenile gynaecomastia without local protrusion.*

Treatment of the Secondary Gynaecomastia

If a cause for the gynaecomastia is identified, it will resolve with treatment of the underlying abnormality or withdrawal of the offending drug. If, for some reason, the disease is not amenable to treatment or, if continuation of a drug is essential and treatment of gynaecomastia is still considered necessary, the plan for treatment of primary gynaecomastia may be followed with advantage. Three injections of nandrolone 25 mg at 3-week intervals have been recommended for gynaecomastia of the elderly, but we have no experience of this treatment and are not aware of any formal report in the literature.

Other Male Breast Disease

Any disease of the male breast is uncommon. However, most diseases of the breast that afflict women have also been reported in men from time to time. Not surprisingly lesions that have their origin in lobular tissue are excessively rare but may occur in XXY phenotypes and in patients with long-standing raised oestrogen levels.

It has been estimated that of all male breast lesions, 65% are gynaecomastia, 25% malignant neoplasms, leaving 10% for miscellaneous benign disease[5]. However, this autopsy study greatly underestimates the frequency of pubertal gynaecomastia.

Duct Ectasia

This is a rare clinical entity, but Sandison[5] in his postmortem study of 500 men found that 6% of the specimens had histological evidence of duct ectasia. Anderson and Gram[6,9] found 30 examples of ectatic ducts in 100 consecutive male autopsies but in only 7 of these was it diffuse. In none of these patients was there periductal inflammation; there were no clinical associations and they considered that the findings were different from duct ectasia of the female breast. Tedescki and McCarthy[37] described periductal mastitis in a male. Haagensen[38] describes a patient with nipple discharge which was attributed to androgens, although the description of the pathological findings in this case suggests that he had at least some degree of duct ectasia with periductal inflammation. The patient was clearly endocrinologically hypogonadal, following mumps orchitis at the age of four. We have seen a number of cases in the male, some of which have been previously reported[39]. The patients have shown all the features of the condition as seen in women with nipple inversion, nipple discharge, abscess and fistula formation (Figures 16.5 and 16.6). Treatment is by excision of the duct system as performed in postmenopausal women.

Epithelial Hyperplasia

Sandison[5] in his review of 500 postmortems in men records that 11 had significant epithelial hyperplasia, in 3 of whom it was associated with ectatic ducts. The clinical significance of this finding is uncertain. Sandison[5] also records that one of his subjects had a localized fibroadenoma – a surprising finding in view of the absence of lobular activity in the male. Anderson and Gram[9] found 7 cases of epithelial hyperplasia in their postmortem series. Presumably there is a carcinoma *in situ* phase preceding overt male breast carcinoma, but we are not aware of any description of this condition.

Nipple Discharge

Detraux *et al*[40] performed galactography in seven males with unilateral nipple discharge. The lesions causing discharge were two papillomas, two carcinomas, two cases of duct ectasia and one breast abscess.

Treves *et al*[41] collected 42 male patients with a serosanguineous discharge in 23 years and estimated that about 2% of male breast disease had nipple discharge as a symptom. Of their 42 cases 18 were found to have benign disease and in many cases the discharge had been present for several years. The underlying causes in these cases were duct papilloma or gynaecomastia, all instances of blood-stained nipple discharge occurring with papilloma.

Abscess

Inflammatory masses around the nipple occur in men and may be related to breast disease, especially periductal mastitis, but they more commonly represent retention cysts or infection in adjacent skin structures (Figure 16.7).

Adenoma of the Nipple

Azzopardi[8] mentions seven male patients with this condition in the world literature, and records a case of his own. It behaves identically to the same lesion in women.

Mondor's Disease

We have seen but one example of this condition (Figure 16.8)[42] although Oldfield[43] considers that at least a third of the cases occur in men.

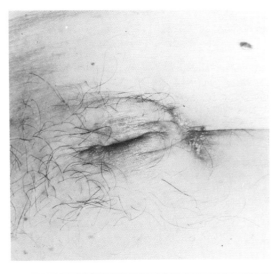

16.5 *Duct ectasia/ periductal mastitis in a male with transverse nipple retraction and a mammary duct fistula following drainage of several subareolar abscesses.*

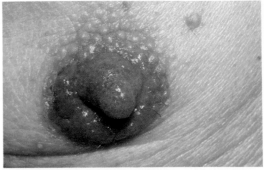

16.6 *A male patient with nipple discharge due to duct ectasia resulting in inflammation of the areolar skin.*

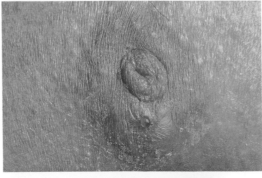

16.7 *Young male with discharge from a retention cyst of an areolar gland – treated by local excision.*

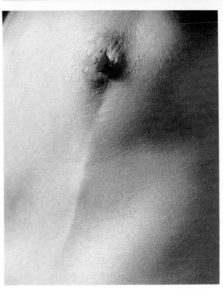

16.8 *A case of Mondor's disease in a male – the appearance is similar to that seen in women.*

REFERENCES

1. Hall R., Anderson J., Smart G. A. & Besser M. *Fundamentals of Clinical Endocrinology*. London, Pitman Medical, 1980.

2. Foot H. Remarks on gynaecomazia. *Dublin Quarterly Journal of Medical Sciences* 1866; **XLI**: 451–453.

3. Gruber F. Uber die gynaecomastie. *Memoires de l'academi du Science de St Petersburg* 7th series t 10, 1866.

4. Karsner H. T. Gynaecomastia. *American Journal of Pathology* 1946: **22**: 235–315.

5. Sandison A. T. *An Autopsy Study of the Human Breast*, Monograph No. 8, National Cancer Institute, US Dept Health, Education and Welfare, 1962.

6. Anderson J. A. & Gram J. B. Gynecomasty: Histological aspects in a surgical material. *Acta pathologica et microbiologica scandinavia* Section A: Pathologica 1982; **90**: 185–190.

7. Smith T. C. G. The breast and its disorders. *Practitioner* 1982; **226**: 1454–1455.

8. Azzopardi J. *Problems in Breast Pathology*. Philadelphia, W. B. Saunders, 1979, p 14.

9. Andersen J. A. & Gram J. B. Male breast at autopsy. *Acta pathologica et microbiologica scandinavia* Section A: Pathologica or Microbiologica immunologica 1982; **90**: 191–197.

10. Carlson H. E. Gynecomastia. *New England Journal of Medicine* 1980; **303**: 795–799.

11. Burke C. W. Gynaecomastia. *Practitioner* 1982; **226**: 1403–1410.

12. Nydick M., Bustos J., Dale J. H. & Rawson R. W. Gynaecomastia in adolescent boys. *Journal of the American Medical Association* 1961; **178**: 449–457.

13. Nuttall F. Q. Gynaecomastia as a physical finding in normal men. *Journal of Clinical Endocrinology and Metabolism* 1979; **48**: 338–340.

14. Dershaw D. D. Male mammography. *American Journal of Roentgenology* 1986; **146**: 127–131.

15. Kapdi C. C. & Parekh N. J. The male breast. *The Radiological Clinics of North America* 1983; **21**: 137–148.

16. Turkington R. W. Serum prolactin levels in patients with gynaecomastia. *Journal of Clinical Endocrinology and Metabolism* 1972; **34**: 62–66.

17. Moore D. C., Schlaepfer L. V., Paunier L. & Sizonenko P. C. Hormonal changes during puberty vs transient pubertal gynaecomastia and abnormal androgen estrogen ratios. *Journal of Clinical Endocrinology and Metabolism* 1984; **58**: 492–499.

18. Lee P. A. The relationship of concentrations of serum hormones to pubertal gynaecomastia. *Journal of Pediatrics* 1975; **86**: 212–215.

19. Pirke K. M. & Doerr P. Age related changes and interrelationships between plasma testosterone, oestradiol and testosterone-binding globulin in normal adult males. *Acta Endocrinologica* 1973; **74**: 792–800.

20. Wilson J. D., Aiman J. & MacDonald P. C. The pathogenesis of gynecomastia. *Advances in Internal Medicine* 1980; **25**: 1–32.

21. Cole E. W. Klinefelter syndrome and breast cancer. *Johns Hopkins Medical Journal* 1976; **125**: 25–43.

22. Gordon G. G., Olivo J., Rafii F. & Southren A. L. Conversion of androgens to estrogens in cirrhosis of the liver. *Journal of Clinical Endocrinology and Metabolism* 1975; **40** 1018–1026.

23. Jacobs E. C. Effects of starvation on sex hormones in the male. *Journal of Clinical Endocrinology* 1948; **8**: 227–232.

24. Gabrilove J. L. & Luria M. Persistent gynaecomastia resulting from scalp inunction of estradiol: A model for persistent gynecomastia. *Archives of Dermatology* 1978; **114**: 1672–1673.

25. Edidin D. V. & Levitsky L. L. Prepubertal gynecomastia associated with estrogen containing hair cream. *American Journal of Diseases in Children* 1982; **136**: 587–588.

26. Bellati G. & Ideo G. Gynaecomastia after spironolactone and potassium canrenoate. *Lancet* 1986; **i**: 626.

27. Myhre S. A., Ruvalcaba R. H. A., Johnson H. R., Thuline H. C. & Kelley V. C. The effects of testosterone treatment in Klinefelter's syndrome. *Journal of Pediatrics* 1970; **76**: 267–276.

28. Eberle A. J., Sparrow J. T. & Keenan B. S. Treatment of persistent pubertal gynaecomastia with dihydrotestosterone heptanoate. *Journal of Pediatrics* 1986; **109**: 144–149.

29. Stephanas A. V., Burnet R. B., Harding P. E. & Wise P. H. Clomiphene in the treatment of pubertal adolescent gynaecomastia: a preliminary report. *Journal of Pediatrics* 1977; **90**: 651–653.

30. Plourde P. V., Kulin H. E. & Santner S. J. Clomiphene in the treatment of adolescent gynecomastia. *American Journal of Diseases of Children* 1983; **137**: 1080–1082.

31. Fusco F. D. & Rosen S. W. Gonadotropin-producing anaplastic large-cell carcinomas of the lung. *New England Journal of Medicine* 1966; **275**: 507–515.

32. Jeffreys D. B. Painful gynaecomastia treated with tamoxifen. *British Medical Journal* 1979; **i**: 1119–1120.

33. Hooper P. D. Puberty gynaecomastia. *Journal of the Royal College of General Practitioners* 1985; **35**: 142.

34. Parker L. N. Gray D. R., Lai M. K. & Levin E. R. Treatment of gynecomastia with tamoxifen: A double blind cross-over study. *Metabolism* 1986; **35**: 705–708.

35. Buckle R. Danazol therapy in gynaecomastia; recent experience and indications for therapy. *Postgraduate Medical Journal* 1979; **55**(suppl 5): 71–78.

36. Malis I., Cooper J. F. & Wolever T. H. S. Breast radiation in patients with carcinoma of the prostate. *Journal of Urology* 1969; **102**: 336–340.

37. Tedeschi L. G. & McCarthy P. E. Involutional mammary duct ectasia and periductal mastitis in a male. *Human Pathology* 1974; **5**: 232–236.

38. Haagensen C. D. *Diseases of the Breast*. Philadelphia, WB Saunders, 1986.

39. Mansel R. E. & Morgan W. P. Duct ectasia in the male. *British Journal of Surgery* 1979; **66**: 660–662.

40. Detraux P., Benmussa M., Tristant H. & Garel L. Breast disease in the male: galactographic evaluation. *Radiology* 1985; **154**: 605–606.

41. Treves N., Robbins G. F. & Amoroso W. L. Serous and serosanguineous discharge from the male nipple. *Archives of Surgery* 1956; **90**: 319–329.

42. Bahal V. & Mansel R. E. Mondor's disease secondary to breast abscess in a male. *British Journal of Surgery* 1986; **73**: 931.

43. Oldfield M. C. Mondor's disease. A superficial thrombophlebitis of the breast. *Lancet* 1962; **i**: 994–996.

17 Miscellaneous Conditions

This chapter brings together a number of conditions which do not conveniently fit elsewhere. They may be classified either as true breast disease or as local manifestations of systemic disease. Their main importance lies in their presentation which often clinically mimics carcinoma. When the breast lesion occurs as part of a widespread process, diagnosis is usually straightforward; when the breast is the first or dominant site of symptoms, diagnosis is less easy. In the past, many such diagnoses have only been made on histological sectioning of the mastectomy specimen; the more rational approach to breast disease that now appertains means the diagnosis should be made before such a tragedy occurs.

Apart from glandular breast tissue and its supporting fibrous stroma blood vessels, nerves, fat and lymphatics may be the primary source of the problem.

Trauma

The breast is relatively infrequently damaged in trauma. Burns of the chest wall are not uncommon in children, usually as a result of scalds. The resulting scars are unsightly and, if the nipple is involved, there may be problems with breast-feeding. Partial thickness burns may be disturbing but are otherwise of little importance. Full thickness burns may lead to failure of development. If the scarring is severe, plastic surgery may play a useful role in management[1], and pressure garments may help to minimize scarring.

In adult life blunt trauma is the most usual form. Even a clear history of injury, such as that obtained in car accidents, with bruising does not exclude the possibility of an underlying carcinoma[2]. The introduction of seat belt legislation has led to a number of reports of breast injury due to seat belts, sometimes sufficient to cause complete disruption of the breast[3]. The typical injury in a severe case is a furrowed deformity in the line of the seat belt. This may be masked initially by haematoma and soft tissue oedema, but as this resolves the defect in the breast may be seen and palpated. The architectural disturbance may be revealed on mammography. In less severe cases, the clinical features of fat necrosis are evident – but beware, the accident may only have served to draw attention to a pre-existing carcinoma.

Fat Necrosis

The most common sequel to trauma that gives rise to clinical problems is fat necrosis. This is one of those uncommon lesions which is perversely known to all medical students as a condition which simulates cancer. In spite of the universal teaching that fat necrosis may simulate cancer, procrastination with cancer still occurs because doctors accept a history of trauma from the patient and accept the possibility of a condition so familiar to them.

It would be better if the condition were unknown, for it is sufficiently rare in its classic form that no-one would be disadvantaged if the condition were unrecognized. Breast cancer is 40 times more common in Haagensen's experience[4]. We would put the figures even higher. The situation would have been very different in 1920 when Lee and Adair[5] first reported it, for radical mastectomy was then commonly performed on clinical appearance alone. Sandison[6] found evidence of fat necrosis in only 2 of his 800 autopsies.

Clinical Features

It is not widely recognized that there are two quite distinct forms of fat necrosis: one simulates cancer, the other simulates simple cysts, unusual because of the added symptom of a dull aching pain.

The first form is common in elderly patients – perhaps because they injure themselves more frequently and the involuted breast tissue is less able to absorb a sudden blow.

The diagnosis is aided by the presence of skin ecchymosis or reddening, although this is not always present. The actual lump is usually small and attached to surrounding tissue. Later a more florid, inflammatory picture may produce skin fixity and oedema, resembling both cancer and the chronic form of periductal mastitis. Mammography in this group may show features consistent with carcinoma. In these cases, section shows a small cavity with thick necrotic material and often white fat necrosis on the edge of the cavity. Other cases merge into a picture of haematoma with some fat necrosis around the edge. The pathology is that of a chronic inflammatory reaction with marked histiocytic reaction and peripheral fibrosis which increases with time.

The second type has been seen in our experience in younger women in their forties who represent with tender swellings after quite severe trauma such as a car accident. Nothing is noted on inspection, but palpation reveals one or more tender cystic structures which feel just like ordinary cysts but with a sensation of slight thickening around the wall. Mammography shows striking cystic translucent areas (Figure 17.1).

The diagnosis of the first type cannot be made safely without biopsy for we have seen several cases where fat necrosis and cancer have been adjacent to each other. Mammography and cytology may both be helpful but needle biopsy is mandatory. Excision will be neccessary where necrotic material is present. Because the necrosis is usually sterile, the wound may be closed primarily with suction drainage but in case of any doubt the surgeon need have no hesitancy in packing the wound and allowing it to granulate. The technique of managing the granulating wound with Silastic foam dressings is particularly satisfactory allowing rapid painless and convenient convalescence.

The second type is readily diagnosed by mammography and cured by aspiration removing clear oily fluid.

Paraffinoma

Contemporary reconstructive procedures are relatively safe and any problems are outlined in Chapter 15. Earlier attempts at augmentation using injections of silicone and paraffin had disastrous results with chronic discharging lesions which may appear at sites remote from the

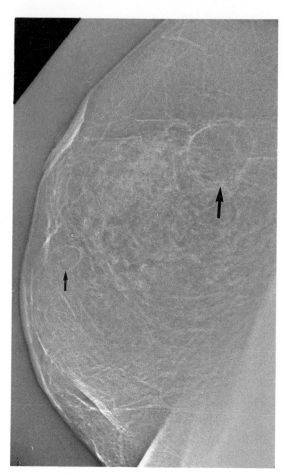

17.1 *A mammogram showing oily cysts following traumatic fat necrosis.*

breast[7,8]. The diagnosis is not always immediately apparent because intervals of up to 35 years may occur between the injection and re-presentation[7]. Alagaratnam and Ong[7] recognized two modes of presentation: painless hard mass clinically resembling cancer and hard masses with ulceration or sinus formation usually associated with lymphadenopathy. A further aid to diagnosis is the mammographic finding of a characteristic honeycomb appearance.

In the first group, treatment is by local excision without entering the paraffin, which is found to have remained liquid and which, if spilt, will lead to recurrence of the problem. The cosmetic deformity may be considerable but is preferable to a simple mastectomy. When the skin ulceration is extensive, simple mastectomy may become necessary although, in less severe cases, excision of the secondarily infected mass may be sufficient. Migratory masses should be removed in continuity with the breast mass. Some patients will request further reconstructive surgery. Those who have experience of this problem advise that reconstruction should be delayed until it is clear that the original problem will not recur.

Radiation Damage

Radiotherapy is often used in the management of malignant breast disease. Most ulcerating lesions that subsequently occur will prove to be due to recurrent disease, but this requires histological confirmation because some of these will be radionecrosis. The patient has usually had radical surgery and radiotherapy often some years previously. The presentation is of a clinically discharging ulcer most frequently on the medial half of the chest wall (Figure 17.2). Examination will usually reveal necrotic underlying costal cartilage. Occasionally, severe bleeding will occur from the internal mammary artery. The only satisfactory treatment is surgical with debridement of the ulcer and removal of the underlying necrotic costal cartilage. It is impracticable to excise the whole of the irradiated area, so skin and subcutaneous tissue need only to be excised until good bleeding is seen. Because of their poor blood supply, the whole of the involved (and infected) costal cartilage will need to be removed. The underlying pleura is usually markedly thickened and the pathology lends itself to excisional surgery and reconstruction[9]. The defect may be covered by a variety of means but, if available, a latissimus dorsi myocutaneous flap will provide not only skin cover but an excellent new blood supply to facilitate healing.

Lipoma

It is not surprising that lipomas are sometimes found in the breast. Haagensen[4] describes a series of 186 patients with a mean age of 45. The clinical features are those of lipoma – a smooth, slightly lobulated mobile mass. Their main importance lies in distinguishing them from a clinical variant of carcinoma: the pseudolipoma. This condition is produced by shortening of Cooper's ligaments as a carcinoma infiltrates. The intervening fat lobules are compressed and 'bunched up', so that they take on a lobulated form as seen in lipoma, at the same time concealing the small underlying cancer. As lipomas occur in the cancer age group they require careful evaluation to exclude this possibility. The mammographic features are typical producing a circumscribed translucent area compressing the surrounding structures. If there is any doubt about the diagnosis, the lesion is better removed.

Adenolipoma (Hamartoma)

Haagensen[4] and Azzopardi[10] both regard this as a variant of lipoma which has incorporated epithelial elements. These tend to occur at a younger age group than lipomas which they clinically resemble. Mammographically, however, they have a typical appearance of a smooth mass with a fat halo[11]. At operation they appear well encapsulated although no capsule is found on histology (Figure 17.3). The epithelial elements may contain a whole spectrum of patterns of ductal and lobular involution.

An alternative view is to regard this lesion as a hamartoma. A review of the literature of hamartomas and adenolipomas leaves no real doubt that this is a single condition masquerading as two entities. Arrigoni et al[12] have presented a convincing case for regarding this lesion as hamartoma. This condition is probably more common than is generally recognized.

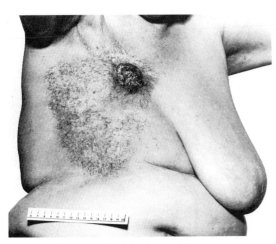

17.2 *Radiation necrosis of the chest wall. There is no recurrent tumour in this case, in spite of the malignant appearance of the ulcer.*

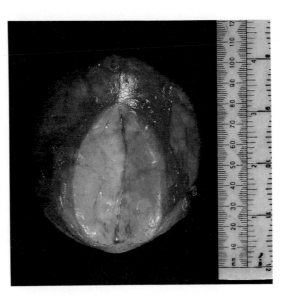

17.3 *Fibroadenolipoma of the breast.*

Mondor's Disease

Superficial thrombophlebitis over an area of the breast was described several times before Mondor's paper in 1939[13]; the earliest appears to be in 1869, but his name is now firmly attached to the condition[14]. It is one of those rather rare conditions that every doctor has heard about as a medical student, and this carries two risks. The rarity of the condition may lead to unnecessary biopsy to avoid missing cancer or in the desire to recognize a condition long known about but never encountered; alternatively an atypical cancer may be described as Mondor's disease: the latter is much the more serious error, for cancer is common but Mondor's disease is rare.

Clinical Features

Females are affected considerably more commonly than males. The patient develops a dull aching pain over the breast or hypochondrium and notices a tender elongated mass in the region (Figure 17.4). Palpation reveals a tender narrow cord just below the skin. This is the thrombosed vein attached to the skin so that elevation of the arm produces a narrow furrow over the vein, accentuated by traction from either end. The furrow is more obvious over the breast. It contracts to a hamstring if the thrombosed vein extends across the submammary fold to the epigastrium. The vein usually affected is the thoraco-epigastric vein which runs from the hypochondrium up across the lateral aspect of the breast to the anterior axillary fold. As with spontaneous thrombophlebitis elsewhere, any vein may be affected – less rare examples are a vein from the epigastrium over the lower medial quadrant of the breast and one extending vertically down from the nipple.

The thrombophlebitis follows a similar pattern to that elsewhere. The pain settles over 10 days or so, a process accentuated by rest. The tender

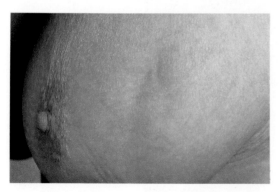

17.4 *Mondor's disease, with skin retraction simulating dimpling due to cancer.*

cord resolves more slowly taking from 2 to 12 weeks until finally no evidence remains of the lesion.

An important variant is when a short segment of vein is affected giving local dimpling which may suggest a cancer. Of greater importance is the fact that a wedge-shaped area of ductal cancer may suggest the diagnosis of Mondor's disease to an inexperienced observer.

Pathology and Pathogenesis

The pathology has been illustrated by Hughes[15]. It shows the typical stages of thrombophlebitis – a thrombosed thickened area with surrounding thrombosis.

Many cases appear to be spontaneous, a situation analogous to thrombophlebitis elsewhere. A variety of aetiological factors have been described. Unusual exercise usually involving the arms above the head is commonest. Operative trauma is well recognized – the condition developing distal to the scar 2 or 3 weeks after biopsy of a benign condition. Direct trauma is of greater importance in males[16].

Treatment

Provided the clinician is familiar with the condition and the clinical features are classic, the patient may be treated conservatively. If there is the slightest doubt, mammography should be performed.

The condition will resolve spontaneously without treatment, but symptomatic relief can be obtained with general measures appropriate to the management of thrombophlebitis – rest to the arm and support for the breast. Simple analgesics are inadequate; phenylbutazone is effective. Anticoagulants are not necessary.

Some authors have recommended introducing active approaches to management. Abramson[17] recommended disruption of the cord by forcible distraction from the ends. Millar[18] divided the cords under local anaesthesia and found symptoms relieved immediately. We have no experience of such methods but they are worth consideration in particularly painful cases.

Oedema of the Breast

The breast may become oedematous due to heart failure and inanition. The changes in the skin of the breast are those of *peau d'orange* which may progress to ulceration so a provisional diagnosis of carcinoma is made even though no mass is palpable. General examination usually reveals evidence of generalized oedema due to either heart failure[19] or the nephrotic syndrome[20]. The so-called nursing home breast represents another variant of this problem[21].

We have seen a case in which the cardiac failure went unrecognized, a clinical diagnosis of carcinoma was made and the patient treated with tamoxifen in spite of negative biopsies. Mammography revealed skin oedema but no focal lesion. The clinical and radiographic signs of malignancy resolved upon appropriate treatment of her heart failure.

Fibrous Disease of the Breast

This is a rarely recognized clinical entity without a clear pathological basis. In this way it resembles painful nodularity and indeed parallels this condition in a number of ways. It is a reflection of normal physiological processes proceeding to excess, in this case, the involutional replacement of lobules by dense fibrous tissue (*see* Chapters 1 and 3). This proceeds to an excessive degree in one area of the breast, presenting clinically as a mass, yet the pathological changes are no different to those occurring during involution in a clinically inconsequential breast.

The clearest description is that of Haagensen[4] and we have a small parallel experience of this as a clinical entity. It is uncommon – in Haagensen's experience, 1 case for every 10 carcinomas. We recognize it considerably less commonly. All but a few of Haagensen's patients were premenopausal although ranging in age from 24 to 72 (average 42). Our experience is mainly of patients in the fifth and sixth decades. It is difficult to explain its occurrence in the young patients, yet involutional changes can commence quite early in the breast and one can only speculate that such changes occur earlier than usual in a particular part of the breast – perhaps a further putative example of local end-organ failure to respond to hormonal stimulation, which may ultimately prove to be the cause of much obscure breast disease.

It presents as a painless, well-defined mass but without a clear edge – it merges into surrounding breast tissue. It is usually in the upper, outer quadrant and firm rather than hard. This consistency (there is no suggestion of cragginess at all) does not raise an expectation of cancer in an experienced examiner. The modest degree of fixity to the breast tissue and the absence of skin retraction also help in the differentiation. Aspiration is possible, but an attempt at Trucut needle biopsy produces a characteristic result – bending of the cutting obturator. If resected, the tissue is dense white with an abnormally tough consistency; in fact, exactly the finding in involutional nodularity but to a more marked degree. Like this condition, it is diffuse, merging gradually with surrounding breast tissue. Hence, excision, if carried out, must be based on preoperative palpatory assessment of the extent of the disease and not on the macroscopic appearance of the breast tissue. Ignoring this will lead to a subcutaneous mastectomy.

The clinical management of this condition raises a problem, for clearly it is best if excision can be avoided. Our approach is to leave the condition if mammography convincingly excludes malignancy, as is often the case in the older patient. Where malignancy cannot be excluded, biopsy must be carried out, and the decision between incisional and excisional biopsy is made according to individual circumstances.

Fibromatosis (Desmoid Tumour)

Fibromatosis of the breast needs to be considered in the differential diagnosis of fibrous disease. Rosen et al[22] collected 15 cases. The condition is analogous to desmoid tumour of the abdominal wall and, like that condition, can be seen in association with colonic polyps in cases of Gardner's syndrome. The disease process is much more extensive than in fibrous disease and fixes the breast to underlying tissues, such as the pectoral muscle. The radiographic appearances have been described[23].

A recent useful publication is that of Wargotz et al[24]. They describe the clinical and pathological findings of 28 examples of fibromatosis of the breast not involving the deep fascia or chest wall. Five of the 20 lesions treated by local excision recurred, usually within a few months but in one case after 6 years. The lesions which recurred had been inadequately excised initially because surgical margins showed fibromatosis. Histological features such as cellularity, atypia and mitotic figures did not help in predicting recurrence. Wide local excision appeared to have been adequate in the majority of patients, stressing the importance of documentation of free tissue margins.

Diabetes

Two groups[25,26] have described a variant of fibrosis in the breast which appears to be confined to young women with juvenile-onset, insulin-dependent diabetes. Most, but not all, of the patients had other complications of diabetes, most commonly retinopathy. The patients had had the initial diagnosis at least 6 years before presenting with a discrete lump which required assessment to exclude malignancy. Byrd et al[26] reported eight such patients who presented with a firm to hard discrete nodule suggestive of cancer, with mammographic changes in some consistent with cancer. One patient had three biopsies for the same condition over 13 years. The pathological changes described were of dense fibrotic tissue with an irregular perivascular lymphatic infiltrate and lymphocytic vasculitis – changes similar to the microangiopathy seen in diabetic retinopathy.

Sarcoid

Sarcoid is rarely recorded in the breast. Haagensen[4] documents three cases from the literature, two from the UK and one from Denmark, and mentions two further cases, one his own and another from Australia. The most recent reviews bring the number of reported cases of sarcoid of the breast to 14[27,28]. In all but two of the cases, there was evidence of systemic sarcoid at the time of diagnosis; in one the diagnosis became apparent 5 years later; in the other no further disease has yet appeared so that this may be an example of non-specific granulomatous mastitis[28].

Amyloid

Amyloid deposits, mimicking the clinical presentation of cancer have been recorded on several occasions[29-32]. The cases usually present with a lump clinically and mammographically diagnosed as a carcinoma. Extensive amyloid deposits are usually found elsewhere and usually antedate the breast lesion. A case of amyloid of the nipple which presented with pruritis has also been reported[33].

Granular Cell Myoblastoma

This is a rare condition of the breast and most reported cases have occurred in the overlying skin. Clinically, lesions of the breast parenchyma present as tumours and may be fixed to pectoral fascia so that a diagnosis of malignancy is made in spite of the young age of many of the patients[10]. Azzopardi[10] reviewed the literature to 1979; McCracken et al[34] have added two cases to the literature since then. The histological features are similar to those occurring in skin and elsewhere.

They are benign and only require local excision. It is considered most likely that myoblastoma is of Schwann cell origin.

Vasculitis

It is not surprising that multifocal arteritis should occasionally afflict the breast; it is perhaps surprising that it seems to be such a rare occurrence. The clinical manifestations mimic carcinoma – a particular problem if the breast is the first site of disease to present. Giant cell arteritis[35], polyarteritis nodosa[36] and Wegener's granulomatosis[37] have all be reported, but even together there are less than 20 cases reported in the literature.

Aneurysm of the Breast

A single case of an aneurysm of a vessel within the breast has been reported[38]. The diagnosis was made by auscultation and confirmed by Doppler flowmetry of the lump. It was successfully treated by local excision.

Infarction

The breast may occasionally undergo infarction – an event first described in 1894[39]. The best review of this subject is that of Robitaille et al[40] who divide such events into those that mimic carcinoma and those that do not. Infarction of fibroademona has been previously described in Chapter 7, and infarction of duct papilloma in Chapter 12.

Spontaneous mammary infarction is a rare event usually occurring in lactating women. The clinical finding is of a tender nodule in the breast rather suspicious of lactational cancer – a diagnosis which may be apparently confirmed on frozen section[10].

Haemorrhagic Necrosis Complicating Anticoagulant Therapy and Spontaneous Haematoma

Since the first report by Flood et al[41] in 1943, there has been a steady flow of papers reporting single cases of this syndrome. It may occur with any anticoagulant[10]. The sequence of events is obscure. It seems likely to start as a spontaneous haematoma but the final picture is of aseptic ischaemic necrosis. Treatment is by debridement of the affected tissue; if the subsequent cosmetic defect is severe, secondary plastic surgery may be indicated, if the underlying condition permits.

Spontaneous haematoma is also sometimes seen (Figure 17.5). Although concealed trauma or factitial disease cannot be excluded with certainty, there is no reason to question the patient's claim that it has appeared spontaneously. Our cases have been followed by slow but uneventful resolution. Mammography is always performed to exclude an underlying carcinoma.

Non-specific Granulomatous Disease

Keisler and Wolloch[42] described a granulomatous condition of the breast that did not appear to be related to an infective process or to other systemic granulomatous diseases. Fletcher et al[43] described a further seven cases and described the typical histology (discrete granulomata occurring in the lobules) and clinical features – a painful extra-areolar swelling of young parous women with the most recent pregnancy within the previous 6 years. Fletcher et al[43] speculated on the possible aetiology of this syndrome, which they regard as an immunological reaction analogous to granulomatous thyroiditis – this appears to be the most attractive theory.

Going et al[44] have recently reviewed a further nine cases, with similar clinical features to the previous two papers. These are similar to the case illustrated earlier in Chapter 11 of this book. Going et al[44] agree that there is overlap with duct ectasia/periductal complex but consider it to be a specific condition – especially because of its tendency to persist or recur. This may be because of inadequate treatment, so we believe that local excision should be combined with major duct excision. They suggest a trial of steroid therapy.

Collagenous Spherulosis of the Breast[45]

This is a histological finding in breast biopsies with intraluminal clusters of esinophilic spherules within areas of benign epithelial hyperplasia. The condition is mainly of interest to histopathologists, because it may lead to a mistaken diagnosis of malignancy. The histological details are given in the above paper.

Benign Disorders of the Breast in Non-Western Populations

Reports of benign breast conditions seen among non-European races, such as Indians, Chinese and Africans, suggest that there are basic differences in the spectrum of disease seen in these countries. The commonest condition of the breast appears to be fibroadenoma. This is not only much commoner than carcinoma but occurs in large numbers in young girls, is frequently of large size and also multiple and bilateral. There appears to be a corresponding decrease in the proportion of presentation due to disorders of involution such as cysts and cyclical nodularity, but this may reflect cultural differences and limitation of medical services. A recent paper[46] gives a survey of breast disease in Nigeria and reviews publications from other non-European populations.

Artefactual Disease of the Breast

Artefactual or factitial disorders are ones which are created by the patient often through complicated and repetitive actions. All reviews in the literature refer only to hospitalized patients – it is impossible for us to estimate the number of patients who have artefactual illnesses who are never suspected or who are treated as outpatients. Such disorders involving the female breast have only rarely been reported even though recognized by Hippocrates: 'It is a sign of madness when blood congeals on a woman's nipples'[47]. Sampson[48] described a case of dermatitis artefacta in

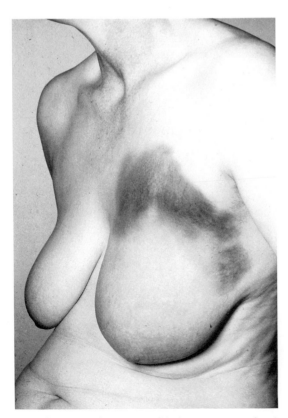

17.5 *Spontaneous haematoma of the breast – no cause found.*

which the woman had her left nipple excised for intermittent profuse bleeding. One month later she had a large tender hard mass above the incision which was found to be a pocket containing multiple small stones, gravel and sand. General reviews of dermatitis artefacta sometimes include cases affecting the nipple[49-51]. We have reported three patients with this condition[52]. One complained of intermittent bleeding from her right nipple which eventually led to simple mastectomy. She was then referred to us because of bleeding which soon started from the opposite breast (Figure 17.6). A second case was one of persistent eczema of the nipple and a third was a woman who had recurrent breast abscesses resistant to all the standard methods of treatment for duct ectasia and periductal mastitis (Figure 17.7). The organisms grown were faecal in nature suggesting deliberate infection. After a number of years a period in hospital with occlusion of the breast led to healing only to be followed after discharge by a similar problem appearing on the opposite side.

Such patients have usually had many investigations and operations before the nature of the underlying mechanism is recognized. Even so, establishing the diagnosis may be difficult and time consuming. Although the self-induced nature of the problem may be suspected, it is usually difficult to prove. The disorders may extend over a long period of time, may be recurrent and may result in long-term disability or cosmetic problems from tissue destruction; they are occasionally life threatening. The patients are usually young to middle-aged women, often in medically related jobs[50]. The patients are often pleasant and co-operative and do not appear to be bizarre or psychologically disturbed, but they tend to be

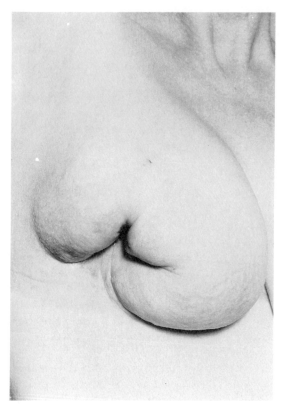

17.7 *Artefactual disease: this patient had multiple operations at many hospitals throughout the country for recurrent persistent sepsis in the right breast. Typical bowel organisms were grown from the discharge.*

immature and do have problems with their sexuality. A husband who appears to be unusually concerned may hide underlying marital stress but this is hardly specific to artefactual disease. Sometimes, as in two of our cases, patients will actively and without appropriate affect seek mastectomy – this should alert the clinician to the possibility of artefactual disease. The diagnosis is difficult to establish but artefactual disease should be considered where the clinical situation does not

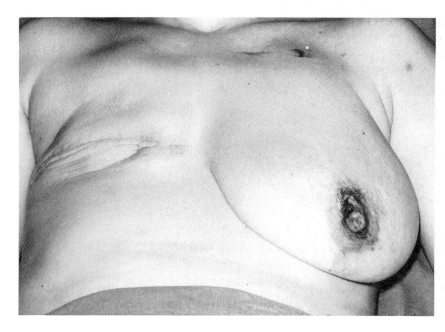

17.6 *Artefactual disease: the patient had multiple operations on the right breast for recurrent severe bleeding from the right nipple, culminating in a simple mastectomy. The condition promptly occurred on the left side and has all the hallmarks of artefactual injury.*

conform to common appearances or pathological processes. Unusual infections need to be considered such as tuberculosis, fungal infection or chronic subareolar abscess. A number of cases where self-injury has been suspected have cleared satisfactorily when appropriate attention was paid to this latter diagnosis.

It is difficult to give specific recommendations regarding treatment. Psychiatric consultation is often helpful in elucidating a personality disorder consistent with a diagnosis of artefactual breast disease. Direct confrontation of the patient is probably not worth while but may be considered in association with psychiatric help. These problems are difficult to manage and may extend over a long period of time. They tend to resolve if the patient is strongly reassured and attention withdrawn. Unnecessary and repetitive surgery must be avoided.

Mammalithiasis

In his postmortem series, Sandison[6] noted four examples (0.5%) of laminated concretions in the breast which were either intramammary or intraductal. The nature of this rare condition is obscure – we have not seen an example.

Hidradenitis Suppurativa of the Breast

Aprocrine sweat glands are found predominantly in the axilla and inguinoperineal regions but are described in a number of other sites. In relation to the breast, they are described in the areola and in the chest wall, particularly in the inter- and inframammary folds[53]. Hidradenitis has been described as involving the breast – in most series only one or two cases, but in a series from the Mayo Clinic, it was reported in 8% of 177 women with the disease[54]. We have not been able to find a paper which details the site of the disease, but most papers suggest it is the areola. Our experience is different. We have seen it mainly in the inter- and inframammary folds, usually in obese patients. In an experience of over 150 patients requiring surgery for hidradenitis, and many more with mild disease, we have not seen a single case involving the areola. We suspect that the reported cases reflect misdiagnosis of recurrent subareolar abscesses (Chapter 11) because these reports arose at a time when this condition was not widely recognized.

Patients with extensive hidradenitis elsewhere will sometimes have an individual or a few lesions scattered on the lower part of the breast (Figure 17.8). However, we have now seen five patients

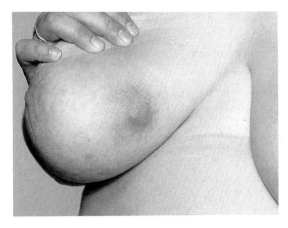

17.8 *Localized lesion of hidradenitis suppurativa of the breast, in a patient with the disease elsewhere.*

with severe and extensive disease in the inter- and inframammary folds. These patients often have scattered lesions on the lower half of the breast, although it is sometimes difficult to differentiate these from cystic acne – the two conditions frequently coexist. The distribution of the true hidradenitis lesion suggests that pressure is an aetiological factor. The worst lesions are seen under the strap of the brassière and on the skin surfaces where the undersurface of the breast and the chest wall are in contact and rub together.

Treatment is unsatisfactory, in contrast to surgical excision of hidradenitis in other sites[55]. We recommend conservative excision for local areas of disease, recognizing that recurrence is very likely (Figure 17.9). Local recurence has been seen in 50% of our cases, even after radical excision (Figure 17.10). Even though wounds such as this will granulate to give a very satisfactory linear scar (Figure 17.11), local recurrence is usual (Figure 17.12). Some patients with recurrent disease benefit from conservative therapy with an anti-androgen/oestrogen combination, such as cyproterone acetate and ethinyloestradiol, as used for severe acne. There are no reports as yet of properly controlled trials in hidradenitis with adequate follow-up. In our experience, about half the patients benefit but are more likely to do so if they have mild disease, or the worst affected areas are first excised surgically.

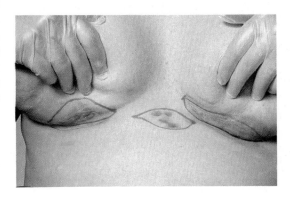

17.9 *Local clusters of lesions are best treated by local excision, followed by conservative therapy for recurrence.*

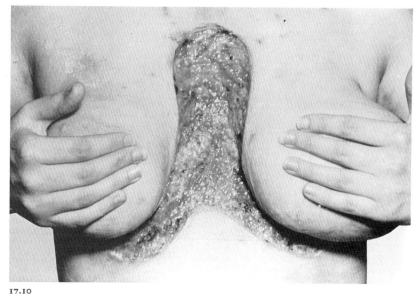

17.10

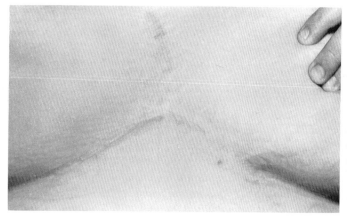

17.11

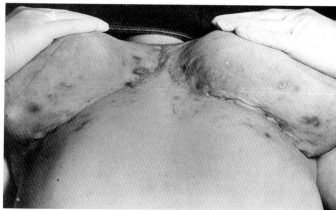

17.12

17.10 *Radical excision of extensive hidradenitis of the inter- and inframammary fold.*

17.11 *The wound was allowed to heal by granulation and gave a satisfactory scar.*

17.12 *Same patient as Figure 17.11. Within 2 years there were multiple recurrent lesions of hidradenitis.*

REFERENCES

1. Neale H. W., Smith G. L., Gregory R. O. & McMillan B. G. Breast reconstruction in the burned adolescent female. An 11 year, 157 patient experience. *Plastic and Reconstructive Surgery* 1982; **70**: 718.
2. Dawes R. F. H., Smallwood J. A. & Taylor I. Seat belt injury to the female breast. *British Journal of Surgery* 1986; **73**: 106–107.
3. Eastwood D. S. Subcutaneous rupture of the breast: a seat belt injury. *British Journal of Surgery* 1972; **59**: 491–492.
4. Haagensen C. D. *Disease of the Breast*, 3rd edn. Philadephia, W. B. Saunders, 1986.
5. Lee B. J. & Adair F. E. Traumatic fat necrosis of the female breast and its differentiation from carcinoma. *Annals of Surgery* 1920; **37**: 189.
6. Sandison A. T. An autopsy study of the adult human breast. *National Cancer Institute Monograph 8*, US Dept Health, Education and Welfare, 1962.
7. Alagaratnam T. T. & Ong G. B. Paraffinoma of the breast. *Journal of the Royal College of Surgeons of Edinburgh* 1983; **28**: 260–263.
8. Raven R. W. Paraffinoma of the breast. *Clinical Oncology* 1981; **7**: 157–161.
9. Hughes L. E. Repair of the chest wall defects after irradiation for breast cancer. *Annals of the Royal College of Surgeons (England)* 1976; **58**: 140–143.
10. Azzopardi J. *Problems in Breast Pathology*. London, W. B. Saunders, 1979.
11. Crothers J. G., Butler N. F., Fortt R. W. & Gravelle I. H. Fibroadenolipoma of the breast. *British Journal of Radiology* 1985; **58**: 191–202.
12. Arrigoni M. G., Docherty M. B. & Judd E. S. The identification and treatment of mammary hamartoma. *Surgery, Gynecology and Obstetrics* 1971; **133**: 577–582.
13. Mondor H. Tronculite Sous-cutanée subaigue de la paroi thoracique antero-laterale. *Memoires Academies de Chirurgie* 1939; **65**: 1271.
14. Thomford N. R. & Holadya W. J. Mondor's disease (phlebitis of the thoraco epigastric vein). *Annals of Surgery* 1969; **170**: 1035–1037.
15. Hughes E. S. R. Sclerosing peri-angiitis of the lateral thoracic wall. *Australia and New Zealand Journal of Surgery* 1952; **22**: 17–24.
16. Oldfield M. C. Mondor's disease. A superficial phlebitis of the breast. *Lancet* 1962; **i**: 994–996.
17. Abramson D. J. Mondor's disease and string phlebitis. *Journal of the American Medical Association* 1966; **196**: 1087.
18. Millar D. M. Treatment of Mondor's disease. *British Journal of Surgery* 1967; **54**: 76–77.

19. McElligott G. & Harrington M. G. Heart failure and breast enlargement suggesting cancer. *British Medical Journal* 1986; **292**: 446.

20. Muller J. W. T. & Koehler P. R. Cardiac failure simulating inflammatory cancer of the breast. *Fortschrift beb Rontgenstr Nuklearmedizin, Erganzeousband* 1984; **140**: 441–444.

21. Kaufman S. A. Nursing home breast. *Archives of Surgery* 1984; **119**: 615.

22. Rosen Y., Papasozomenos S. & Gardner B., Fibromatosis of the breast. *Cancer* 1978; **41**: 1409–1413.

23. Hermann G. & Schwartz I. S. Focal fibrous disease of the breast: Mammographic detection of an unappreciated condition. *American Journal of Roentgenology* 1983; **140**: 1245–1246.

24. Wargotz E. S. M., Norris H. J., Austin R. M. & Enzinger F. M. Fibromatosis of the breast. A clinical and pathological study of 28 cases. *American Journal of surgical Pathology* 1987; **11**: 38–45.

25. Soler N. G. & Khardori R. Fibrous disease of the breast, thyroiditis, and cheiro arthropathy in type I diabetes mellitus. *Lancet* 1984; **i**: 193–194.

26. Byrd B. F., Hartmann W. H., Graham L. S. & Hogle H. H. Mastopathy in insulin dependent diabetes. *Annals of Surgery* 1987; **205**: 529–532.

27. Ross M. J. & Merino M. J. Sarcoidosis of the breast. *Human Pathology* 1985; **16**: 185–187.

28. Fitzgibbons P. L., Smiley D. F. & Kern W. H. Sarcoidosis presenting initially as breast mass: report of two cases. *Human Pathology* 1985; **16**: 851–852.

29. Fernandez B. B. & Hernandez F. J. Amyloid tumour of the breast. *Archives of Pathology* 1973; **95**: 102–105.

30. Sadeghee S. A. & Moore S. W. Rheumatoid arthritis, bilateral amyloid tumours of the breast and multiple cutaneous amyloid nodules. *American Journal of Clinical Pathology* 1974; **62**: 472–476.

31. Hardy T. J. Diffuse parenchymal amyloidosis of lungs and breast. *Archives of Pathology and laboratory Medicine* 1979; **103**: 583–585.

32. Lew W. & Seymour A. E. Primary amyloid of the breast. Case report and literature review. *Acta Cytologica* 1985; **29**: 7–11.

33. Ganor S. Amyloidosis of the nipple presenting as pruritus. *Cutis* 1983; **31**: 318.

34. McCracken M., Hamal P. B. & Benson E. A. Granular cell myoblastoma of the breast: a report of 2 cases. *British Journal of Surgery* 1979; **66**: 819–821.

35. Stephenson T. J. & Underwood J. C. E. Giant cell arteritis: an unusual cause of palpable masses in the breast. *British Journal of Surgery* 1986; **73**: 105.

36. McCarthy D. J., Imbrigia J. & Hung J. K. Vasculitis of the breasts. *Arthritis and Rheumatism* 1968; **11**: 796–801.

37. Paterson A. G., Fortt R. W. & Webster D. J. T. Wegener's granulomatosis. An unusual cause of a breast lump. *Journal of the Royal College of Surgeons of Edinburgh* 1985; **30**: 332–335.

38. Dehn R. B. & Lee E. C. G. Aneurysm presenting as a breast mass. *British Medical Journal 1986*; **292**: 1240.

39. Schneck J. A case of grangenous necrosis of the mammary gland. *Journal of the American Medical Association* 1894; **23**: 181.

40. Robitaille Y., See Mayer T. A., Thelmo W. L. & Cumberlidge M. C. Infarction of the mammary region mimicking carcinoma of the breast. *Cancer* 1974; **33**: 1183–1189.

41. Flood E. P., Redish M. H., Bociek S. J. & Shapiro S. Thrombophlebitis migrans disseminata: report of a case in which gangrene of a breast occurred. *New York State Journal of Medicine* 1943; **43**: 1121–1124.

42. Kessler E. & Wolloch Y. Granulomatous mastitis: a lesion clinically simulating carcinoma. *American Journal of Clinical Pathology* 1972; **58**: 642–646.

43. Fletcher A., McGrath I. M., Riddell R. H. & Talbot I. C. Granulomatous mastitis: a report of seven cases. *Journal of Clinical Pathology* 1982; **35**: 941–945.

44. Going J. J., Anderson T. J., Wilkinson S. & Chetty U. Granulomatous lobular mastitis. *Journal of Clinical Pathology* 1987; **40**: 535–540.

45. Clement P. B., Young R. H. & Azzopardi J. G. Collagenous spherulosis of the breast. *American Journal of Surgical Pathology* 1987; **11**: 411–417.

46. Oluwole S. F., Fadiran O. A. & Odesanmi W. O. Diseases of the breast in Nigeria. *British Journal of Surgery* 1987; **74**: 582–585.

47. Radice B. (Ed.) *Hippocractic Writings*. Harmondsworth, Penguin Classics, 1983, p. 225.

48. Sampson D. An unusual self inflicted injury of the breast. *Postgraduate Medical Journal* 1975; **51**: 116–118.

49. Carney M. W. P. & Brown J. P. Clinical features and motives among 42 artefactual illness patients. *British Journal of Medical Psychology* 1983; **56**: 57–66.

50. Reich P. & Gottfried L. A. Factitious disorders in a teaching hospital. *Annals of Internal Medicine* 1983; **99**: 240–247.

51. Sneddon I. & Sneddon J. Self-inflicted injury. A follow up study of 43 patients. *British Medical Journal* 1975; **3**: 527–530.

52. Rosenberg M. W. & Hughes L. E. Artefactual breast disease: a report of three cases. *British Journal of Surgery* 1986; **72**: 539–541.

53. Craigmyle M. B. L. *The Apocrine Glands and the Breast*. Chichester, John Wiley & Sons, 1984.

54. Jackman R. J. & McQuarrie H. B. Hidradenitis suppurativa: its confusion with pilonidal disease and anal fistula. *American Journal of Surgery* 1949; **77**: 349–351.

55. Harrison B. J., Mudge M. & Hughes L. E. Recurrence after surgical treatment of hidradenitis suppurativa. *British Medical Journal* 1987; **294**: 487–489.

18   Operations

The detailed indications for various operations have been outlined in previous chapters dealing with individual conditions. The general indications, detailed technique and complications of each operation are gathered together in this chapter.

Needle Biopsy

Two forms of needle biopsy need to be differentiated: fine needle aspiration for cytology and core needle biopsy for definitive histology.

Fine needle aspiration (FNA) is simple, causes little discomfort and can be used to sample lesions of all sizes. It is unlikely to spread tumour cells or lead to implantation along the needle track. Accurate interpretation is critically dependent on the availability of a skilled experienced cytologist.

Core needle biopsy is easily performed under local anaesthesia, but can cause some discomfort. The coarser instrument is efficient in obtaining satisfactory specimens from carcinomas of 2 cm diameter or more but it is more difficult to locate small lesions than is the case with FNA, and the rubbery fibrotic tissue typical of benign breast conditions rarely gives a good tissue core. An adequate core can provide definitive histology equivalent to that from an open biopsy. There is a small risk of needle track implantation from carcinoma. With both techniques, the benefit lies only in obtaining a positive diagnosis and little credence should be placed on a negative result because of sampling errors.

Fine Needle Aspiration

Indications

This technique[1] is used with advantage in every lump or suspected lump with the exception of classic fibroadenoma under the age of 25 years (where it is unnecessary because the clinical diagnosis is usually obvious, cancer is excessively rare, and cytology may be difficult to interpret). It should also be used for diffuse nodularity if a particular area stands out, or for a fibroadenoma in a young girl which is not classic in its physical characteristics.

Important Principles

1. Use a fine needle without local anaesthetic.
2. Make sure the technique used is that approved by your cytologist.
3. Ignore a negative result.

Technique

The equipment necessary for making satisfactory smears should be available (Figure 18.1). No anaesthetic is required. The skin is cleansed with a spirit-based antiseptic and a 21-gauge needle attached to a syringe is inserted into the lump which is steadied between two fingers of the second hand. The syringe should be large enough to aspirate the total volume if it proves to be a

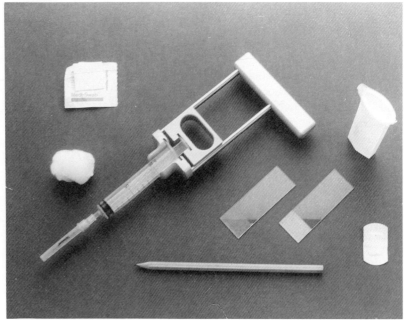

18.1   *The instruments and equipment needed for fine needle aspirtion.*

cyst. The consistency of the breast tissue, and of the lump in particular, is 'sensed' with the needle point: no resistance of fat, toughness of fibrous tissue, the characteristic gritty sensation of cancer, and firmness followed by a sudden 'give' as the needle enters a cyst.

If the lesion proves to be a cyst, a record should be made of the site, colour and quantity of the aspirate. Unless the fluid is blood stained, cytology is not indicated. Measurement of electrolyte content[2] may give some indication of likelihood of recurrence, but is not used routinely. Cysts may be deeper than suggested by palpation, so if no cyst is located on the first needle pass, it is worth while exploring a little deeper. After withdrawing the needle, the area is palpated to ensure that the lump has disappeared completely.

If the lesion proves to be solid, the needle should be moved in and out of the mass in several directions while maintaining negative pressure. The negative pressure is released before removing the needle from the lump. The needle is disconnected, the syringe filled with air and the needle replaced to expel the contents onto a labelled microscope slide. Expulsion should be repeated several times before it is assumed that no specimen is present – a completely dry aspirate is rare. Gross blood contamination interferes with cytology so that, if a blood vessel is hit, it is usually best to repeat the procedure later. Exact technique and the method of fixing the specimen needs to be discussed with the cytologist. The specimens may be fixed immediately in alcohol as for cervical smears or air-dried prior to fixation. Some cytologists prefer that a small amount of heparinized saline be in the syringe. A special syringe holder (CAMECO) is available to facilitate one-handed manipulation. An adhesive dressing is placed over the puncture site.

Complications

This simple procedure should be free of complications. However, occasionally, small haematomas are encountered and pneumothorax occurring after aspiration has been reported. We have seen two cases of pneumothorax in several thousand aspirations. Sometimes a cyst will become inflamed after aspiration, either from infection, or more often when cyst contents leak into the surrounding breast.

Core Needle Biopsy

Indications

An attempt should be made to obtain a core biopsy in any solid mass more than 1 cm in diameter.[3] Needle biopsy can cause sufficient tissue

oedema to obscure mammographic detail, hence biopsy should be deferred until after mammography, or mammography deferred for 1 week after biopsy. While most patients readily tolerate needle biopsy, some find that it causes considerable pain, so it should be used with discretion for tender masses or those deep to the areola. We generally use it together with, and following, FNA cytology.

Important Principles

1. Use local anaesthetic but avoid this form of biopsy if the lump is particularly painful.
2. Develop a one-hand technique for needle manipulation so the other hand can stabilize the lump.
3. Insert the closed needle into the lump to avoid bending the trocar at its weak point.
4. Apply pressure after biopsy for at least 3 minutes, to minimize early and late bleeding.

Technique

A number of biopsy needles are available. Our preference for breast biopsy is a short (3 inch; 7.6 cm) Trucut needle (Travenol) because short needles are easier to control. The equipment necessary for the procedure (Figure 18.2) should be available and a sterile no-touch technique should be used, although gloves are unnecessary. After cleansing the skin, a small intradermal weal of local anaesthetic (1% lignocaine) is raised at the biopsy site – Figure 18.3. The proposed line of the needle should also be infiltrated down to the lesion to be biopsied, but excessive infiltration is to be avoided because it will obscure the position of the underlying mass. Using a sterile technique, a small nick is made in the skin and through to the subcutaneous fat with a pointed disposable scalpel blade (No. 11 or 15; Figure 18.4) and the closed Trucut needle inserted through this

18.2 *The instruments and equipment needed for core needle biopsy using a Trucut needle.*

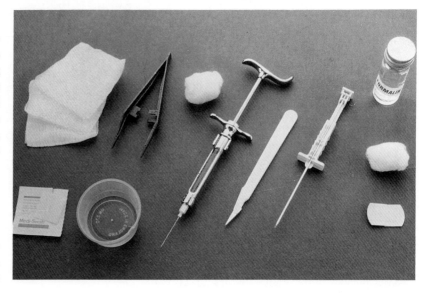

until it abuts against the lesion (Figure 18.5). The closed needle is advanced into the mass (Figure 18.6a); sometimes a rotating action is needed. The cutting sheath is then withdrawn to allow tissue to prolapse into the notch (Figure 18.6b) in the trocar and the cutting sheath is advanced over the trocar to obtain the specimen (Figure 18.6c). The needle is withdrawn in the closed position and the core of the tissue placed straight into formalin. With practice the needle can be manipulated with one hand leaving the second hand free to steady and manipulate the mass. If necessary, further cores of tissue can be taken until a satisfactory specimen is obtained. A general guide to the nature of the specimens can be obtained by examining the cores. If these float on the formalin they are likely to be fat only. If they sink, they are likely to be breast tissue. Bleeding is not uncommon, so haemostasis is secured by firm digital pressure over the area for several minutes. The small skin incision is then covered with an occlusive dressing. The needles cuts malignant tissue much more readily than benign fibrotic tissue, so that an adequate biopsy specimen is not often obtained with a fibrotic benign breast lump.

Complications

Haematoma may occur when a vascular lesion has been biopsied or a subcutaneous vein punctured and moderate bruising is common, hence the need for local pressure for at least 3 or 4 minutes. The 'complication' of missed diagnosis can be avoided by ignoring inadequate or negative biopsies.

Open Biopsy Procedures

Open biopsy covers a number of procedures, including excision biopsy, incision biopsy, removal of a fibroadenoma and biopsy under radiological control. Each procedure carries different indications and requires a special technique.

Excision Biopsy

Indications

This is indicated for removal of any persistent undiagnosed discrete lump in the breast, as outlined in Chapter 5.

Wounds in young girls may be complicated by hypertrophic scars and this is particularly frequent and noticeable in the upper inner quadrant of the

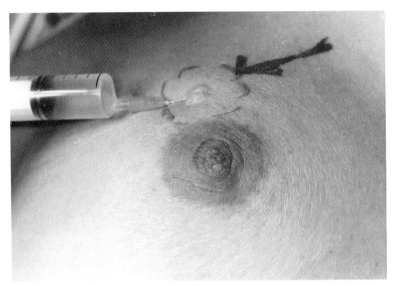

18.3 *Infiltration of skin and underlying tissues with local anaesthetic.*

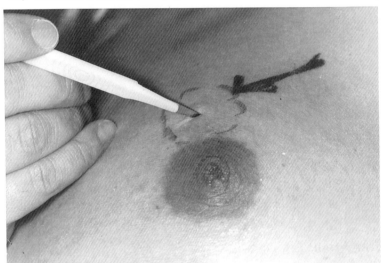

18.4 *A small stab incision is made through the skin and subcutaneous tissue wth a fine pointed scalpel.*

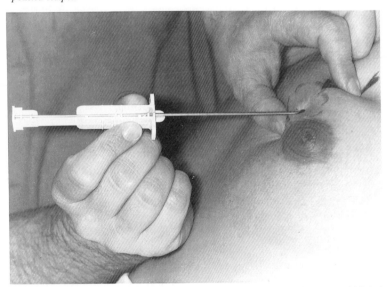

18.5 *The closed needle is held in one hand and inserted down to the mass, which is held and manipulated by the other hand. In this figure, the detail of the needle is shown. In practice, the needle is held in the palm to keep it closed, and manipulated by the fingers of the same hand.*

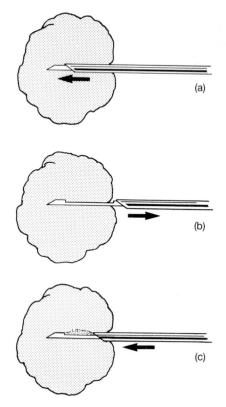

18.6 *(a) The needle is advanced into the mass in the closed position. (b) The sheath is withdrawn to allow some breast tissue to prolapse into the notch of the needle. (c) The sheath is advanced over the notch to cut off the enclosed tissue. The whole needle is then withdrawn.*

breast. Account should be taken of this before recommending biopsy in young girls where the indications may be equivocal.

Important Principles

1. Think carefully before excising breast lumps under local anaesthetic, especially in young girls, where breast tissue is dense and deep lumps may feel superficial.
2. Never biopsy a lump before inserting a needle – it may be a cyst.
3. Define the lump carefully before operation. Avoid the temptation to keep removing fibrotic breast tissue which looks and feels 'abnormal' at operation – this can lead to inadvertent subcutaneous mastectomy.
4. Be careful with haemostasis – vessels in fibrotic breast tissue are difficult to control.
5. Mark the site of the lump before operation with the patient in the position in which she will be placed on the operating table.

Technique

This procedure usually requires a general anaesthetic. Local anaesthetic is an option recommended by many authorities but the possible disadvantages should be considered. The major problems with local anaesthesia are: the mass is

often deeper in the breast than seems to be the case on palpation; a small mass may be obscured by local infiltration of anaesthetic and infiltration of dense fibrotic breast tissue is often ineffective. All these disadvantages are more noticeable when operating on younger women and this technique is certainly suited only to those experienced in breast surgery. Despite careful technique with local anaesthetic the procedure is often uncomfortable for the patient.

Periareolar incisions are preferred for all masses within 5 cm of the areola and curved incisions parallel to the circumference for more peripheral masses (Figure 18.7). In general, the blood supply to the breast is so profuse that ischaemia need not cause concern except in extensive periareolar incisions. However, subcutaneous mastectomy or reduction mammoplasty may cause problems after multiple previous biopsies. The blood supply of the breast and it implications for biopsy are discussed by Robertson[4]. Where cancer is suspected, the incision should be planned to take into account the possibility of proceeding to mastectomy. A horizontal incision is appropriate in a peripheral breast lump to allow re-excision within a transverse mastectomy incision. In re-excising a biopsy wound for malignancy, the whole of the wound and contaminated tissue should be removed without re-entering the original wound, so a badly orientated biopsy wound may necessitate excessive sacrifice of skin at the second procedure (Figure 18.8).

The skin incision is deepened to the subcutaneous fat and veins divided and ligated. Lesser bleeding is controlled by a self-retaining retractor. Most discrete lumps will prove to be a prominent area of fibrotic nodularity. This is invariably a diffuse process and the lump palpated can rarely be defined visually. It must be carefully defined by palpation – both preoperatively and through

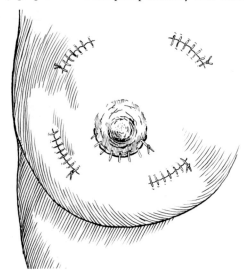

18.7 *Incisions for breast biopsy for benign conditions. Where the mass lies within 5 cm of the areola, a periareolar incision is used. For more distant masses, a curved incision parallel to the areola is used.*

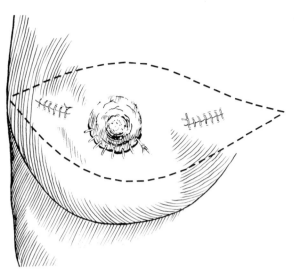

18.8 *In patients of the cancer age group, biopsy incisions should be sited in such a way as to be readily re-excised within the skin island of a mastectomy wound, should this be necessary.*

the wound. The further one goes into the breast, the more difficult it is to define the mass precisely. It is sometimes useful to insert a needle into the mass at an early stage to ensure that the area which was felt preoperatively is the area that will be excised. The mass is grasped with an Allis forceps and excised with a scalpel, suppressing any impulse to continue excising the surrounding breast tissue which may look the same as the palpable nodule. Pursuit of all apparently abnormal tissue will lead to an inadvertent subcutaneous mastectomy. Bleeding is often troublesome because the small vessels lie embedded in the dense fibrous tissue.

As this operation is usually carried out to exclude the possibility of malignancy, it is important that diathermy is not used on tissue which may be needed for histology or oestrogen receptor analysis. It is better to pick up the vessels with mosquito forceps and diathermy them after the lesion has been removed. Because of the tendency for oozing from this fibrotic tissue we believe that suction drainage is usually advisable, although one randomized trial reported no difference in haematoma rate between wounds drained or not drained[5]. There is a difference of opinion as to whether the defect in the breast tissue should be closed. This will require an absorbable suture on a heavy cutting needle because of the fibrous nature of the breast tissue. Such suturing may lead to further haematoma formation. On the other hand, large defects may persist and leave a palpable ridge which is prone to be mistaken for a further lump. Neither situation is satisfactory. Our practice is to use suction drainage alone in small wounds, but with wedge excisions we close the defect with interrupted ooo catgut sutures.

The skin should be closed with a very fine intracuticular suture: 4/o prolene is satisfactory or 5/o polydioxanone (PDS) which obviates the need for suture removal.

Complications

The only complication seen with any frequency is haematoma formation. If care is taken to obtain meticulous haemostasis, haematoma should be a rare event. If it occurs, it is better to return the patient to theatre and evacuate the clot than wait for spontaneous resolution.

Postoperative Care

Provided drainage is minimal and there is no haematoma formation, a drain may be removed the following day and the patient allowed home. The subcuticular sutures are removed at 7 days. At this time a check should be made that the pathology has been reviewed and arrangements made for further management and follow-up depending on the diagnosis.

Many surgeons routinely carry out breast biopsy on a day patient basis; others (like ourselves) do this selectively. This has obvious advantages, but requires monitoring of results to ensure that results and complications are within acceptable limits.

Incision Biopsy

Since incision biopsy is used mainly to confirm the diagnosis of large carcinomas and to obtain material for oestrogen receptor analysis, it is largely outside the scope of this book. As a general rule, a diagnosis should be made before definitive treatment is planned for large masses of obscure aetiology. This can usually be achieved by cytology or needle biopsy. In the rare instances where neither technique has been satisfactory, it is better to perform an incision biopsy than to do a very wide excision for a lump which may prove to be no more than fibrous tissue. Large fibroadenoma, in an older patient, and fibromatosis are uncommon examples. Details of the technique are given under excision biopsy (p. 190).

Removal of a Fibroadenoma

The early stages of the operation are the same as those described under open biopsy. However, fibroadenoma in young women usually lies within a well-defined capsule and can be enucleated easily. The pedicle may require ligation or diathermy (Figure 18.9) and the base of the pedicle may require excision if this is broad because there

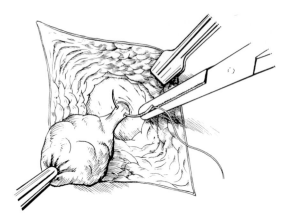

18.9 *Removing a fibroadenoma. The blood supply comes only through the pedicle so this should be ligated if it is substantial.*

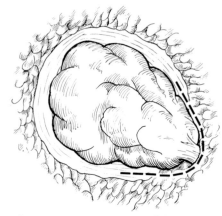

18.10 *There is sometimes extension of fibroadenomatous tissue in the pedicle so that, where this is broad, an area adjacent to the base should be removed to minimize recurrence.*

may be some extension of fibroadenomatous tissue into the area of the capsule (Figure 18.10). Bleeding is minimal and there should be no need to insert a drain into the cavity if haemostasis of the vascular pedicle has been obtained. Because the parenchyma of the breast is hardly disturbed, there is no need to close the defect in the breast tissue which will soon disappear.

In older women, a fibroadenoma usually presents as a dominant mass in an involuting breast. These fibroadenomas often do not enucleate satisfactorily and are best removed by the technique of excision biopsy described earlier.

Radiologically Controlled Biopsy

Indications

This procedure is indicated to remove a lesion seen on mammography but which cannot be felt clinically. The commonest indication is a small area of microcalcification or trabecular distortion for which the differential diagnosis usually lies between early carcinoma – *in situ* or invasive – and sclerosing adenosis. Because these two conditions cannot be differentiated radiologically, excision biopsy is indicated. We do not believe that ultrasound-guided FNA cytology is yet sufficiently reliable to replace radiologically controlled open biopsy.

Principles

1. Close co-operation is required between surgeon, radiologist and pathologist.
2. The radiological abnormality is localized by the radiologist in the radiology department (Figure 18.11).

3. Excision biopsy by surgeon under general anaesthetic (Figures 18.12 and 18.13).
4. Immediate specimen radiology by the radiologist to confirm that the area in question has been removed (Figure 18.14).
5. Further tissue excision is performed if the abnormal area was not located in this specimen.
6. Dissection of the specimen by the radiologist to isolate the radiological abnormality.
7. Rapid paraffin section.

Technique

Radiological localization

A number of techniques have been described, the commonest being double dye localization and the hooked needle technique – *see* Chapter 6. In the former, the radiologist injects 0.5 ml of a mixture of 1 ml 25% Hypaque and 2 drops of Patent Blue Violet dye into the breast at the site where he calculates the radiological abnormality will lie. Further mammography is then performed in two planes to determine the relationship between the Hypaque dye and the radiological lesion. This information is sent with the mammograms and the patient to theatre. The surgeon undertakes a biopsy procedure in the same way as described under open biopsy but following the dye into the breast. The relationship of the dye to the radiological lesion is used to define the area to be excised. The specimen is subjected to immediate soft tissue radiology either in the theatre or the radiology department, depending on the facilities available. The radiologist confirms that the lesion is question has or has not been excised.

If the radiological lesion is identified, the surgeon closes the wound in the usual way. If it has not been identified, a further biopsy is taken and the procedure repeated until radiological confirmation of the abnormality is obtained. The radiologist uses further soft tissue radiography to localize and excise the portion of tissue containing the radiological abnormality and this, and the remainder of the biopsy, are sent to the pathologist as separate labelled specimens. The pathologist then submits the material to rapid paraffin section and appropriate treatment is determined by definitive histology[6].

Many units prefer a hooked needle technique as outlined in Chapter 6. When used, it is important that adequate fixation prevents movement of the needle during transport to the theatre. Preference for one or other technique is largely due to personal familiarity and experience.

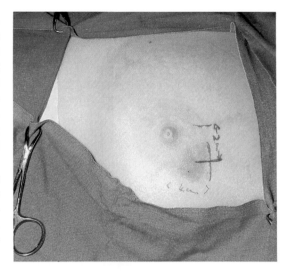

18.12   *A skin incision is made in relation to the dye at the skin puncture point and taking account of the relationship of the radiological abnormality to the dye on the mammograms.*

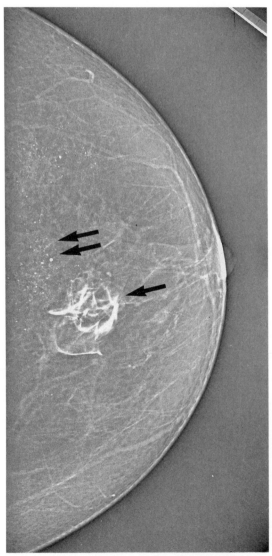

18.11   *A subclinical radiological lesion (↑↑) has been localized and dye (↑) inserted into the breast. A mammogram is then taken to show the relationship of the dye to the lesion (this is done in two planes).*

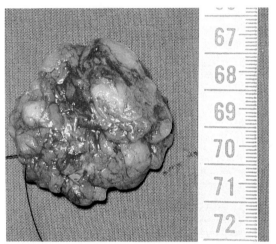

18.13   *The area considered to be abnormal is removed and sent for immediate soft tissue radiology.*

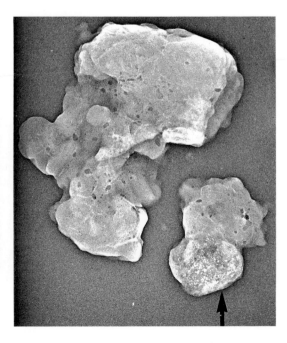

18.14   *The specimen radiology confirms the presence of the suspected lesion and localizes the piece (arrow) for special attention by the pathologist.*

Removal of a Giant Fibroadenoma

In a Young Patient (< 20 years)

A giant fibroadenoma is usually defined as a lesion more than 5 cm in diameter. These lesions may lie close to the surface of the breast and may then be removed in the same way as a smaller fibroadenoma. Larger lesions tend to lie deeper in the breast and are best approached from behind through a submammary incision which will give a better cosmetic result than one located on the breast.

Technique

A submammary incision (Figure 18.15) is taken down to the fascia over the serratus anterior and pectoralis major muscles and dissection is carried upwards in this largely avascular retromammary plane (Figure 18.16). The fibroadenoma is then pushed through the posterior aspect into the wound, the capsule incised (Figure 18.17) and the tumour shelled out in the usual way. A suction drain is inserted into the retromammary space and the wound closed with subcuticular prolene. This approach to the back of the breast through the submammary fold was described by Gaillard-Thomas in 1892.

It is important that more radical procedures are avoided in young girls and that no attempt is made to close the cavity, and even more important that no complex reconstructive procedures are used – for reasons given in Chapter 7 (p. 60).

In an Older Patient

Giant fibroadenema in older patients differs from those in young girls in a number of ways (*see* Chapter 7). They vary in the degree of malignancy, and may not shell out from surrounding involuting breast tissue. Hence, they are best managed by incision biopsy to provide definitive histological assessment before planning management, which is usually by a wide local excision or by simple mastectomy.

Microdochectomy

Indications

This operation is indicated for blood-stained or serous discharge from a solitary duct when the opening of the affected duct on to the nipple can be identified. We practise this operation for patients under the age of 40, preferring the operation of major duct excision for blood-stained nipple discharge in patients over this age – *see*

Chapters 11 and 12. No attempt should be made to express discharge from the nipple for several days prior to operation so that some discharge is present to identify the duct at operation. Alternatively, the nipple may be sprayed with Nobecutane 2 or 3 days before operation to ensure retention of secretion.

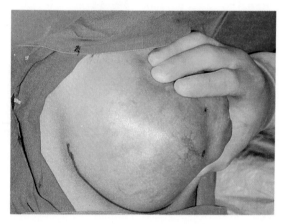

18.15   *The Gaillard–Thomas incision for giant fibroadenoma.*

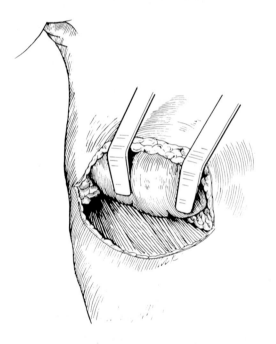

18.16   *The dissection is carried upwards in the submammary plane at the level of the pectoral fascia.*

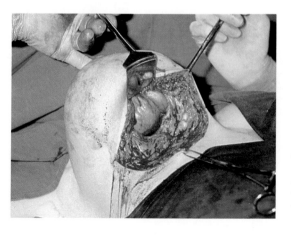

18.17   *The fascial layer on the posterior aspect of the breast is incised and the fibroadenoma enucleated and delivered through this wound.*

Operative Principles

1. Avoid expressing fluid for a few days before operation.
2. Radial or periareolar incisions are both satisfactory.
3. Identify the duct with a lacrimal probe.
4. Excise all dilated parts of the duct system which contain blood.

Operative Technique

The orifice of the affected duct is identified by squeezing the nipple to express a drop of discharge. A lacrimal probe is inserted into the duct and passed as far into the breast tissue as possible (Figure 18.18). This should be done gently to avoid creating a false passage. The probe will frequently pass only 1–2 cm because passage along the duct may be blocked by little pockets which tend to occur as the duct dilates around a papilloma. This distance is sufficient to demonstrate the direction of the duct and, after making the incision, the dark fluid in the dilated duct is usually visible.

Using the direction of the lacrimal probe as a guide, a racquet-shaped incision is carried out to enclose the immediate termination of the duct with a minimal amount of surrounding nipple tissue and carried radially across the areola and on to the breast skin for a total distance of 5 cm (Figure 18.19). The skin flaps are raised over a

short distance and the whole of the affected duct and its branching system dissected out in segmental fashion for a distance of at least 5 cm from its orifice (Figure 18.20). The main portion of the duct can usually be identified for about 2.5 cm. It is dissected carefully to interfere as little as possible with surrounding ducts, although if a central duct is affected, some damage to the adjacent ducts may be inevitable. A further segmental area of breast tissue about 2.5 cm long is

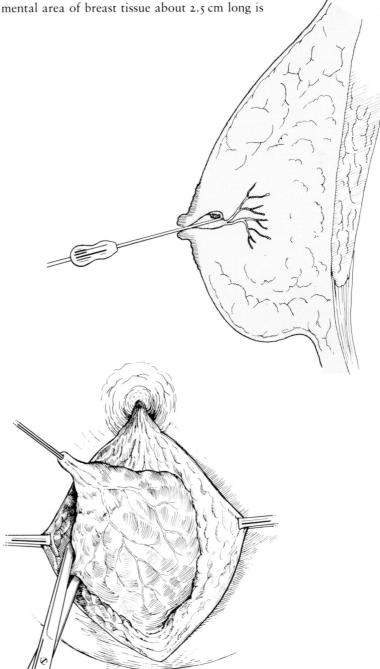

18.18 *A lacrimal probe is passed into the affected duct to find its direction within the breast. It often will not go very far because it catches in small pockets of the dilated duct.*

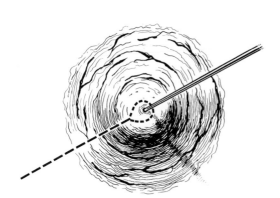

18.19 *The incision for microdochectomy – the skin surrounding the terminal duct is removed in continuity within the duct.*

18.20 *The segment drained by the duct is dissected back into the breast for a distance of 2–3 cm, but further if the ducts remain dilated at this level.*

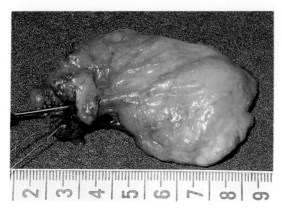

18.21 *A typical specimen following microdochectomy from a large breast.*

removed in continuity with the duct (Figure 18.21). A length of 5–6 cm of the duct system will usually remove any papillomas present because these are lesions of the large duct.

However, if the duct remains dilated beyond 5 cm, it should be followed further into the periphery of the breast. Peripheral dilatation of ducts is rarely seen in older patients and is readily recognized at operation by the dark fluid within the ducts, oozing out when they are damaged. Normally a duct is only dilated between the papilloma and the nipple. So, if peripheral ducts are dilated, peripheral papillomas – benign or malignant – should be anticipated and a segmental resection of the breast carried out to encompass all dilated, blood-filled ducts.

Haemostasis is secured and the specimen removed. The terminal portion of the duct is marked with a silk suture to help the pathologist orientate the tissue. Having done this, the duct system may be opened and inspected for the presence of a papilloma. However, macroscopic papilloma is found in only about half the cases, others being due to duct ectasia. A suction drain is inserted and the skin closed with fine sutures.

Variations of Technique

Several variations have been described for this procedure. The tissues around the duct may be infiltrated with saline containing 1:300 000 adrenaline solution to help maintain haemostasis and allow more exact dissection. The use of binocular magnifying loops will also help precise dissection.

Some surgeons (e.g. Haagensen[7]) prefer to use a periareolar incision, dissecting the flap upwards in the same manner as described under major duct excision. The dilated duct is then dissected to its entry onto the nipple. The peripheral flap is raised to allow segmental excision of the duct drainage area. Haagensen advocates this incision on cosmetic grounds, although we find a radial incision gives a satisfactory cosmetic result. The radial incision has the advantage that it can more readily be extended where this is necessary, so is particularly appropriate in the older patient.

Excision of Mammary Duct Fistula

Indications

1. Established duct fistula with a single opening.
2. A localized abscess which always presents at the same spot.
3. In a patient who does not seek correction of an inverted nipple.

Important Principles

1. Conservative drainage of periareolar abscess as an acute procedure if the fistula is not established.
2. The central (nipple) opening of the duct must be excised.
3. Healing by granulation gives the most reliable method of obtaining a satisfactory result but the wound must be well shaped and managed correctly.

Fistulotomy or Fistulectomy?

In his original description, Hedley Atkins[8] simply laid the fistula open and allowed it to granulate (fistulotomy). This is probably a satisfactory procedure, but we have preferred fistulectomy because it ensures that the central portion of the duct is excised (important in minimizing recurrence), removes some of the ductal system and leaves healthy tissue to granulate. This operation is described, but similar principles apply to fistulotomy. A probe is passed into the external opening of the fistula and passes easily out of the duct opening on to the nipple (Figure 18.22). The skin incision encompasses the fistula and an ellipse of skin is removed which needs be only about 1 cm wide at its maximum (Figure 18.23). More important is that the incision includes the whole of the affected lactiferous sinus and the opening on to the nipple – this is the portion of terminal duct lined by squamous epithelium. The ellipse and underlying tissue also include a centimetre or two of the duct system distal to the fistula. The incision is deepened through subcutaneous fat

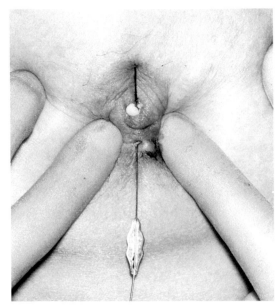

18.22 *A probe is passed through the duct fistula and out through the nipple.*

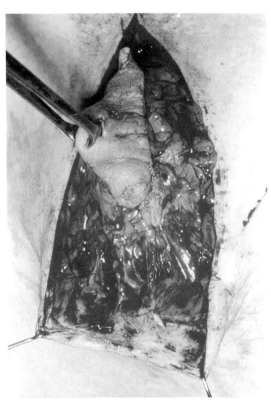

18.24 *The underlying tissue is excised conservatively.*

into the breast tissue just below the affected duct (Figure 18.24).

If the wound is allowed to granulate, healing will be rapid and certain, provided that the wound is well shaped (Figure 18.25) and does not close prematurely. The disadvantage of granulation lies in the pain associated with wounds in the nipple region with conventional gauze dressings, and the longer period of hospitalization associated with this technique. Both these disadvantages can be avoided by using a non-adherent dressing such as Silastic Foam, which causes no pain on dressing change and can be managed by the patient at home, so hospitalization is frequently shorter than with primary wound closure.

Our practice is to suture a pack soaked in proflavine/paraffin emulsion *in situ* for 3 days (Figure 18.26) to produce wound edges which are firm and maintain the shape of the wound. After this period the gauze pack is replaced by Silastic Foam dressing (Figure 18.27) which can be

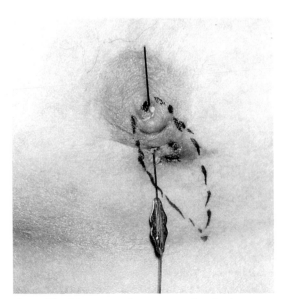

18.23 *The skin excision for mammary duct fistula.*

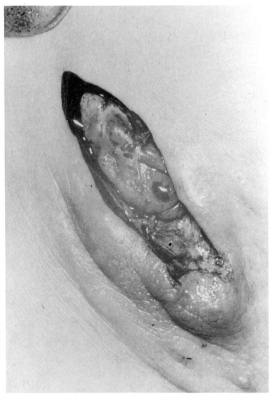

18.25 *The resulting wound is boat shaped – as broad as it is deep so that it will heal from below.*

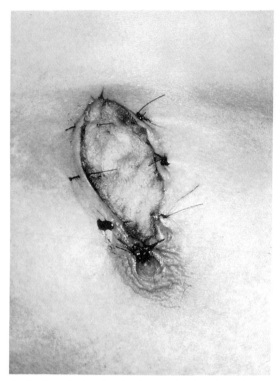

18.26 *A proflavine dressing is sewn in place for 3 days to provide stiff walls to the wound so that they will not collapse and close prematurely.*

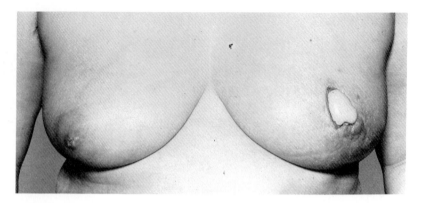

removed and replaced painlessly. The patient can be discharged home for self-care of the wound and dressing[9]. An alternative is to close the wound primarily under antibiotic cover[10]. This is a new approach with as yet insufficient follow-up to show whether it will produce sound long-term results.

Major Duct Excision (Adair/Urban/Hadfield)

This important procedure has an interesting history for it was first reported in 1960 by Hadfield[11], based on 31 cases. In the UK, the operation is commonly referred to as Hadfield's procedure. In his paper he paid tribute to Adair and Urban of the Memorial Hospital, New York for having taught him the operation. Three years later, Urban described his technique[12] reporting 167 operations. Hence, the operation is also frequently known as Urban's duct excision but in his own paper, Urban assigns his own precedence to Adair whose first operation preceded Urban's by 2 years, although he published no account of his technique.

Indications (*see* Chapter 11 for details)

1. Serosanguineous discharge in a patient over the age of 40 years. Here is is preferred to microdochectomy because of the more generous pathological material provided in a patient with a significant risk of cancer (Urban found 41 unsuspected cancers in 434 duct excision operations mainly in the older age groups), and more certain control of symptoms should the symptoms prove to be due to duct ectasia.
2. Non-sanguineous discharge sufficiently copious to be an embarrassment to the patient. If the discharge is milky, prolactinoma should first be excluded.
3. Subareolar abscess, selected according to the criteria discussed in Chapter 11, or a peripheral mass or abscess with central major duct ectasia, when the mass and major ducts can be excised in continuity.
4. The operation is *not* necessary for biopsy for small areas of periductal mastitis with moderate duct ectasia. These are satisfactorily managed by local excision biopsy.

Principles of Operation

1. The areolar flap is dissected in a plane deep to the venous plexus to avoid ischaemia.
2. The under surface of the nipple is bared completely:
   (a) to remove all terminal duct tissue;
   (b) to ensure that no ducts are missed at the back of the duct cone.
3. Remove the central portion of the nipple if the nipple does not evert easily.
4. Ignore peripheral dilated ducts.
5. Submit all excised tissue to histology.

Technique

Incision
The ducts are approached through a periareolar incision extending no further than 50% around the circumference. It is usually based inferiorly but may be centred anywhere towards localized pathology. It should be placed accurately at the

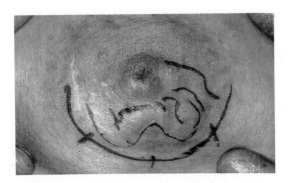

18.28 *Incision for major duct excision – exactly at the areolar margin.*

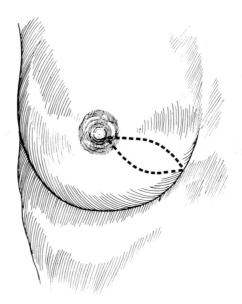

18.29 *The alternative incision, for major duct excision advocated by Urban[12].*

areolar margin to obtain maximum cosmetic benefit (Figure 18.28).

Urban[12] recommended a radial incision removing an ellipse of skin stopping short of the nipple. He found it easier to repair the oval-shaped defect in the breast tissue (Figure 18.29). We advise this approach where there is severe scarring from periareolar sepsis, because it allows easy entry to the subareolar plane through relatively normal tissue, instead of through dense scar tissue. It has the disadvantage that it may encourage the surgeon to leave small amounts of terminal duct on the undersurface of the nipple.

A 'Z'-shaped incision transecting the nipple has been recommended. We quickly abandoned this approach because it proved tedious, was more destructive and presented no advantages.

Dissection

The incision is deepened until the prominent radially running subcutaneous veins are reached. These are divided and ligated with fine (0000) catgut and the plane of dissection developed immediately deep to these veins (Figure 18.30). By preserving the vascular plexus of the areola, the viability of nipple and areolar is assured. The penalty for neglecting this careful definition of tissue planes is shown in Figure 18.31.

The areolar flap is dissected in this plane until half the areaola has been elevated and the cone of fibroductal tissue passing to the nipple is reached. A subareolar tunnel is then developed behind the ductal cone by blunt dissection with a haemostat working from each side (at 3 o'clock and 9 o'clock, respectively) to meet in the middle behind the ducts (Figure 18.32). This can be done in the correct plane without great difficulty because both the ductal tissue and the skin of the areola are tough structures and the subcutaneous fat represents the path of least resistance.

The core of ductal tissue is grasped by a Kocher forceps passed through the subareolar tunnel. The ducts are divided on the forceps to ensure that an inverted nipple is not damaged by this manoeuvre (Figure 18.33). With retraction on the Kocher forceps, the ductal mass is dissected back into the breast for a distance of 3 cm or so and then

18.30 *The areolar flap is elevated in the subvenous plane.*

18.31 *Partial nipple necrosis due to dissection of the flap in too superficial a plane.*

18.30

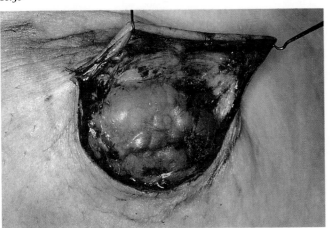

18.31

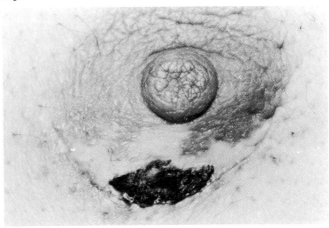

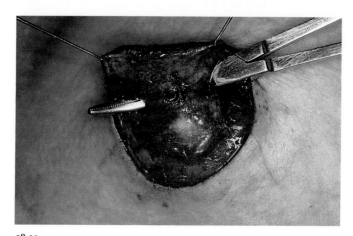

18.32

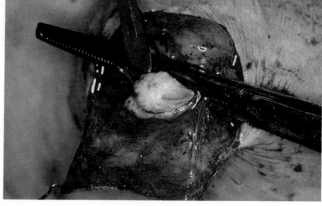

18.33

transected. During this process, any bleeding vessels should be caught and ligated before they retract back into the breast substance.

It is not uncommon for ducts to remain dilated at the site of transection. Hadfield recommends that they be ligated with fine catgut, but this is not easy because they are embedded in fibrous tissue. Urban recommended that dissection be extended into the breast until the ducts are of normal size – but this will sometimes result in a major defect, little short of subtotal mastectomy. There seems to be no disadvantage in ignoring the transected dilated ducts, as recommended by Haagensen, and wounds without overt sepsis can be expected to heal in spite of some continuing leakage of duct contents.

Attention is drawn to the under-surface of the nipple to ensure that the terminal ducts are removed completely. The nipple is fully inverted and stretched over the tip of the index finger and the remaining duct tissue excised with scissors (Figure 18.34). This manoeuvre also ensures that no ducts are missed as can happen if the tunnelling traverses the duct mass rather than the subcutaneous plane – leaving some ducts at the far side of the incision.

If dissection is complete the nipple will usually

resume the everted position. If there is any tendency to re-invert, a further examination should be made to ensure that all ductal tissue has been excised and a loose purse-string suture of fine PDS may be placed around its base (a tight purse-string suture may produce nipple ischaemia). Sometimes the centre of a deeply inverted nipple is thickened, keratotic and contains dilated terminal ducts, and cannot be inverted satisfactorily after duct division. It may then be best to excise, in conservative fashion, the central portion of the nipple and close the defect with one or two fine sutures. This central portion needs to be 5 mm or so in diameter.

Drainage and closure
In the abscence of infection a small suction drain should be inserted and the wound closed with fine silk sutures or a subcuticular prolene suture. Some authors recommend obliteration of the subareolar cavity by a series of approximating purse-string sutures. We omit this step and have not found it to be a disadvantage. The cosmetic result of this operation is excellent when there has been little or no tissue destruction before surgery (*see* Figure 11.21). When the operation is

18.32 *A subareolar tunnel is formed behind the ducts by blunt dissection, and a Kocher forceps passed through the tunnel to grasp the ducts.*

18.33 *The ducts are divided immediately below the nipple by cutting onto the Kocher forceps.*

18.34 *Any residual terminal duct tissue is removed after inverting the nipple over the index finger.*

18.35 *Severe wound infection resulting from ill-advised closure following major duct excision in the presence of active infection.*

18.34

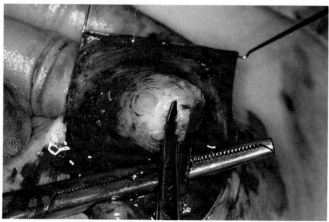

18.35

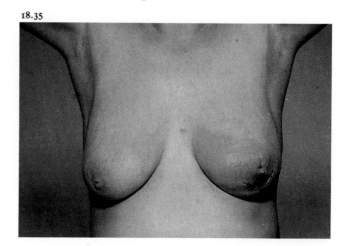

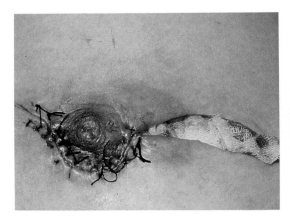

18.36 *In cases with extensive incision for recurrent sepsis, partial closure may be appropriate.*

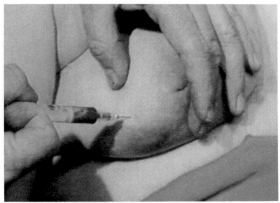

18.37 *The presence of pus should always be confirmed by needle aspiration before proceeding to open drainage of an abscess*

performed after extensive sepsis the cosmetic result is likely to be less satisfactory.

In the presence of overt or recent infection, the wound should not be closed primarily because of a considerable risk of postoperative infection (Figure 18.35). This predisposes to nipple necrosis or chronic infection leading to sinus formation. It is best to pack the wound with gauze soaked in proflavine and paraffin emulsion and subsequently allow the wound to granulate using a Silastic Foam dressing. In some situations where extensive sepsis extends into the breast, it may be satisfactory to close the pariareolar portion of the incision and leave a radial portion of the incision open for counter-drainage (Figure 18.36).

The increasing evidence for a role for bacterial infection in some of these abscesses, particularly recurrent ones, raises the question of whether they may be safely closed primarily in the presence of adequate antibiotic therapy. We consider this remains an open question, but if it is to be tried, the minimum spectrum of cover should be that of anaerobic organisms and Gram-positive cocci – metronidazole and flucloxacillin or erythromycin seems to be a satisfactory combination. On balance, our experience leads us to prefer continuation of our policy of open granulation. However, where the infection has been well controlled by antibiotics and prior drainage so that only a track remains, we are willing to close the wound after excision of this tract under antibiotic cover. Hence out preference for two-stage management of abscesses where possible – preliminary conservative drainage, followed by major duct excision 6–8 weeks later with primary closure under antibiotic cover.

There does not seem to be any carcinogenic risk from leaving the peripheral ducts *in situ*. Urban found only 7 cancers developing in his 434 patients having duct excision and followed for 2–14 years. Three were *in situ* and four infiltrating.

Drainage of a Lactational Breast Abscess

This should be performed under general anaesthetic. Antibiotic cover is given if there is surrounding widespread cellulitis – otherwise it is unnecessary. In the vast majority of cases, a curvilinear incision parallel to the areola should be made over the area of maximum tenderness after confirmation of the presence of pus by needle aspiration (Figures 18.37 and 18.38). The abscess is usually multilocular and these loculi will need to be broken down with the finger but without unnecessary disturbance of the uninvolved breast tissue (Figure 18.39). The skin incision should be adequate – at least three-quarters of the diameter of the abscess. The cavity is then lightly packed with gauze soaked in proflavine/paraffin emulsion and the wound left open (*see* Figure 18.26). Tight packing must be avoided as it interferes with drainage. After a day or two, the pack should be replaced by a Silastic Foam dressing, which will eliminate pain from the wound dressing, give excellent drainage and allow the patient to manage her own wound at home. This can only be

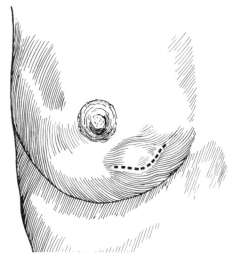

18.38 *The incision for abscess drainage. It should be of generous proportion.*

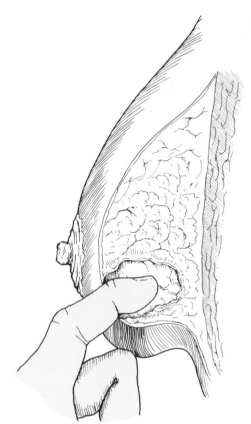

18.39 *All loculi must be broken down with an exploring finger.*

used if the incision is generous and the wound cavity well shaped (Figure 18.40). The cavity rapidly fills and healing is usually complete by 2–3 weeks (Figure 18.41). Treated in this way there is surprisingly little deformity of the breast. If, for any reason, the incision does not provide dependent drainage, an independent counter incision can be made and tube drain brought out through this. In these cases, the skin edges of the original incision may be loosely opposed with interrupted sutures – provided the skin edges are healthy. However, if the initial incision is well placed and adequate in size, counter drainage should rarely be necessary. An alternative

approach to the drainage of breast abscess is that of Benson and Goodman[13] – curettage and primary closure under antibiotic cover. The abscess cavity is opened as before, and emptied, and the lining of granulation tissue curetted out. The cavity is then closed primarily with interrupted vertical mattress sutures which pass deep to the cavity. These authors recommend removing the sutures on the fourth day. We have no experience of this technique.

Subcutaneous Mastectomy in Male Patients

This is indicated in a minority of patients with gynaecomastia, where gross degrees of breast enlargement are causing cosmetic and psychological trauma, and in cases where there is no underlying correctable cause and which have not responded to hormone therapy (*see* Chapter 16).

Important Principles

1. Submammary incision should be used for very large volumes of breast tissue.
2. Periareolar incisions are preferred for moderate gynaecomastia.
3. Splitting the breast tissue down to the pectoral fascia gives mobility which facilitates dissection.
4. Leave a modest amount of subcutaneous fat and adherent breast tissue and close as a separate layer beneath the nipple.

Technique

A periareolar incision is made around the lower half of the circumference. It is often necessary to extend this laterally for adequate haemostasis. Alternatively, an inframammary incision may be used, although this is cosmetically less satisfactorily, especially in young patients who have a

18.40 *A satisfactory, well-shaped wound following removal of a proflavine emulsion pack from a very large abscess.*

18.41 *Successive Silastic foam dressings as the wound healed over 5 weeks – same patient as Figure 18.40.*

18.40

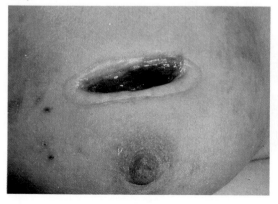

18.41

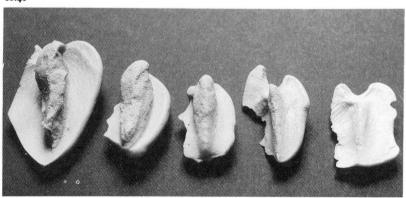
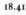

greater tendency to keloid formation. In practice the periareolar incision is best in young patients and a submammary incision in elderly obese patients with dependent breast tissue.

The nipple is elevated with much greater difficulty than is the case in the female breast because the fibroglandular tissue of gynaecomastia is adherent to the areola. A small amount of subcutaneous fat and adherent breast tissue is left behind the nipple – both to avoid damage to the nipple (much more easily done than might be thought) and to improve the cosmetic result by preserving normal nipple protrusion. The amount of tissue left behind the nipple is a matter of judgement and experience.

The flaps are dissected only a small distance upwards and downwards in a deep subcutaneous plane, so that a considerable thickness of subcutaneous fat is retained. The breast cone is then grasped and split tranversely down to the pectoral fascia (Figure 18.42). Upper and lower halves are dissected from the pectoral fascia upwards and downwards, respectively, so that the flap dissection is completed with a much more mobile breast cone[14]. With very marked gynaecomastia, the breast cone can be quartered rather than halved and this further facilitates dissection through a small periareolar incision. It is important to dissect superficial to the pectoral fascia, as its preservation ensures that the skin retains its mobility. Haemostasis is obtained as the dissection proceeds because it is difficult to obtain adequate access to the periphery of the depth of the wound once the tissues have retracted after the breast has been removed. Haematomas are a common complication of this procedure when done through a subareolar incision and, in cases where haemostasis is excessively difficult, a lateral extension of the wound should be made to give adequate access (Figure 18.43). Suction drains (two) are then inserted and the wound closed either with subcuticular prolene or with interrupted silk sutures. Saline should be instilled into the wound while it is being closed to prevent clot formation with blockage of the suction drains.

The drains can be removed as soon as drainage is reduced to a small quantity, usually on the first postoperative day.

Subcutaneous Mastectomy in Women

Important principles

1. Think carefully, twice or even three times, about the validity of the indication for the operation.

2. Accept the risk of skin or nipple necrosis where many previous biopsy scars are present.

3. Use an incision which will allow removal of all breast tissue – including the axillary tail.

4. Warn the patient that silicone prosthesis reconstruction is associated with considerable long-term problems.

This operation is very rarely indicated (*see* Chapter 4) and should not be undertaken lightly. There are many possible complications, especially in the breast scarred by numerous previous biopsies. Incision needs to be planned to take account of these scars which may predispose to skin necrosis. A submammary incision is used most commonly. However, it should be recognized that total excision of the breast tissue (especially the axillary tail) is not achieved through a small submammary incision. For this reason, we prefer a periareolar incision with a lateral extension because it is important that all breast tissue be excised, particularly when the operation is being

18.42 *Excision of gynaecomastia through a periareolar incision is facilitated by splitting the breast tissue cone into two (or four) pieces.*

18.43 *A lateral extension to a periareolar wound impairs cosmesis, but may be necessary to give adequate access.*

18.42

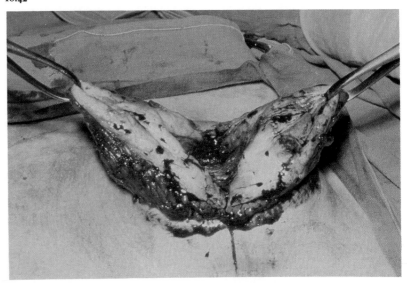

18.43

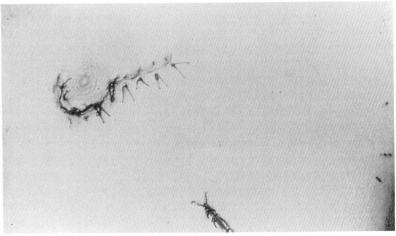

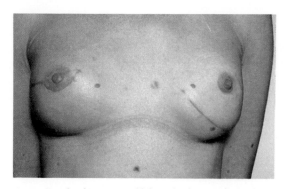

18.44 *Result of insertion of bilateral subpectoral prostheses following subcutaneous mastectomy. Previous biopsy incisions have been utilized and extended to ensure that all breast tissue has been removed.*

carried out for pre-neoplastic states. The procedure differs from the operation in the male in that all the tissue behind the nipple needs to be removed, and preferably the central core of the nipple should be taken as well to eliminate the terminal ducts. Fortunately, the areola can be elevated without difficulty in the female and this part of the procedure does not differ from major duct excision. The plane between the subcutaneous tissue and the breast tissue is more easily found with scissors than with a scalpel. It is important that all breast tissue be removed and this extends further medially, superiorly and laterally than may be anticipated. The most troublesome part of the dissection is the axillary tail and breast tissue is very often left in this region. The axillary tail is best defined by blunt dissection and its limit defined by palpation. A curved haemostat should be placed around the axillary tissue at its upper level and tied after the pedicle has been divided. It is advisable to insert at least two suction drains at the completion of this procedure. In appropriate cases, a silicone gel prosthesis may be inserted into the subpectoral pocket. The skin is closed with either subcuticular prolene or with interrupted silk.

The main complication of subcutaneous mastectomy is haematoma formation, resulting from inadequate haemostasis associated with the use of small incisions. Skin flap or nipple necrosis is not uncommon, particularly in patients who have had multiple previous biopsies.

The inevitable consequence of leaving adequate tissue under the nipple is the risk of cancer developing in the major ducts, a risk which is by no means only theoretical[15]. Similarly, the development of late cancer due to residual breast tissue left in the periphery of the breast is a significant problem. Where the operation is being done for putative prophylaxis against the development of cancer, this possibility should be considered carefully at the time of surgery, for total removal of breast tissue is necessary but not easily achieved through conventional cosmetic incisions.

There are many complications of silicone gel reconstruction, which are dealt with in plastic surgery textbooks.

In spite of these problems, a modest result is often satisfactory to the patient (Figure 18.44), although individual patients will react very differently to similar cosmetic results.

Inverted Nipple

A surgeon setting out to correct congenital inverted nipples, or secondarily inverted nipples, has a wide variety of procedures from which to choose. So wide a choice makes it difficult to choose any individual technique and also suggests that no particular method is satisfactory. This is confirmed by the sparsity of papers reporting large series of cases with long-term follow-up.

On general principles, one would expect that a successful procedure would need to deal with the underlying pathology – which is poor development or fibrotic shortening of the major ducts. This can only be corrected by transecting the ducts completely.

Reported techniques fall into two main groups:

1. Those which correct by pulling on the ducts and attempt to hold them out – by sutures or by providing an underlying buttress of tissue.
2. Those that divide the ducts completely and then use one of the methods in (1) to hold the nipple everted[16,17]. Although these reports are of small numbers with little follow-up, they at least meet the basic principles.

In our experience, major duct excision, combined if necessary with excision of the central core of the nipple, will cure inverted nipples without any additional buttressing procedures. Hence out recommendation is that this operation, performed as described earlier in this chapter, is the procedure of choice – provided the patient is aware that they will be unable to breast-feed following this procedure. It is possible that simple division of the ducts by transfixion may be satisfactory[18], but we have no experience of this technique. We prefer to do a conservative major duct excision.

In the absence of long-term follow-up, those procedures which do not divide the ducts must be considered unproven. It is also possible that some conservative procedures divide the ducts without recognizing it, so details of subsequent breast-feeding should accompany long-term results of operation for nipple inversion.

REFERENCES

1. Duguid H. L. D., Wood R. A. B., Irving A. D. *et al.* Needle aspiration of the breast with immediate reporting of material. *British Medical Journal* 1979; ii: 185–187.
2. Dixon J. M., Scott W. N. & Miller R. W. Natural history of cystic disease: the importance of cyst type. *British Journal of Surgery* 1985; 72: 190–192.
3. Roberts J. G., Preece P. E., Bolton P. M., Baum M. & Hughes L. E. The Trucut biopsy in breast cancer. *Clinical Oncology* 1975; i: 297–303.
4. Robertson J. L. A. The choice of incision for biopsy in large breasted women. *South African Journal of Surgery* 1980; 18: 9–12.
5. Wheeler M. H. & Lakhany Z. Breast biopsy – A trial of wound drainage. *Americal Journal of Surgery* 1976; 31: 581–582.
6. Preece P. E., Gravelle I. H., Hughes L. E., Baum M., Fortt R. W. & Leopold J. G. The operative management of subclinical breast cancer. *Clinical Oncology* 1977; 3: 165–169.
7. Haagensen C. D. *Diseases of the Breast*, 3rd edn. Philadelphia, W. B. Saunders, 1986.
8. Atkins H. J. B. Mammillary fistula. *British Medical Journal* 1955; 2: 1473–1474.
9. Wood R. A. B., Williams R. H. P. & Hughes L. E. Foam elastomer dressing in the management of open granulating wounds: experience with 250 patients. *British Journal of Surgery* 1977; 64: 554–557.
10. Bundred N. J., Dixon J. M., Chetty U. & Forrest A. P. M. Mammillary fistula. *British Journal of Surgery* 1987; 74: 466–468.
11. Hadfield G. J. Excision of the major duct system for benign disease of the breast. *British Journal of Surgery* 1960; 47: 472–477.
12. Urban J. A. Excision of the major duct system of the breast. *Cancer* 1963; 16: 516–520.
13. Benson E. A. & Goodman M. A. Incision with primary suture in the treatment of acute puerperal breast abscess. *British Journal of Surgery* 1970; 57: 55–58.
14. Von Kessel F., Pickrell K. L., Huger W. E. & Matton G. Surgical Treatment of Gynaecomastia: An analysis of 275 cases. *Annals of Surgery* 1963; 157: 142–151.
15. Srivastava A. & Webster D. J. T. Isolated nipple recurrence 17 years after subcutaneous mastectomy for breast cancer – a case report. *European Journal of Surgical Oncology* 1987; 13: 459–461.
16. Hartrampf C. R. & Schneider W. J. A simple direct method for correction of inversion of the nipple. *Plastic and Reconstructive Surgery* 1976; 58: 678–679.
17. Broadbent T. R. & Woolf R. M. Benign inverted nipple. Trans nipple areola correction. *Plastic and Reconstructive Surgery* 1976; 58: 673–677.
18. Crestinu J. M. The inverted nipple – a blind method of correction. *Plastic and Reconstructive Surgery* 1987; 79: 127–130.

Index

A-cells, 8
Abscess, 143–147
    drainage, 201–202
Abscess, recurrent subareolar, 147, *see also*
        Mammary duct fistula; Periductal mastitis
Accessory breasts, 45, 159–160
Actinomycosis, 148
Adenolipoma, 177
Adenoma, syringomatous, 153
Adenosis, erosive, of nipple, 152–153
Amastia, 47, 161–162
Amenorrhoea-galactorrhoea syndrome, 86
American Cancer Society Consensus Statement, 29
American College of Pathologists (ACP) study, 29
Amyloid, 180
ANDI, *see* Aberrations of normal development and
        involution (in text)
Androgen in gynaecomastia, 168
Aneurysm, 180
Antibiotics
    for breast abscess, 145
    for breast lumps, 123
Apocrine metaplasia, cancer risk, 31
Apocrine metaplastic epithelium, 95
Aerola
    disorders, 151–156
    eczema, 120, 153–154
Artefactual disease, 181
Aspiration cytology, 43–44
Asymmetry, breast, 162–163
Athelia, 162

B-cells, clear basal, 8
Bacteroides spp., 111, 147
BBD, *see* Breast, disorders, benign
Beta human chorionic gonadotrophin, 94
Biopsy
    needles, 188
    open procedures, 190–192
    radiologically controlled, 192–193
    wound edge, 45
Blood supply, breast, 7
Blood-milk barrier, 11
Blue-domed cyst of Bloodgood, 93
Blunt duct adenosis
    histology, 36
    low cancer risk, 30

Brassiere for mastalgia, 82
Breast
    aberrations of normal development and
            involution (ANDI), 2, 15–25
    abscess, 111
        formation, 117
        lactational, 144–146
            drainage, 201–202
        in male, 173
        neonatal, 146
        non-lactational, 146–147
    accessory, 45, 159–160
        recurrent subareolar, 124–125, 196–198
    actinomycosis, 148
    adenoma, 66
    adolescent hypertrophy, 20, 24, 163–165
    adolescent masses, 47–48
    anatomy and physiology, 5–12
    aneurysm, 180
    artefactual disease, 181–183
    assessment, follow-up, 46–47
    asymmetry, 162
    augmentation, 164
        complications, 164–165
    cancer, non-histological risk factors, 34
    carcinoma, relative risk, 29
    changes at puberty, 6
    collagenous spherulosis, 181
    cosmetic aspects, 164
    cyclical change, 17
        disorders, 20–21, 24
        in epithelium, 10
    cyst, 93–100
        fluid, 35
    development, 5, 16–17
    developmental anomalies, 159
    disorders
        benign, 2, 15–25
            cancer risk assessment, 28–38
            epidemiology, 27–30
            management, 24–25
            pathogenesis framework, 23
            population incidence, 27–28
        clinics, 2
        concept and nomenclature, 1–3, 15
        of development, 20
        with high cancer risk, 33–34
        history, 2–3

emptying, 146
fascia, 8
fibroadenosis, 1, 2, 16, *see also* ANDI
   premalignant potential, 1
fibrous disease, 179
fusion, 162
histological changes and clinical symptoms, 16
hormone-controlled processes, 16
hypertrophy
   in pregnancy, 163
   treatment, 163–164
imaging methods, 49–56
infarction, 180
infection, 143–149
   lactational, 143–146
involution, 12, 17–19
   disorders, 21
   excessive postlactational, 164
lesion, subclinical, 52
lobule involution, 16
lymphatics, 7
male, 167–173
microscopic anatomy, 8–9
neonatal enlargement, 162
nerve supply, 7–8
nodularity, 20–21, 24
   and mastalgia, 75–90
normal, 17
normal involuting, 18
normal microanatomy, 9
normal pregnant, 18
normal/abnormal borderline, 15–16
oedema, 178–9
operations, 187–204
pain, *see* Mastalgia
palpation, 42–43
perimenarchal, 17
physiological and structural changes, 3
postlactational, 18
postmenopausal, 18, 19
premalignant potential assessment, 16
prepubertal, 5
residual ducts, 128
screening, 34–35
skin lesions, 149
stroma, 9–10
supernumeracy, 45, 159–160
syphilis, 148
trauma, 175
tuberculosis, 147
vascular anatomy, 7
Breast-feeding, *see* Lactation
Bromocriptine
   for lactation suppression, 146
   for mastalgia, 84, 85, 88
   for nipple discharge, 122
   for periductal mastitis, 122
Burns, 175

Caffeine/methylxanthine theory of benign breast
   disease, 86, 122
Cancer risk, of BBD, 30–34
Cancer risk after duct excision, 126–127
Carcinoembryonic antigen (CEA), 94
Carcinoma, incision biopsy, 191
Cardiff BBD study, 29, 60, 65
Cardiff Mastalgia Clinic, 84, 85, 87, 90
Cardiff Mastalgia Protocol, 76

Cellulitis, 145
Collagenous spherulosis, 181
Colostrum
   cells, 110
   in new-born, 5
Comedo mastitis, 108
Computerized tomography, 53
Condyloma accuminatum, 156
Contraceptive pill
   and benign breast disorders, 28
   and mastalgia, 83
Cooper, Sir Astley, 1, 2, 93, 148
Cooper's ligaments, 42, 43
Core needle biopsy, 188–190
Cosmesis of duct surgery, 125–126
Cracked nipple, 152
Cyclical nodularity
   cancer risk, 30
   description, 46
Cyclical pain, treatment, 88
Cyclist's nipple, 154
Cyst, fine needle aspiration, 188
Cystic lobular involution, 94
Cystic papillary tumours, 97, 100
Cystosarcoma phyllodes, *see* Phyllodes tumour
Cysts, 24, 93–100
   aetiology, 18, 21
   aspiration, 97–98
   biochemistry, 35
   blue-domed, of Bloodgood, 93
   clinical features, 96
   description, 46
   fluid
      colours, 94
      Na^+/K^+ ratio, 95
   formation, 18, 21, 96
   incidence, 94
   investigation, 97
   management, 97
   multiple, 94
   natural history, 97
   nipple discharge in, 138
   palpation, 42–43
   pathogenesis, 94–96
   recurrent, 98–99
   sites, 144
   treatment, 145–146
   types, 93
Cytology of nipple discharges, 139

Danazol
   Cardiff trial, 90
   for cysts, 99
   for gynaecomatia, 171
   for hypertrophy, 163
   for mastalgia, 84–85, 88
Dermatitis artefacta, 182
Desmoid tumour, 179
Diabetes, 179–180
Diaphanography, 53
Diuretics, for mastalgia, 83
Domperidone
   and galactorrhoea, 136
   test, 82
Doppler ultrasound scanning, 53
Drug-induced galactorrhoea, 136
Drugs
   excretion into milk, 11–12

adverse effects, 11
and gynaecomastia, 170
Duct
  continuity restoration after division, 126
  dilatation, 115
  distal, persistent, 129
  excision, indications for, 123
  injection, for nipple discharge, 139
  major
    excision, 198–201
      breast problems after, 127
    papilloma
      benign, 23
      focal-solitary, 31–32
      infarction, 137
      multiple, 137–138
      solitary, 136–137
    proximal, persistent, 128
    terminal, benign papilloma, 153
Duct ectasia, 2, 16, 19, 21
  indications for surgery, 124
  low cancer risk, 31
  in male, 120, 172–173
  neonatal, 120
  nipple discharge in, 138
  pathogenesis, diagram, 22
  pathology, 109–110
  surgical complications, 127–128
  surgical results, 125–130
Duct ectasia/periductal mastitis complex, 107–130,
    138
  breast masses in, 116–118
  frequency, 121
  historical survey, 107–109
  in male, 172
  management, 122–123
  pathogenesis, 112–115
  radiology, 121–122
  surgery, 123–125
Duct excision, 194, 196, 198
  results of, 125–130
Ductal carcinoma in site (DCIS), 33, 65–66
Ductal hyperplasia, moderate cancer risk, 32–33
Ductogram, 135
Ductography, 49–50

Eczema, 120, 125, 153–154
  duct excision for, 125
Endocrine abnormalities and mastalgia, 80–81
Epithelial hyperplasias, 16, 19, 22–23, 25
  assessment, 37–38
  classification, 32
  florid, cancer risk, 32
  in male, 173
  with moderate cancer risk, 32–33
  simple, cancer risk, 31–32
  terminology, 35
Epithelial stromal junction, 9
Epitheliosis, 32, 33
  histology, 36–37
Erosive adenomatosis, 152
Evening primrose oil (EPO) for mastalgia, 85, 88
Excision biopsy, 190
Extralobular terminal ductule, 8

Factitial disease, see artefactual disease
Family history of breast disease, 34

Fascia, breast, 8
Fat lobule, 45
Fat necrosis, 175–176
  cystic, 97
Fetoprotein, 94
Fibroadenoma, 20, 59–60
  aetiology, 20
  assessment, 45–46
  cancer in, 65–66
  clinical features, 62–63
  cytology, 64
  giant, see Giant fibroadenoma
  groups, 60–61
  histological variations, 65–66
  hormonal therapy, 64
  incidence, 61
  infarction, 65
  mammography, 63
  palpation, 42–43
  and race, 62, 63
  recurrence after surgery, 64–65
  recurrent and progressive, 69
  removal, 191–192, 194
  steroid receptors in, 61
  ultrasonography, 64
Fibroadenosis, see ANDI
Fibrocystic disease, see ANDI
Fibrocystic dieease of breast, see Breast,
    fibroadenosis
Fibroepithelial polyp, simple, 153
Fibromatosis, 179
Fibrous disease of breast, 179
Filaria, 148
Film-screen mammography, 49
Fine needle aspiration, 187–188
Fistulectomy
  recurrent disease causes, 128
  results, 127
  for subareolar abscess, 125
  technique, 196–197
Fistulotomy
  results, 127
  for subareolar abscess, 125
Foam cells, 8
Foetal mammary ridge, 5
Foreign bodies in breast, 147

Gaillard-Thomas incision, 68, 194
Galactocele, 46, 97, 99–100
Galactorrhoea, 135–136
  causes, 136
  management, 141
Giant fibroadenoma, 2, 66–69
  of adolescence, 66–69
  definition, 66
  management, 68
  nomenclature, 66
  perimenopausal, 69
  removal, 194
Gigantomastia, 163
Granular cell myoblastoma, 180
Granulomatous disease, non-specific, 181
Guinea-worm infection, 148
Gynaecomastia, 47–48, 167–172
  assessment, 170
  drug therapy, 171
  histology, 167–168
  incidence, 168

mastectomy, 202–203
mammography, 171
mastectomy for, 203–204
physiological, 169
radiotherapy, 172
secondary, 169–170
surgery, 171–172
treatment, 171

Hadfield's procedure, 198–201
Haematoma
    after biopsy, 190, 191
    and breast abscess, 147
Haemorrhagic necrosis, 180–181
Hamartoma, 177
Helminthic infection, 148
Herpes viral infections of nipple, 156
Hidradenitis suppurativa, 149, 183–184
Hooked needle technique, 52, 193
Hormonal defect in gynaecomastia, 168–169
Hydatid disease, 148
Hyperplasia
    assessment, 37
    definition, 35
Hypertrophy
    adolescent, 20
    virginal, 163–165
Hypoplasia, 161–162

Impalpable lesions, localization techniques, 52–53
Incision biopsy, 191
Infection, recurrent, 128
Intraduct hyperplasia, 32, 33
Intraductal papilloma, 100
    macroscopic, assessment, 37–38
Intralobular terminal ductule, 8

Jogger's nipple, 154
Juvenile fibroadenoma, 65, 66
Juvenile papillomatosis, 38

Klinefelter's syndrome, 169–170

Lactation
    after duct excision, 126
    established, 11
    and galactocele, 99
    and inverted nipples, 160–161
    suppressive, 146
Lactational breast abscess, 144–146
    drainage, 201–202
Lactational mastitis, 143
Leiomyoma of nipple, 154
Lignocaine for non-cyclical mastalgia, 86, 89
Linear analogue scale (VLA), 84
Lipoma, 177
Liver failure and gynaecomastia, 170
Lobular carcinoma *in situ* (LCIS), 33, 65
Lobular hyperplasia
    assessment, 37
    moderate cancer risk, 32–33
Local anaesthetic, 188, 189, 190
Lumps
    assessment and management, 41–48

causes, 41
clinical assessment, 41–44
fine needle aspiration, 187–188
inspection, 42
in older women, 48
palpation, 42–43
as presenting symptom, 28
recurrent, management, 47
Lymph node, intramammary, 45
Lymphatics of breast, 7

Macrocyst, 19
Macroscopic cysts, cancer risk, 30–31
Magnetic resonance imaging, 53
Major duct excision, 198–201
Male breast, 167–173
Mammalithiasis, 183
Mammary duct fistula, 23, 109, 111, 114, 118–119
    excision, 196–198
Mammillary fistula, *see* Mammary duct fistula
Mammography, 34, 44, 49–50
    in benign disorders, 53–55
        indications, 54–55
    for nipple discharge, 138–139
    in nipple retraction, 151
Mammoplasty
    augmentation, 164
    reduction, 163, 165
Marijuana-induced gynaecomastia, 170
Mastalgia, 20–21, 75–90
    aetiology, 79–82
        hypotheses and treatments, 83
    in breast cancer, 76
    cancer risk, 30
    cyclical, 24
        pattern, 76–77
    drug choice and side-effects, 89
    drug treatment length, 89–90
    and duct ectasia, 120
    frequency, 75–76
    natural history, 87
    non-cyclical, 77–78
        treatment, 86–87
    and reassurance, 82–83
    surgical excision, 86–87
    treatment principles, 88
    trigger spot, 86
Mastectomy, 34
    for cysts, 99
    for mastalgia, 86–87
    in males, 202–203
    subcutaneous, 202–204
Mastitis
    periductal, 16, 19, 21
        diagram, 22
        low cancer risk, 31
Mastitis obliterans, 108, 110
Mastodynia, *see* Mastalgia
Menstrual cycle
    and breast, 17
    tissue changes, 10
Metoclopramide and galactorrhoea, 136
Microcystic/macrocystic formation, 19
Microdochetomy, 137, 139, 140
    technique, 194–196
Microscopic anatomy of breast, 8–9
Milk
    drug excretion into, 11–12

secretion, 11
Mitral valve prolapse and hypoplastic breasts, 161
Molluscum contagiosum, 156
Mondor's disease, 173, 178
Montgomery's glands, 6, 7, 154–155
    retention cyst, 156
Multiple duct papilloma, 137–138
Mycobacterial infection, 148
Mycotic infections, 148
Myoblastoma, granular cell, 180
Myoepithelial cells, 9

Needle
    biopsy, 44, 187
    fine, aspiration, 187–188
Neonatal breast abscess, 146
Neonatal enlargement of breast, 162
Nephrotic syndrome, 179
Nerve supply of breast, 7–8
Nipple
    adenoma, in male, 173
    areolar complex, 6–7
    congenital inversion, 111, 114, 115, 119
    cracked, 152
    crusting, 152
    cyclist's, 154
    discharge, 21, 112–113, 115–116, 133–141
        blood and serosanguineous, 133–134
        blood-stained, of pregnancy, 134–135
        bloody, 124
        causes, 134
        coloured opalescent, 135
        hormone therapy, 122
        incidence, 133
        investigation, 138–139
        in male, 173
        management, 124, 140–141
        milk, see Galactorrhea
        non-bloody, 124
        operations for, 194–199
        type and diagnosis, 134
        watery, 135
    disorders, 151–156
    eczema, 153–154
    genital warts, 156
    imperforate, 162
    inversion, 23, 24, 114, 151, 160
        after periductal inflammation, 161
        and breast-feeding, 160–161
        congenital, 160
        correction, 124, 204
        and cosmesis, 161
        persisting after duct excision, 129–130
        surgery, 204
    jogger's, 154
    Paget's disease, 152, 153, 155
    retraction, 21, 24, 114, 115, 119–120, 151
        assessment, 151
    sebaceous cyst, 155–156
    sensation after surgery, 126
    supernumeracy, 160
    surgery, 194–196
    traumatic lesions, 154
Nodularity, assessment, 44–48
Non-cyclical pain, treatment, 88–89
Non-lactational breast abscess, 146–147
Non-organoid hyperplasia, histology, 36–37
Nottingham Breast Clinic, 87

Nursing home breast, 179

Oedema, 178–179
Organoid hyperplasia, 36
Oxford-FPA contraceptive study, 27, 28

Paget's disease, 152, 153, 155
Pain in breast problems, 28
Papillary cystadenoma, 100
Papillary tumours, in cysts, 100
Papilloma, microscopic, assessment, 38
    multiple, 137
Papillomatosis, 32, 33
    erosive, 137
    histology, 36–37
    juvenile, 38
Paraffinoma, 176
Peau d'orange, 42, 178
Peptostreptococcus spp., 111
Periductal fibrosis, 112–113
Periductal inflammation, 110
    and inverted nipples, 161
Periductal mastitis
    bacteriology, 111–112
    breast abscess in, 146–147
Periductal mastitis, see Duct ectasia/periductal
        mastitis complex
Perimenarchal breast, 17
Perimenopausal giant breast tumours, 69–72
Phyllodes tumour, 59, 66, 67, 69–72
Pilonidal abscess, 149
Plasma cell mastitis, see Duct ectasia/Periductal
        mastitis
    radiology, 122
Pneumocystography, 50, 100
Pneumothorax after aspiration, 188
Poland's syndrome, 161
Polymastia, 159–160
Polythelia, 160
Postlactional involution, 12
Postmenopausal hormone therapy and breast
        lumps, 48
Postmenopausal involution, 12
Prednisolone for non-cyclical mastalgia, 66, 89
Pregnancy
    after duct excision, 126, 130
    anatomical changes, 10
    epithelial hyperplasia, 23
    fibroadenoma in, 65
    nipple discharge, 134
    physiological changes, 11
Proflavine dressing, 197, 202
Progestogens and mastalgia, 83–84
Prolactin and mastalgia, 80–81
Prolactinoma, 136
Prosthesis
    capsular contraction, 165
    deflation, 164–165
    migration, 165
Protozoan infections, 148
Pseudoretraction of nipple, 42
Psychoneurosis and mastalgia, 80
Ptosis, correction, 165
Pubertal assymmetry, 163
Puberty, breast changes, 6
Public health education and referral rates, 28
Puerperal breast infection, incidence, 143

Pyridoxine for mastalgia, 86

Race
    and benign breast disorders, 181
    and fibroadenomas, 63, 67–68
Radiation damage, 177
Radiologically controlled biopsy, 192–193
Raynaud's phenomenon, 154
Recurrent subareolar abscess, 147
Relaxin, 94
Retroareolar mass, diagnosis, 124
Rib, prominent, 45
Royal College of General Practitioners study, 28

Sarcoid, 180
Sclerosing adenoma, and trauma, 78–79
Sclerosing adenosis, 21, 24, 103–105
    description, 46
    in fibroadenoma, 65
    histology, 36
    low cancer risk, 30
    with neural invasion, 103
    radiological criteria, 104
Seat belt injury, 175
Sebaceous cyst
    infected, 149
    of nipple, 155–156
Secretory atrophy after duct excision, 126
Silastic Foam dressing, 197, 200, 201, 202
Spironolactone and gynaecomastia, 170
Squamous metaplasia, 110–111
Staphylococcus aureus, 143
Starvation re-feeding and gynaecomastia, 170
Subareolar abscess, 109, 111, 115, 124–125
    recurrent, treatment, 125
Subareolar glands, anatomy, 155
Syphilis, 148
Syringomatous adenoma, 153

Tamoxifen
    for gynaecomastia, 171
    for mastalgia, 85–86
Terminal ductal lobular units (TDLU), 8, 22
    hyperplastic lesions, 29
Testicular failure and gynaecomastia, 170
Thelache, prepubertal, 163
Thermography, 53
Thrombophlebitis, 178
Thyrotrophin-releasing hormone (TRH) test, 81
Tietze's syndrome, 78, 79
Trauma, 175
    and breast abscess, 147
    and sclerosing adenoma, 78–79
Trucut needle biopsy, 188–190
Tuberculosis, 147
Tumours and gynaecomastia, 169
Typhoid, 144

Ultrasound, 44
    examination, 50–51
Urban's duct excision, 198–201

Vasculitis, 180
Viral infections, 148–149
    of nipple, 156
Virginal hypertrophy, 163
Vitamin B6 for mastalgia, 86

Water retention and mastalgia, 79–80
Witch's milk, 5, 136
Wolfe parenchymal patterns, 55–56
Woolwich shield, 161

Xeromammography, 49, 54